Prevention of Type 2 Diabetes

Prevention of Type 2 Diabetes

Edited by
Dr Manfred Ganz, M.D.

Specialist Internal Medicine, Diabetologist (DDG)
Associate Professor of Medicine
Campus Biomedico, University of Rome, Italy

John Wiley & Sons, Ltd

Copyright © 2005 John Wiley & Sons Ltd,
The Atrium, Southern Gate, Chichester,
West Sussex PO19 8SQ, England

Telephone (+44) 1243 779777

Email (for orders and customer service enquiries): cs-books@wiley.co.uk
Visit our Home Page on www.wileyeurope.com or www.wiley.com

Reprinted August 2005

Other Wiley Editorial Offices

John Wiley & Sons Inc., 111 River Street, Hoboken, NJ 07030, USA

Jossey-Bass, 989 Market Street, San Francisco, CA 94103-1741, USA

Wiley-VCH Verlag GmbH, Boschstr. 12, D-69469 Weinheim, Germany

John Wiley & Sons Australia Ltd, 33 Park Road, Milton, Queensland 4064, Australia

John Wiley & Sons (Asia) Pte Ltd, 2 Clementi Loop #02-01, Jin Xing Distripark, Singapore 129809

John Wiley & Sons Canada Ltd, 22 Worcester Road, Etobicoke, Ontario, Canada M9W 1L1

British Library Cataloguing in Publication Data

A catalogue record for this book is available from the British Library

ISBN 10: 0-470-85733-1 (H/B)
ISBN 13: 978-0-470-85733-5 (H/B)

Typeset by in 10.5/13pt Times by Thomson Press (India) Limited, New Delhi
Printed and bound in Great Britain by Antony Rowe Ltd, Chippenham, Wiltshire
This book is printed on acid-free paper responsibly manufactured from sustainable forestry in which at least two trees are planted for each one used for paper production.

For my loving family: my wife Helmi
with Nicholas, Fabian, Simon, Angela,
our foster child Christina, my parents
Rosa-Maria and Josef for their lifelong support

Contents

Preface

Diabetes mellitus Type 2 is growing worldwide with epidemic dimensions. Still most societies in the world act on an acute care approach when dealing with diabetes. Although there is evidence from health economic data that a long-term approach with preventive elements pays off over time, most governments and payers are still reluctant to invest heavily in preventive diabetes care.

The intention of this book is to provide a comprehensive synopsis on prevention of Type 2 diabetes. Earlier attempts either mixed Type 1 and Type 2 or did not cover the broad range from screening to prevention.

Renowned authors describe the 'Problem' in the first section, mainly the underlying social and socio-economic changes in 'modern' lifestyle with the sequels of sedentary life- and work style and over- and malnutrition. My emphasis lies on the global perspective, including the views of WHO, IDF and other major diabetes authorities, as well as the advent of 'a novel disease': Type 2 diabetes in children and youth, a new threat of eventually pandemic impact, unless interventions are put into place.

Section 2 covers the field of 'Screening' as one optional prerequisite of prevention. Current activities as well as future approaches ('genetic testing') are described here. One of the beauties is the coexistence of global perspective on the one hand and local problem solving on the other, for example described in the New Zealand Community Screening Initiative.

This is followed by Section 3 on primary prevention with Section 4 on secondary and tertiary prevention, although epidemiologists no longer use this discrimination, described here as 'Prevention of Complications'.

I would like to take the opportunity to warmly thank all my authors from Germany, the Netherlands, Denmark, the UK, Finland, Switzerland, Italy, Belgium, the United States, Australia and New Zealand for their outstanding contributions, and Joan Marsh and Andrea Baier from the publisher, John Wiley and Sons, for using the right balance between push and encouragement for me and the authors to get this book done in time.

Manfred Ganz
Summer 2004

Foreword

This book is centred on the prevention of the most common form of the condition, Type 2 diabetes. It covers screening and primary prevention, as well as the secondary prevention of the devastating complications of diabetes. Its perspective is worldwide with contributions from experts drawn from across Europe, North America and Asia–Pacific.

I sincerely hope that this timely publication will attract not only the interest of the physicians and scientists who form its primary audience, but also the attention of health policy and decision makers working at national, regional and international levels, so that it can play a part towards advocating change, encouraging action and promoting increased awareness of a condition that can be treated but not as yet cured.

As stated elsewhere in this book, it is through the promotion of diabetes prevention that the International Diabetes Federation (IDF) strives to ensure that the millions who are living with diabetes today will not face a future decline in the quality of their care as a result of the many more millions who are predicted to develop the condition. At the same time, IDF is working to increase global access to and bring about improvements in the quality of available care.

IDF has redefined its mission in order to reflect more closely the activity in which it is involved and in particular to reflect the growing concern with the prevention of diabetes that is influencing the activities of diabetes representative organizations throughout the IDF membership network.

In line with our vision of *living in a world without diabetes*, the new mission of the IDF is *to promote diabetes care, prevention and a cure worldwide.*

My deep hope is that through this book diabetes prevention receives a boost in attention and activities among all the partners involved globally.

Although IDF does not support research directly, through awareness and education it encourages the efforts of those who are working towards a better understanding of the causes of the various forms of diabetes and ultimately towards a cure.

As we often say at IDF, *the time has come to act... NOW!*

Pierre Lefèbvre

President International Diabetes Federation

List of Contributors

Ayad Al-Bermani Specialist Registrar in Ophthalmology, Royal Victoria Infirmary, Newcastle upon Tyne NE1 4LP, UK

Bruce Arroll Department of General Practice and Primary Health Care, School of Public Health, University of Auckland, Private Bag 92019, Auckland, New Zealand

Knut Borch-Johnsen Steno Diabetes Centre, Niels Steensensvej 2, 2820 Gentofte, Denmark

Adrian Cameron International Diabetes Institute, 260 Kooyong Road, Caulfield, Victoria 3162, Australia

Stephen Colagiuri Department of Medicine, Prince of Wales Clinical School, 1st Floor, Edmund Blacket Building, Prince of Wales Hospital, Randwick NSW 2031, Australia

Michael Faust Klinik II und Poliklinik für Innere Medizin, Universität zu Köln, Joseph-Stelzmann-Strasse 9, 50924 Köln, Germany

Charlotte Glümer Steno Diabetes Centre, Niels Steensensvej 2, 2820 Gentofte, Denmark

Reinhard Griebenow Klinik II und Poliklinik für Innere Medizin, Kliniken der Stadt Köln, Köln Merheim, Ostmerheimer Strasse 200, Köln, Germany

Markolf Hanefeld Centre of Clinical Studies, Institute of Technology and Science Transfer, Technical University Dresden, Fiedlerstrasse 34, 01307 Dresden, Germany

Tim Kenealy Division of General Practice and Primary Health Care, The University of Auckland, Private Bag 92019, Auckland 1020, New Zealand

Thomas Konrad Institute for Metabolism Research, Heidelberger Strasse 13, 60327 Frankfurt, Germany

Pierre Lefèbvre International Diabetes Federation and Department of Medicine (B35), C.H.U. Sart Tilman 4000 Liege 1, Belgium

Hermann Liebermeister Executive Committee of the German Diabetes Union, Schlesierweg 2, Neunkirchen/Saar, 66538, Germany

Carl Erik Mogensen Department of Medicine, M, Aarhus Kommunehospitalet and University Hospital, 8000 Aarhus C, Denmark

Peter Müller DD-E, Roche Diagnostics GmbH, Sandhofer Strasse 116, D-68305 Mannheim, Germany

Paolo Pozzilli Department of Endocrinology and Diabetes, University Campus Bio-Medico, Via E Longoni, 83, 00155 Rome, Italy

Thomas Reinehr Vestische Kinder- und Jugendklinik, University of Witten-Herdecke, Dr F Steiner Strasse 5, 45711 Datteln, Germany

Gojka Roglic Diabetes Program, World Health Organisation, 20 avenue Appia, 1211 Geneva 27, Switzerland

Richard R. Rubin The Johns Hopkins University School of Medicine, 500 West University Parkway, Suite 1-M, Baltimore, MD 21210, USA

Jonathan Shaw International Diabetes Institute, 260 Kooyong Road, Caulfield, Victoria 3162, Australia

Anders A. F. Sima Departments of Pathology and Neurology and Morris Hood Jr Diabetes Center, Wayne State University, Detroit, MI 48201, USA

Frank J. Snoek Department of Medical Psychology, Diabetes Research Group, VU University Medical Centre, Van der Boechorststraat 7, 1081 BT Amsterdam, The Netherlands

Roy Taylor School of Clinical Medical Sciences, Medical School, Framlington Place, Newcastle upon Tyne NE2 4HH, UK

Jaakko Tuomilehto Diabetes and Genetic Epidemiology Unit, Department of Epidemiology and Health Promotion, National Public Health Institute, Mannerheimintie 166, FIN-00300 Helsinki, Finland

Martin Wabitsch Pediatric Endocrinology, Department of Pediatrics and Adolescent Medicine, University of Ulm, Prittwitzstrasse 43, 89075 Ulm, Germany

Sabine Wiedenmann Klinik II und Poliklinik für Innere Medizin, Kliniken der Stadt Köln, Köln Merheim, Ostmerheimer Strasse 200, 51058 Köln, Germany

Rhys Williams The Clinical School, University of Wales Swansea, Singleton Park, Swansea SA2 8PP, UK

Paul Zimmet International Diabetes Institute, 260 Kooyong Road, Caulfield, Victoria 3162, Australia

1 The Diabetes Epidemic: Description of the Problem

1

The Diabetes Epidemic: Genes and Environment Clashing

Paul Zimmet, Adrian Cameron and **Jonathan Shaw**

Introduction

Diabetes mellitus affects large numbers of people from a wide range of ethnic groups and at all social and economic levels throughout the world.[1] The last few decades of the 20th century saw an explosive increase in this disorder globally, mainly in the number of people with Type 2 diabetes. At the present time it is estimated that 190 million people worldwide have diabetes and that this will increase to 324 million by 2025.[2] The epidemic is taking place in both developed and developing nations.

Over the last 40 years, there have been dramatic changes in the human environment, behaviour and lifestyle. These changes have resulted in escalating rates of both obesity and diabetes.[3] There is every reason to believe that over the next decade the epidemic of Type 2 diabetes will continue to escalate. It is for this reason that the emphasis of this chapter is on Type 2 diabetes. It has now become one of the major threats to human health in the 21st century.

An Epidemiological Perspective

The dramatic increase in the prevalence of diabetes (mainly Type 2) world-wide is a matter of enormous concern to individuals and public health authorities in both developed and developing nations and the World Health Organization (WHO).

Prevention of Type 2 Diabetes Edited by Manfred Ganz
 ISBN: 0-470-85733-1

Globally, the percentage of Type 2 diabetes is greater than 90 per cent. Type 1 diabetes is relatively uncommon in many populations, particularly Asian, Middle Eastern, the Pacific Islands and African.[1] Not only is the prevalence increasing, but the age of onset of Type 2 diabetes is becoming younger with an increasing, but so far poorly quantified, number of children and adolescents now being diagnosed.[4]

The changing perception of diabetes as a global public health threat relates partly to a better appreciation of its devastating complications, but mainly to the rapid, and unanticipated, rise in its prevalence that has occurred in the latter part of the 20th century. The evidence for this global rise is now clear. In Native American and Pacific Island populations, Type 2 diabetes now affects up to 40 per cent of adults,[5,6] but was virtually unknown 50 years ago.

There has been an overwhelming number of studies of diabetes prevalence in the last few decades, again underlining the increasing interest in this chronic disease. Just to cite a few striking examples:

- Between 1976 and 1988, the prevalence of diabetes rose from 11.4 per cent to 14.3 per cent in the USA among people aged 40–74 years.[7]

- Two cross-sectional studies in an urban south Indian population showed that the prevalence in the over-20s had risen from 8.3 per cent in 1989 to 11.6 per cent in 1995.[8] For the year 2000, the prevalence in six major cities across India was reported to be 12.1 per cent.[9]

- In China, the prevalence of 3.1 per cent in 1994 in the over-25 age group was almost two and a half times higher than a figure from the Chinese province of Da Qing eight years earlier.[10] By 2001, the prevalence amongst those aged 35–74 had further risen to 5.5 per cent.[11]

- European studies are few, but Drivsholm and coworkers reported a 38 per cent rise in the prevalence of diabetes over 22 years.[12]

- In Latin American countries, the crude prevalence of Type 2 diabetes in the year 2000 ranged from 1.2 per cent in Chile to 8.2 per cent in Argentina.[13]

- In Africa, diabetes prevalence ranges from 0.7 per cent in rural Tanzania to 10.0 per cent in the Northern Sudan.[14]

- In Australia, 7.4 per cent of adults now have diabetes compared with an estimated 3.4 per cent in 1981.[15] Almost one in four Australians aged 25 years and over has either diabetes or a condition of impaired glucose metabolism. The prevalence has trebled over the last 20 years. Approximately 20 per cent of the population are affected by their late 60s.[15]

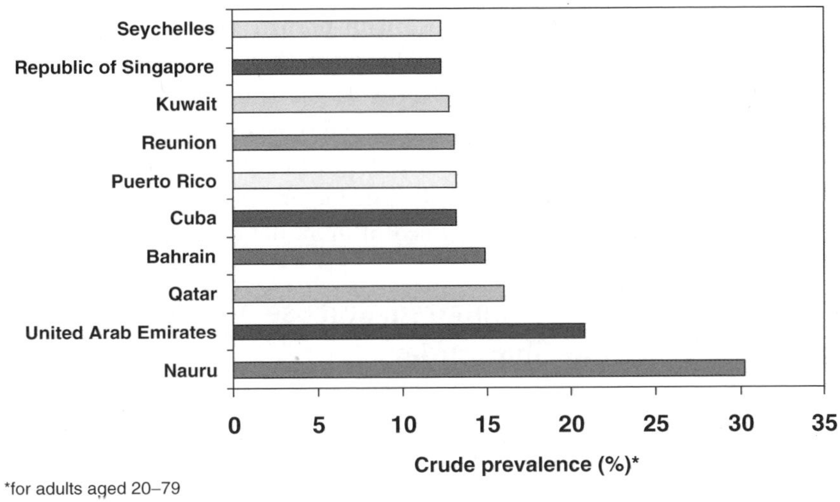

FIGURE 1.1 The top 10 countries for diabetes prevalence (modified from reference 2)

It should be noted that many of the high prevalence figures reported in Pacific Island communities, including Asian Indians in Fiji, were from surveys performed over 15 years ago, yet these rates still remain amongst the highest yet recorded.[16] More recently, a study during 1998 and 2000 by Colagiuri and coworkers revealed a prevalence of diabetes in Tonga of 15.1 per cent, of which 80 per cent was undiagnosed.[17] A similar survey in 1973 reported a 7.5 per cent prevalence, indicating a doubling of diabetes over the past 25 years in this Polynesian paradise!

We have recently undertaken an analysis of worldwide data on diabetes prevalence rates. Figure 1.1 shows the top 10 countries for diabetes as reported in the *Diabetes Atlas* 2003.[2]

A particularly worrying feature of the epidemic of diabetes has been the concurrence of glucose intolerance with other cardiovascular disease (CVD) risk factors. In the Australian Diabetes, Obesity and Lifestyle Study (or AusDiab), the presence of obesity, hypertension, elevated LDL cholesterol, low HDL cholesterol and elevated triglycerides (shown in Table 1.1) were dramatically increased in the

TABLE 1.1 Prevalence (%) of CVD risk factors in Australia stratified by glucose tolerance status[18]

	NGT	IFG	IGT	Diabetes
Obesity (BMI $\geq$ 30 kg/m^2)	16.2	29.9	31.4	46.2
Hypertension ($\geq$ 140/90 mm Hg)	21.1	44.4	51.1	68.6
LDL $\geq$ 3.5 mmol/l	47.3	69.9	62.1	63.8
HDL $<$ 1.0 mmol/l	14.9	27.1	22.5	39.1
Triglycerides $\geq$ 2.0 mmol/l	19.6	39.9	38.8	56.7

Data are not age or sex adjusted. Reproduced with permission from Shaw, JE and Chisholm DJ[18].

diabetic population compared with those with normal glucose tolerance.[18] This concern regarding CVD risk becomes even greater when one considers that people with a lesser abnormality of blood glucose levels (impaired glucose tolerance (IGT) and impaired fasting glucose (IFG)) have a substantial increase in CVD risk factors and an approximate doubling of cardiovascular risk.[1,18] The association of glucose intolerance with other key CVD risk factors is known as the metabolic syndrome and this association is discussed in more detail later.

The Hidden Epidemic – Impaired Glucose Tolerance and Impaired Fasting Glycaemia

Worldwide it is estimated that more than 350 million people have IGT or IFG.[2] The Australian AusDiab Study recently surveyed the glycaemic status of a population of 11 247 adults.[15] The combined prevalence of IFG and IGT was 16.4 per cent. These glucose-intolerant, but non-diabetic, individuals represent a large reservoir of potential new diabetes cases.

Impaired glucose tolerance was considered a separate class in the previous WHO classification but is now categorized as a stage in the natural history of disordered carbohydrate metabolism.[19] Impaired fasting glycaemia (IFG) is now formally recognized, as these people also are at greater risk for progression to diabetes and macrovascular disease, although prospective data are sparse and early data suggest a similar risk of progression to diabetes as exists for IGT.[20,21] IFG refers to fasting glucose concentrations that are lower than those required to diagnose diabetes mellitus but higher than the 'normal' reference range.[19] IGT and IFG are not clinical entities in their own right but rather risk categories for future diabetes and/or cardiovascular disease.[22] They represent impaired glucose regulation, which refers to a metabolic state intermediate between normal glucose homeostasis and diabetes. Both IGT and IFG are often associated with the metabolic syndrome.[22]

The American Diabetes Association (ADA) has recently considered whether the lower limit for IFG should be reduced from 6.1 mmol/l (110 mg/dl).[23] The ADA, on reviewing the data, suggested that the cut point for IFG should be reduced from 6.1 mmol/l (110 mg/dl) to 5.6 mmol/l (100 mg/dl), and that IFG should be redefined as an FPG of 5.6–6.9 mmol/l (100–125 mg/dl). If an OGTT is performed, some individuals with IFG will have IGT. Some may have diabetes, but this cannot be determined without an OGTT. If resources allow, it is recommended that those with IFG have an OGTT to exclude diabetes.[22,23]

Glucose Intolerance and the Metabolic Syndrome

The metabolic syndrome, also known as syndrome X[24] and the insulin resistance syndrome,[25] is a cluster of metabolic abnormalities (glucose intolerance, hyperinsulinaemia/insulin resistance, central obesity, dyslipidaemia and hypertension) that occur together in an individual more often than might be expected by chance. They are associated with increased CVD risk, and in two studies from Europe[26,27] the presence of the syndrome predicted increased cardiovascular and coronary heart disease mortality. Insulin resistance has been suggested as a single common cause for all of the components of the syndrome, and some studies have implicated it in this role, but this has not been confirmed in other work.

The putative central role of insulin resistance led to the labelling of the insulin resistance syndrome,[25] whose features include insulin resistance, central obesity, dyslipidaemia (especially elevated triglycerides and reduced HDL-cholesterol), hypertension, hyperuricaemia and increased plasminogen activator inhibitor-1. The causative mechanisms involved have still not been precisely defined but one possibility is that central obesity and excess lipid availability constitute a major mechanism for many or all of these abnormalities.

There are currently several definitions of the syndrome in use, making it difficult to compare prevalence rates between countries. The World Health Organization (WHO) definition[19] and the European Group for the Study of Insulin Resistance (EGIR)[28] require glucose intolerance or insulin resistance as an essential component. However, for the ATPIII definition developed by the American National Cholesterol Education Program (NCEP),[29] this is not the case. The cut points for each component and the means of combining components also differ.

A comparison of prevalence, applying the WHO definition of the metabolic syndrome[19] among various populations worldwide[30–34] is shown in Table 1.2. Even where studies involve participants within the same age range, there is a wide variation in prevalence between countries. A consistently higher prevalence is seen

TABLE 1.2 Prevalence of the metabolic syndrome according to the WHO definition[19]

Country	Age group (years)	Reference	Prevalence (%) Men	Women
Australia	>24	unpublished	25.2	16.7
Denmark	60	35	38.0	22.0
France	35–64	30	23.0	12.0
Italy	40–81 M, 40–55 F	35	34.5	18.0
Sweden	46–68	35	43.3	26.3
Mauritius	>24	32	20.9	17.6
Occupied Palestinian Territories	30–65	36		Total = 17
Ireland	50–69	37	24.6	17.8
USA	40–74	33	41.3	32.7
USA	30–79	34	30.3	18.1
USA (non-Hispanic white)	30–79	34	24.7	17.2
USA (Mexican American)	30–79	34	32.0	28.3

among men, with almost all studies finding a prevalence higher than 20 per cent. For women, most populations had a prevalence of less than 20 per cent.

Globalization – Its Impact on Human Health

Globally there has been a small but important increase in the incidence of Type 1 diabetes (which will be discussed elsewhere in this issue) but a massive explosion of Type 2 diabetes.[2] What is the reason for this phenomenal increase? Although we do not have all the molecular answers, the epidemiological data seem clear. Type 2 diabetes is a lifestyle disorder, and during the last 30–40 years there have been dramatic changes in the human environment, behaviour and lifestyle, which have resulted in escalating rates of obesity and diabetes.[1,38] More recently, the term diabesity has become fashionable to describe the association of obesity and Type 2 diabetes.[1]

Genetic influences are clearly important, with a strong familial tendency and also major ethnic differences in prevalence.[16,39] In the Pacific region, the Micronesians in Nauru, Polynesians in Samoa[39] and Tonga[17] and our own Australian indigenous population have especially high risk.[40] Asian Indian and Chinese who have moved to urban centres or to developed nations also have a relatively high risk, though the particular predisposing genes have defied identification.[39] The highest rates in the world have been consistently found among Native American populations.[41]

The genetic aspect forms a background to massive changes in the human environment. A favoured theory to explain the unduly high risk in some populations relates to a 'thrifty genotype'. Historically, this genotype permitted populations such as the Polynesians in the Pacific to survive long famines, unfavourable environments and migration by favouring energy conservation and fat accumulation.[42,43] The proposal is that these communities had genes that allowed increased fat storage in times of feast, but result in obesity, hyperinsulinaemia and Type 2 diabetes in the transition to a modern lifestyle characterized by sedentary activity and relative over-nutrition.[43] The Western lifestyle appears to unmask the effects of pre-existing genes because the consistent result has been diabetes within a few decades.[43] An alternative theory, proposed by Hales and Barker,[44] suggests that foetal nutritional deprivation, with low birth weight, is a major predisposing factor to the later development of the insulin resistance syndrome and Type 2 diabetes. Their proposal remains controversial as statistically it may explain only a small proportion of the diabetic risk. Also, the association of low birth weight with diabetic risk in later life could be related more to genetic rather than nutritional factors, in fact another example of the thrifty gene scenario.[43]

Jared Diamond, a leading American biologist and author, has suggested that the lifestyle-related diabetes epidemic in Native Americans and Pacific Islanders probably results from the collision of our old hunter–gatherer genes with the new 20th century way of life.[45] He has recently taken this further, raising the question of why it is that while Type 2 diabetes is exploding in prevalence, despite its obvious selective disadvantage, some human populations are much more affected than others.[46] The epidemic seems well established in most parts of the world except in Europe.[2] Diamond suggests that part of the answer may lie in Europe's recent food history and the genetic and evolutionary consequences of geographic differences in food history.[46]

Type 2 Diabetes in Children and Adolescents

One of the most alarming consequences of the diabetes epidemic is the appearance of Type 2 diabetes in children and adolescents.[2,47] Until a decade or so ago, Type 2 diabetes was regarded as a disease of the middle aged and elderly. While it still is true that this age group maintains a higher relative risk (in relation to younger adults), there is accumulating and disturbing evidence that onset in the 20–30 age group is increasingly seen.[47,48] Now, even children are becoming caught up in the Type 2 diabetes epidemic. Although Type 1 diabetes remains the main form of the disease in children worldwide, it is more than likely that within 10 years Type 2 diabetes will be the more prevalent form in many ethnic groups, potentially including Europid groups. There are now numerous reports of Type 2 diabetes in children from countries including Japan, the United States, Pacific Islands, Hong Kong, Australia, the United Kingdom and Taiwan.[47–51] Dabelea and coworkers have reported on changes in rates of diabetes in Pima Indian children over a 30 year period.[52] They have demonstrated rising rates of glucose intolerance with time, and age as well as a female preponderance. From 1967–76 to 1987–96 the prevalence of Type 2 diabetes in children markedly increased from 2.4 per cent in males and 2.7 per cent in females to 3.8 per cent in males and 5.3 per cent for females.

The emergence of Type 2 diabetes in children brings a serious new aspect to the diabetes epidemic and heralds an emerging public health problem of major proportions in the paediatric area. The rise of Type 2 diabetes in this age group is mainly due to the increase of time spent on sedentary activities such as television and computer usage, either for games or school-work, with consequent reduction in sports. Add to this the increasing availability of energy-dense foods, high in saturated fats, and we have a 'witches' brew' to promote obesity and Type 2 diabetes. Type 2 diabetes in children is usually associated with obesity and a strong family history, and often with acanthosis nigricans and polycystic ovarian syndrome. Among children in Japan, Type 2 is already more common than Type 1 diabetes, accounting for 80 per cent of childhood diabetes; the incidence almost doubled between 1976–80 and 1991–5.[48] The rising prevalence of obesity and Type 2 diabetes in children is yet another symptom of the effects of globalization and industrialization affecting all societies, with sedentary lifestyle and obesity the predominant factors involved.[1]

This fall in the age of onset of Type 2 diabetes is an important factor influencing the future burden of the disease. Onset in childhood heralds many years of disease and an accumulation of the full range of both micro- and macrovascular complications.[1] The ADA and the American Academy of Pediatrics have published a consensus statement on the problem.[49] A key area raised in this report is the issue of poor compliance in diet and in tablet and insulin therapies. Recently, a number of pharmaceutical companies have embarked on clinical trials of oral hypoglycaemic agents to check their safety and efficacy in this age group, as they may face up to 40–50 years of therapy. Another worrying aspect is the high risk of, and early appearance of, long-term micro- and macrovascular complications in the adolescent and early adult years. The socio-economic and public health impact of this shift toward younger disease onset will be considerable through effects on the size of the fit and able work-force, premature morbidity and mortality and the negative impact on fertility and reproduction.

Prevention – The Reality and the Challenge

It does not come as a surprise, given the dramatic increase in Type 2 diabetes and its complications, and its socio-economic impact worldwide, that there is now a major interest in primary prevention. A number of studies discussed elsewhere in this book have clearly demonstrated that lifestyle modification (weight reduction and increased physical activity) can dramatically reduce the incidence of Type 2 diabetes in high-risk subjects. Unfortunately, the intensity of effort and associated costs in the two major studies in developed countries, the Finnish Diabetes Prevention Study.[53] and the American Diabetes Prevention Program,[54] may not permit implementation on a community-wide basis.

The use of pharmacological agents for Type 2 diabetes prevention is also being explored and, while contrary to an appropriate community-based lifestyle intervention strategy, may be contemplated where lifestyle intervention fails or is difficult from a socio-cultural perspective.[55] Although preventive action will not be easy or cheap, the magnitude of the problem we face with diabetes and its complications demands serious action.

References

1. Zimmet P *et al.* Global and societal implications of the diabetes epidemic. *Nature* 2001; **414**: 782–787.
2. Sicree R *et al.* The global burden of diabetes. In *Diabetes Atlas* 2nd edition, Gan D (ed.). 2003. Brussels: International Diabetes Federation, pp. 15–71.

3. Zimmet P. Globalization, coca-colonization and the chronic disease epidemic: can the doomsday scenario be averted? *J Internal Med* 2000; **247**: 301–310.
4. Fagot-Campagna A *et al.* Type 2 diabetes among North American children and adolescents: an epidemiologic review and a public health perspective. *J Pediatr* 2000; **136**: 664–672.
5. Knowler W *et al.* Diabetes mellitus in the Pima Indians: incidence, risk factors and pathogenesis. *Diab Metabol Rev* 1990; **6**: 1–27.
6. Dowse G *et al.* Decline in incidence of epidemic glucose intolerance in Nauruans: implications for the thrifty genotype. *Am J Epidemiol* 1991; **133**: 1093–1104.
7. Harris M *et al.* Prevalence of diabetes, impaired fasting glucose, and impaired glucose tolerance in U.S. adults. The Third National Health and Nutrition Examination 1988–1994. *Diabetes Care* 1998; **21**: 518–524.
8. Ramachandran A *et al.* Rising prevalence of NIDDM in an urban population in India. *Diabetologia* 1997; **40**: 232–237.
9. Ramachandran A *et al.* High prevalence of diabetes and impaired glucose tolerance in India: National Urban Diabetes Survey. *Diabetologia* 2001; **44**: 1094–1101.
10. Gu D *et al.* Prevalence of diabetes and impaired fasting glucose in the Chinese adult population: International Collaborative Study of Cardiovascular Disease in Asia (InterASIA). *Diabetologia* 2003; **46**: 1190–1198.
11. Pan X-R *et al.* Prevalence of diabetes and its risk factors in China. *Diabetes Care* 1997; **20**: 1664–1669.
12. Drivsholm T *et al.* Increasing prevalence of diabetes mellitus and impaired glucose tolerance among 60-year-old Danes. *Diabetic Med* 2001; **18**: 126–132.
13. Aschner P. Diabetes trends in Latin America. *Diabetes Metab Res Rev* 2002; **18** (Suppl. 3): S27–S31.
14. Motala A *et al.* High risk of progression to NIDDM in South-African Indians with impaired glucose tolerance. *Diabetes*, 1993; **42**: 556–563.
15. Dunstan D W *et al.* The rising prevalence of diabetes and impaired glucose tolerance: the Australian Diabetes, Obesity and Lifestyle Study. *Diabetes Care* 2002; **25**: 829–834.
16. Zimmet P *et al.* The epidemiology and natural history of NIDDM – lessons from the South Pacific. *Diabetes/Metab Rev* 1990; **6**: 91–124.
17. Colagiuri S *et al.* The prevalence of diabetes in the kingdom of Tonga. *Diabetes Care* 2002; **25**: 1378–1383.
18. Shaw JE and Chisholm DJ. Epidemiology and prevention of Type 2 diabetes and the metabolic syndrome. *Med J Aust* 2003; **179**: 379–383.
19. World Health Organization. (1999). *Definition, Diagnosis and Classification of Diabetes Mellitus and its Complications; Part 1: Diagnosis and Classification of Diabetes Mellitus.* Geneva: Department of Noncommunicable Disease Surveillance.
20. Shaw J *et al.* Impaired fasting glucose or impaired glucose tolerance. What best predicts future diabetes in Mauritius? *Diabetes Care* 1999; **22**: 399–402.
21. Qiao Q *et al.* Progression to clinically diagnosed and treated diabetes from impaired glucose tolerance and impaired fasting glycaemia. *Diabetic Med* 2003; **20**: 1027–1033.
22. Unwin N *et al.* Impaired glucose tolerance and impaired fasting glycaemia: the current status on definition and intervention. *Diabetic Med* 2002; **19**: 708–723.
23. The expert committee on the diagnosis and classification of diabetes mellitus. Follow-up report on the diagnosis of diabetes mellitus. *Diabetes Care* 2003; **26**: 3160–3167.
24. Reaven G. Role of insulin resistance in human disease. *Diabetes* 1988; **37**: 1595–1607.
25. DeFronzo R and Ferrannini E. Insulin resistance. A multifaceted syndrome responsible for NIDDM, obesity, hypertension, dyslipidemia and atherosclerotic cardiovascular disease. *Diabetes Care* 1991; **14**: 173–194.

26. Lakka HM *et al.* The metabolic syndrome and total and cardiovascular disease mortality in middle-aged men. *JAMA* 2002; **288**: 2709–2716.
27. Isomaa B *et al.* Cardiovascular morbidity and mortality associated with the metabolic syndrome. *Diabetes Care* 2001; **24**: 683–689.
28. Balkau B and Charles MA. Comment on the provisional report from the WHO consultation. European Group for the Study of Insulin Resistance (EGIR). *Diabetic Med* 1999; **16**: 442–443.
29. Expert panel on detection, evaluation and treatment of high blood cholesterol in adults. Executive summary of the third report of the national cholesterol education program (NCEP) Expert panel on detection, evaluation, and treatment of high blood cholesterol in adults (Adult Treatment Panel III). *JAMA* 2001; **285**: 2486–2497.
30. Balkau B *et al.* The incidence and persistence of the NCEP (National Cholesterol Education Program) metabolic syndrome. The French D.E.S.I.R. study. *Diabetes Metab* 2003; **29**: 526–532.
31. Marques-Vidal P *et al.* Prevalence of insulin resistance syndrome in southwestern France and its relationship with inflammatory and hemostatic markers. *Diabetes Care* 2002; **25**: 1371–1377.
32. Cameron AJ *et al.* Comparison of WHO and NCEP metabolic syndrome definitions over 5 years in Mauritius. *Diabetologia* 2003; **46**: A3068.
33. Ford ES *et al.* Prevalence of the metabolic syndrome among US adults: findings from the third National Health and Nutrition Examination Survey. *JAMA* 2002; **287**: 356–359.
34. Meigs JB *et al.* Prevalence and characteristics of the metabolic syndrome in the San Antonio Heart and Framingham Offspring Studies. *Diabetes* 2003; **52**: 2160–2167.
35. Balkau B *et al.* Frequency of the WHO metabolic syndrome in European cohorts, and an alternative definition of an insulin resistance syndrome. *Diabetes Metab* 2002; **28**: 364–376.
36. Abdul-Rahim HF *et al.* The metabolic syndrome in the West Bank population: an urban–rural comparison. *Diabetes Care* 2001; **24**: 275–279.
37. Villegas R *et al.* Prevalence of the metabolic syndrome in middle-aged men and women. *Diabetes Care* 2003; **26**: 3198–3199.
38. Zimmet P and Alberti K. The changing face of macrovascular disease in non-insulin dependent diabetes mellitus in different cultures: an epidemic in progress. *Lancet* 1997; **350**: S1–S4.
39. de Courten M *et al.* Epidemiology of NIDDM in ion-Europids. In *International Textbook of Diabetes Mellitus*, Alberti KGMM, Zimmet P, DeFronzo RA and Keen H. (eds). 1997. New York: Wiley, pp. 143–170.
40. O'Dea K. Westernisation, insulin resistance and diabetes in Australian Aborigines. *Med J Aust* 1991; **155**: 258–264.
41. Knowler W *et al.* Diabetes incidence and prevalence in Pima Indians: a 19-fold greater incidence than in Rochester, Minnesota. *Am J Epidemiol* 1978; **108**: 497–504.
42. Neel J. Diabetes mellitus: a thrifty genotype rendered detrimental by 'progress'? *Am J Hum Genet* 1962; **14**: 353–362.
43. Zimmet P. Diabetes epidemiology as a trigger to diabetes research. *Diabetologia* 1999; **42**: 499–518.
44. Hales C *et al.* The thrifty phenotype hypothesis: how does it look after 5 years? *Diabetic Med* 1997; **14**: 189–195.
45. Diamond J. Diabetes running wild. *Nature* 1992; **357**: 362–363.
46. Diamond J. The double puzzle of diabetes. *Nature* 2003; **423**: 599–602.
47. Fagot-Campagna A and Narayan K. Type 2 diabetes in children. *BMJ* 2001; **322**: 377–387.
48. Kitagawa T *et al.* Increased incidence of non-insulin dependent diabetes mellitus among Japanese school children correlates with an increased intake of animal protein and fat. *Clin Pediatrics* 1998; **37**: 111–116.

49. American Diabetes Association. Type 2 diabetes in children and adolescents. *Diabetes Care* 2000; **23**: 381–389.
50. Onyemere KU and Lipton RB. Parental history and early-onset Type 2 diabetes in African Americans and Latinos in Chicago. *J Pediatr* 2002; **141**: 825–829.
51. Chuang LM *et al.* Incidence and prevalence of childhood diabetes in Taiwan – an experience with nation-wide screening. *Diabetes Res Clin Prac* 2002; **56**: S16.
52. Dabelea D *et al.* Type 2 diabetes mellitus in minority children and adolescents. An emerging problem. *Endocrinol Metab Clin North Am* 1999; **28**: 709–729, viii.
53. Tuomilehto J *et al.* Prevention of Type 2 diabetes mellitus by changes in lifestyle among subjects with impaired glucose tolerance. *N Engl J Med*, 2001; **344**: 1343–1350.
54. Knowler WC *et al.* Reduction in the incidence of Type 2 diabetes with lifestyle intervention or metformin. *N Engl J Med* 2002; **346**: 393–403.
55. Simpson RW *et al.* The prevention of Type 2 diabetes – lifestyle change or pharmacotherapy? A challenge for the 21st century. *Diabetes Res Clin Pract* 2003; **59**: 165–180.

2

Type 2 Diabetes Mellitus: Primary and Secondary Prevention The Vision of the International Diabetes Federation

Pierre Lefèbvre

Introduction

Until May 2004 the mission of the International Diabetes Federation was 'to work with its member associations to enhance the lives of people with diabetes'. For the last 50 years, the action of the Federation has been targeted accordingly: recruiting more and more member associations (currently 185 in 145 countries), organizing activities in the Federation's seven regions, increasing awareness about diabetes, promoting solidarity through the associations' twinning programmes, defending the cause of people with diabetes at national, regional and international levels, cooperating with the World Health Organisation and numerous non-governmental bodies, helping to educate health care professionals to improve diabetes management through its Education Foundation, evaluating the cost of diabetes, disseminating information about diabetes through its newsletters, periodicals, nonserial publications, triennal congresses, website and the IDF Atlas. . . .

As evidenced by the information gathered in the preceding chapter, time has come to add *diabetes prevention* to the mission of the Federation.[1] Indeed,

Prevention of Type 2 Diabetes Edited by Manfred Ganz
 ISBN: 0-470-85733-1

estimations and projections all concur to the conclusion that the number of people with diabetes may reach levels in the 20–25 coming years that will qualify diabetes as the largest epidemic humanity has ever experienced. If this indeed occurs, and there is little reason to believe it will not if action is not taken, there is a significant risk that governments and social security systems may fail in ensuring appropriate care to the over 300 million people who will be affected by diabetes in the world at the 2025 horizon, that is tomorrow. By promoting diabetes prevention, the IDF will ensure that those millions who already suffer from diabetes will not face the nightmare of a regression in the quality of care they deserve while, on the contrary, there is a great need in many parts of the world to improve it.

Primary Prevention of Type 2 Diabetes Mellitus

As emphasized in a recent consensus statement,[2] there is strong evidence that genetics plays an important role together with overweight or obesity resulting from excess calorie intake and reduction in physical activity. Furthermore, there is evidence that a low birth weight, as a consequence of poor nourishment of the foetus, significantly increases the risk of Type 2 diabetes mellitus and the related 'metabolic syndrome' in the offspring. Ultimately, some mechanistic studies suggest a relationship between stress and insulinoresistance with predisposition to Type 2 diabetes mellitus. Recent studies, reviewed in detail elsewhere in this book, have shown that lifestyle changes (and also some medications) are effective in preventing Type 2 diabetes in individuals at risk, such as those having impaired glucose tolerance.[3–6] The IDF will promote concerted action by governments and nongovernmental organizations to increase awareness about the seriousness of Type 2 diabetes, promote education at all levels and exercise multisectoral advocacy. A major action in the coming years is the ambitious *Diabetes Action Now* programme elaborated by the WHO Department of Noncommunicable Disease Management in Geneva and the International Diabetes Federation. Supported by the World Diabetes Foundation, this programme aims to enhance awareness about diabetes and its complications amongst the public, health professionals and decision makers, with major emphasis on prevention, particularly in low-income countries. It will support WHO/IDF regions and countries in the reorganization of their health services in response to the current epidemic by developing coordinated programmes for both the promotion of effective management of people with diabetes and the primary prevention of Type 2 diabetes. In these programmes, emphasis will be put on healthy dietary habits, promotion of physical activity and appropriate quantitative and qualitative nutrition of the pregnant mother.

In its recently issued *Global Strategic Plan to Raise Awareness of Diabetes*,[7] the IDF has identified the four following strategic messages:

TABLE 2.1 Example of correlating a 'core strategic message' into 'underlying communication messages' by target audience (from reference 7)

Core strategic message	Underlying communication messages
In some instances diabetes can be prevented.	People with diabetes • Some of your family members may be at high risk of developing diabetes and this can sometimes be prevented. Bring this to their attention. High-risk groups • Appropriate lifestyle changes can reduce your risk of diabetes. Reduce weight if you are overweight or obese. Maintain an appropriate level of physical activity and stay in touch with your health-care provider. General public • Lead a healthy lifestyle. Avoid becoming overweight (or reduce weight if necessary). Maintain an appropriate level of physical activity and seek health-care advice if you think you may be in a high-risk group. Health-care professionals • Recognize people at risk of getting diabetes and recommend the appropriate lifestyle changes. Health decision makers • Assign adequate resources (money and people) to ensure prevention and early diagnosis of diabetes.

1. diabetes is a common condition and its frequency is dramatically rising all over the world;
2. diabetes is a life-threatening condition;
3. diabetes can be detected early and managed effectively;
4. in many instances, diabetes can be prevented.

Target audiences have been defined and specific communication messages have been developed for each unique audience (see Table 2.1 as an example). Relevant tactics have been identified and appropriate measurement methods listed.

Regarding diabetes prevention, the recommendation is made to request health decision makers to assign adequate resources (money and people) to ensure prevention and early diagnosis of diabetes. The present book will be a remarkable source of information in this respect.

Prevention of Complications of Type 2 Diabetes Mellitus

If primary prevention of diabetes must now be considered by the IDF, helping all those affected by diabetes to improve their quality of life, prevent diabetes complications occurring and, if these occur, slow down their progression remains the cornerstone of the action of the Federation. In our times of 'evidence-based medicine', numerous studies performed over the last 20 years, and reviewed in detail in other chapters of this book, have provided strong evidence that strict control of blood glucose reduces the incidence of retinopathy, nephropathy and neuropathy in both Type 1 and Type 2 diabetes mellitus, that control of blood pressure reduces the risk of cardiovascular events and deaths, that intensive treatment of blood pressure reduces the risk of aggravation of nephropathy in subjects with microalbuminuria or *incipiens* renal failure etc. As emphasized by Nathan,[8] the net effect of these controlled clinical trials has been an expansion of lifespan and an improvement in quality of life for persons affected by diabetes. The IDF's role is to disseminate the conclusions of these trials to its member associations and to raise awareness of this progress among the public, health-care providers, social security systems and governments.

THE IDF recognizes some remarkable national programmes against diabetes such as the National Framework Programme on Diabetes in the United Kingdom, the 2000–2010 Development Programme for the Prevention and Care of Diabetes in Finland, the National Plan against Diabetes in France and the soon coming National Prevention Programme for Diabetes in Sri Lanka, to mention only a few.

Through its regions, the IDF has contributed to major programmes in Europe (St Vincent Declaration), North, Central and South America (Declaration of the Americas or DOTA) and the Western Pacific (WP Declaration on Diabetes). It will encourage similar initiatives in other parts of the world.

The Global Issue

As reviewed by P. Zimmet a few years ago,[9] time has come to mobilize politicians, health decision makers and international agencies such as WHO, UNPD, UNICEF and the World Bank as well as other international nongovernmental agencies dealing with noncommunicable diseases to address the socio-economic, behavioural, nutritional and public health issues that have led to the present Type 2 diabetes mellitus epidemic. In this fight against Type 2 diabetes mellitus, which is now seen in children and adolescents, all components of society, including WHO and IDF, will have to counteract the dramatic lifestyle changes that our entire world has seen over the last 30 years by the aggressive promotion of cheap, easily available, high-calorie food and beverages combined with a mechanization of society and sedentary leisure activities such as TV watching and video games. However, it is probably a mistake to consider that diet and exercise alone will prevent Type 2 diabetes mellitus. What is required are major and dramatic changes in the socio-economic and cultural status of people in developing countries, as well as disadvantaged and minority groups in developed nations.[8] Advocating this cause requires intense lobbying of the decision makers. In the year 2000, the European diabetes community was informed that diabetes was no longer a priority of the soon-to-be-introduced Sixth Framework Programme of the European Union. This led to concerted efforts by IDF, its European Member Associations and the European Association for the Study of Diabetes to put diabetes back in the Programme. A broad-based and individually focused campaign of awareness was implemented. It included public relation activities at the European Parliament in Strasbourg and at the European Commission in Brussels. Members of the European Parliament from several countries were asked to defend the cause of diabetes and agreed to do so. On 14 November 2003, which is World Diabetes Day, European Commissioner Philippe Busquin reported the decision to launch a five-year integrated project that will look into the prevention and treatment of obesity, one of the main causes of Type 2 diabetes mellitus. In January 2004, the IDF joined the International Association for the Study of Obesity, the World Heart Foundation, the International Union of Nutritional Sciences and the International Pediatric Association to address the 113th meeting of the Executive Board of WHO to provide active support to the report entitled *Joint WHO/FAO Expert Consultation on Diet, Nutrition and the Prevention of Chronic Diseases*. The proposals detailed in this report are seen to be the first significant opportunity to address the nutritional challenges of the 21st century in a coherent manner and to shape a new vision of public health focused on the prevention of chronic diseases such as diabetes. After some amendments, the report has been approved at the 2004 World Health Assembly.... Preventing diabetes is a big challenge in front of us; the IDF will tackle the problem seriously.

References

1. Lefèbvre P. Diabetes prevention and strategic action. *IDF Diabetes Atlas*. 2003. Brussels: IDF, pp. 301–304.
2. *Consensus on the Aetiology of Type 2 Diabetes Mellitus and Development of a Primary Prevention Strategy for Type 2 Diabetes Mellitus*. 2002. Colombo, Sri Lanka.
3. Pan X-R, Li G-W and Wang J-X *et al.* Effect of diet and exercise in preventing NIDDM in people with impaired glucose tolerance: the Da Quing IGT and Diabetes Study. *Diabetes Care* 1997; **20**: 537–544.
4. Tuomilehto J, Lindström J and Eriksson JG *et al.* Prevention of Type 2 diabetes mellitus by changes in lifestyle among subjects with impaired glucose tolerance. *N Engl J Med* 2001; **344**: 1343–1350.
5. Diabetes Prevention Programme Research Group. Reduction in the incidence of Type 2 diabetes with lifestyle intervention or metformin. *N Engl J Med* 2002; **346**: 393–403.
6. Chiasson J-L, Josse RG, Gomis R, Hanefeld M, Karasik A and Laakso M. For the Stop-NIDDM Trial Research Group. Acarbose for prevention of Type 2 diabetes mellitus: the STOP-NIDDM randomised trial. *Lancet* 2002; **359**: 2072–2077.

7. International Diabetes Federation. Global strategic plan to raise awareness of diabetes; 2003, Brussels: IDF.
8. Nathan DM. The impact of clinical trials on the treatment of diabetes mellitus. *J. Clin. Endocr. Metab* 2002; **87**: 1929–1937.
9. Zimmet P and Lefèbvre P. The global NIDDM epidemic. Treating the disease and ignoring the symptom. *Diabetologia* 1996; **39**: 1247–1248.

3

Type 2 Diabetes Mellitus in Children and Adolescents

Thomas Reinehr and **Martin Wabitsch**

Introduction

Until very recently, Type 2 diabetes has been thought to be a rare occurrence in children and adolescents. However, in the mid-1990s, investigators began to observe an increasing incidence of Type 2 diabetes worldwide.[1] This is particularly the case in the USA[2] but has also been reported in other countries such as Canada, Japan, Austria, the United Kingdom and Germany.[1,3–5]

This observation followed a striking increase in both the prevalence and the degree of obesity in children and adolescents in many populations.[6] Overweight is at present the most common health problem facing children in both developed and developing countries. In some countries, the prevalence of obesity in childhood and adolescence has become higher than that of allergic disorders including both asthma and eczema. Worldwide, approximately 22 million children under the age of 5 years are overweight and the prevalence of overweight in the young is increasing.[7]

Type 2 diabetes is a serious and costly disease. The chronic complications of diabetes include accelerated development of cardiovascular disease, end-stage renal disease, loss of visual acuity and limb amputations. All of these complications contribute to the excess morbidity and mortality in individuals with diabetes. Moreover, the prevalence of Type 2 diabetes in adults is increasing. Superimposed on this disturbing picture in adults are the recent reports of the emerging problem of Type 2 diabetes in children and adolescents.

Prevention of Type 2 Diabetes Edited by Manfred Ganz
 ISBN: 0-470-85733-1

If the incidence and prevalence of Type 2 diabetes in children are increasing and if this increase cannot be reversed, our society will face major challenges. That is, the burden of diabetes and its complications will affect many more individuals than currently anticipated, and the cost of diabetes to our society will cause us to consume enormous resources.

Pathophysiology of Type 2 Diabetes Mellitus in Children and Adolescents

Type 2 diabetes is a complex metabolic disorder of heterogeneous aetiology with social, behavioural and environmental risk factors unmasking the effects of genetic susceptibility.[7] There is a strong hereditary (probably multigenic) component to the disease, with the role of genetic determinants illustrated when differences in the prevalence of Type 2 diabetes in various racial groups are considered. The recent increases observed in diabetes prevalence are too quick to be the result of increased gene frequency and altered gene pool, emphasizing the importance of environmental factors.

Glucose homeostasis depends on the balance between insulin secretion by the pancreatic beta cells and insulin action. It is well recognized that insulin resistance to insulin-stimulated glucose uptake is a characteristic finding in patients with Type 2 diabetes and impaired glucose metabolism. The evolution from normal to impaired glucose tolerance is associated with a worsening of insulin resistance. Impaired glucose tolerance is an intermediate stage in the natural history of Type 2 diabetes and is a strong predictor of the risk of developing diabetes[8] and cardiovascular disease.[9]

For diabetes to develop, insulin resistance alone is not sufficient and inadequate beta cell insulin secretion is necessary. In patients with Type 2 diabetes, impaired insulin action and insulin secretory failure are both present. It has been proposed that hyperglycaemia may worsen both insulin resistance and insulin secretory abnormalities, thus enhancing the transition from impaired glucose tolerance to diabetes.

Puberty appears to play a major role in the development of Type 2 diabetes in children. During puberty, there is increased resistance to the action of insulin, resulting in hyperinsulinaemia.[10] After puberty, basal and stimulated insulin responses decline. Hyperinsulinaemic–euglycaemic clamp studies demonstrate that insulin-mediated glucose disposal is on average 30 per cent lower in adolescents between Tanner stage II and IV compared with prepubertal children and with young adults. Increased growth hormone secretion in puberty is suggested to be responsible for the insulin resistance during puberty. Given this information, it is not surprising that the peak age at presentation of Type 2 diabetes in children coincides with the usual age of mid-puberty.

The adverse effect of obesity on glucose metabolism is evident early in childhood. Obese children are hyperinsulinaemic and have approximately 40 per cent lower insulin-stimulated glucose metabolism compared with non-obese children. Furthermore, the inverse relationship between insulin sensitivity and abdominal fat is stronger for visceral than for subcutaneous fat. In a seven-year longitudinal study of African-American and white young adults 18 years and older, the strongest predictor for increases in both insulin and glucose concentrations was an increase in weight.[1]

It is interesting to note that adipose tissue expanding in the obese state synthesizes and secretes metabolites and signalling proteins such as adiponectin, tumour necrosis factor-alpha, leptin and resistin. These factors are known to alter insulin secretion and sensitivity and even cause insulin resistance under experimental and clinical conditions.

Racial differences in insulin sensitivity are also evident in childhood. African-American 7- to 11-year-old children have significantly higher insulin levels than age-matched white children. These data suggest that minority children may have a genetic predisposition to insulin resistance, which may increase their risk for Type 2 diabetes.

Epidemiology of Type 2 Diabetes Mellitus in Children and Adolescents

The limited amount of information about the epidemiology of Type 2 diabetes in children is in large part due to the relatively recent recognition of its emergence in this age group. In the United States and in Canada Type 2 diabetes in adolescents was found especially in specific ethnic subgroups, being highest in Pima Indians (22.3/1000 in 10–14-year-old children).[2] The estimated prevalence of diabetes (all types) in adolescents has been estimated in the Third National Health and Nutrition Examination Survey (NHANES) to be 0.41 per cent and that of impaired fasting glucose 1.76 per cent. Recently, Sinha *et al.* investigated a multiethnic American cohort of 167 obese children and adolescents and found impaired glucose tolerance in more than 20 per cent of the subjects and silent Type 2 diabetes in four subjects.[11] Finally, in case series, Type 2 diabetes constituted an increasing percentage of incident paediatric cases of newly diagnosed diabetes, with fewer than four per cent reported before the 1990s and up to 45 per cent in recent studies.[2]

The emergence of Type 2 diabetes in children is not limited to North America. Table 3.1 summarizes the studies and reports that provide estimates of the frequency of Type 2 diabetes mellitus in children and adolescents. One epidemiological study of Type 2 diabetes mellitus in Europe reported an incidence rate of 0.25/100 000 children in Austria but many of the children were non-Caucasian or

TABLE 3.1 Estimates of the magnitude of Type 2 diabetes in children (IGT, impaired glucose tolerance T2DM, Type 2 diabetes mellitus)

	Years	Race/ethnicity	Age (years)	Estimates prevalence per 1000
		Population-based studies		
Arizona	1992–1996	Pima Indians	10–14	22.3
			15–19	50.9
Manitoba	1996–1997	First Nations	10–19	36.0
NHANES III	1988–1994	Whites, African-Americans, Mexican Americans	12–19	4.1
Austria	1999–2001	predominantly Caucasian	<15	0.0025
		Clinical-based studies		
Tokyo	1974–1994	Japanese	6–18	0.03
Indian Health Services	1996	American Indians	0–14	1.3
Manitoba	1998	First Nations	5–14	1.0
			15–19	2.3
Cincinnati, OH	1994	Whites, African-Americans	10–19	Incidence 7.2 per 100 000
		Screening studies in obese children		
Yale	2001	Whites, African-Americans	4–10	25% IGT 0% T2DM
			11–18	21% IGT 4% T2DM
Germany	2002	predominantly Caucasian	9–20	7% IGT 1% T2DM
Italy	2002	predominantly Caucasian	6–18	5% IGT

suffered from syndromal obesity.[4] In a screening study of diabetes by using an oral glucose tolerance test in cohort of 520 overweight children and adolescents of Caucasian origin between 9 and 20 years, in eight children (1.5 per cent) diagnosis of diabetes Type 2 was suggested.[5] The overall prevalence of elevated blood glucose levels was seven per cent. Four per cent of these patients had impaired fasting blood glucose and two per cent of the patients showed an impaired glucose tolerance. Based on these data, it could be speculated that up to 15 000 overweight children suffering from Type 2 diabetes might be expected in Germany due to approximately 1 million obese children and adolescents. In contrast to this, only 130 children with Type 2 diabetes are documented in the standardized evaluation program 'dpv', which is used by most paediatric diabetologists in Germany.

Clinical Presentation of Type 2 Diabetes Mellitus in Children and Adolescents

Obesity is the hallmark of Type 2 diabetes. Most children with Type 2 diabetes are overweight or obese at diagnosis and present with glucosuria without ketonuria, absent or mild polyuria and polydipsia and little or no weight loss. Currently, children with Type 2 diabetes are usually diagnosed over the age of 10 years and are in middle to late puberty.

In the mildest Type 2 diabetes form, the diagnosis is made in an asymptomatic child during a routine medical check-up by detection of glycosuria, and subsequent hyperglycaemia. One-third of patients are diagnosed by urinanalysis during routine physical examination.[10] In its severest form, the child presents with evidence of severe insulin deficiency, polyuria, polydipsia and weight loss. Up to 33 per cent in particular ethnic groups have ketonuria at diagnosis and 5–25 per cent ketoacidosis at presentation. With this clinical picture, often the distinction from Type 1 diabetes is not possible until months later, when insulin requirements decline and a non-insulin-dependent course develops without dependence on insulin for survival.

Children with Type 2 diabetes usually have a family history of Type 2 diabetes and those of non-European ancestry (Americans of African, Hispanic, Asian and American Indian descent) are disproportionately represented. Of the patients, 74–100 per cent have a first- or second-degree relative with Type 2 diabetes. Of note, diabetes in the parent or other relative may not be recognized until the child is diagnosed.

Acanthosis nigricans and polycystic ovarian syndrome (PCOS), disorders associated with insulin resistance and obesity, are common in youth with Type 2 diabetes. Acanthosis is a cutaneous finding characterized by velvety hyperpigmented patches most prominent in the intertrigenous area, and is present in up to 90 per cent of children with Type 2 diabetes. It is recognized more frequently in darker-skinned obese individuals. PCOS is a reproductive disorder characterized by hyperandrogenism and chronic anovulation. Lipid disorders and hypertension also occur in children with Type 2 diabetes.

Clinical Features of Caucasian Children with Type 2 Diabetes Mellitus

Until now, there are only a few reports about Caucasian children with Type 2 diabetes in Europe.[5,3,4] The clinical presentation of 16 European Caucasian children with Type 2 diabetes mellitus is presented in Table 3.2 and the data concerning the metabolic presentation in Table 3.3. 75 per cent of these children showed fasting blood glucose above 126 mg/dl and 63 per cent HbA_{1c} above the

TABLE 3.2 Clinical presentation of European Caucasian children and adolescents with Type 2 diabetes mellitus

Age in years	median 14.2 (range 11.0–16.9)
Gender	female > male
SDS height	median 0.0 (range −2.3 to +2.9)
SDS weight	median +2.8 (range +1.6 to +4.2)
BMI kg/m^2	median 33.7 (range 25.4–40.4)
SDS BMI	median +2.8 (range +1.6 to +3.4)
Overweight (BMI > 90th perc.)	12%
Obese (BMI > 97th Perc.)	19%
Extremely obese (BMI > 99.5 perc.)	69%
1st- and 2nd-degree relatives with Type 2 diabete mellitus	75%
Prepubertal	none
Acanthosis nigricans	50%
Asymptomatic	81%
Ketonuria or ketoacidosis	<5%

cut-off point of 6.0 per cent. The two-hour glucose values were always above 200 mg/dl in the oral glucose tolerance test.

The clinical and metabolic presentation of Type 2 diabetes mellitus in Caucasian children differed from reports predominantly of Afro-Americans, Mexicans, Hispanics or Indians (see Table 3.4). In contrast to studies of minorities in the USA with up to 25 per cent ketoacidosis in children with Type 2 diabetes mellitus, only one obese Caucasian adolescent has been published with ketoacidosis at manifestation.[3] Most of the European Caucasian children and adolescents with Type 2 diabetes were asymptomatically at diagnosis. The minority populations

TABLE 3.3 Metabolic presentation of Caucasian children and adolescents with Type 2 diabetes mellitus

	median (range)	norm value
HbA_{1c}	6.9 (4.6–12.0)	<6.0
Fasting blood glucose mg/dl	176 (90–455)	<126
2 hour oGTT mg/dl	229 (206–343)	<140
Insulin μU/ml	19 (8–372)	3–17
C-peptide ng/ml	2.3 (0.9–19.6)	0.6–2.5
Triglycerides mg/dl	175 (60–554)	<150
Triglycerides > 150 mg/dl	56%	
Cholesterol mg/dl	180 (136–260)	<200
Cholesterol > 200 mg/dl	25%	
LDL-cholesterol mg/dl	98 (67–189)	<130
LDL-cholesterol > 130 mg/dl	25%	
HDL-cholesterol mg/dl	39 (24–63)	<40
HDL-cholesterol > 40 mg/dl	50%	

TABLE 3.4 Comparison between Caucasian and non-Caucasian children and adolescents with Type 2 diabetes mellitus (T2DM)

	Caucasian	Non-Caucasian
Number of children and adolescents with T2DM published in the literature	24	>400
Mean age at onset in years	14	12–14
Gender	female > male	female > male
Clinical manifestation	50% asymptomatic 4% ketoacidosis	33% asymptomatic 5–25% ketoacidosis
1st- and 2nd-degree relatives with Type 2 diabetes mellitus	83%	74–100%
Obese	90%	90%
Acanthosis nigricans	50%	90%

demonstrated at manifestation of diabetes frequently more symptoms and higher insulin and C-peptide levels, pointing to greater insulin resistance.[10] African-American children are more insulin resistant than Caucasian children.[12] According to this, acanthosis nigricans, a clinical sign of insulin resistance, occurred more frequently in these populations. Another explanation for these differences may be the fact that most of the Caucasian children with Type 2 diabetes mellitus were detected by screening, in contrast to many of the non-Caucasian children published, who had presented with overt clinical symptoms.[10] The non-Caucasian obese children with Type 2 diabetes mellitus detected by screening in the US had similar levels of insulin and insulin resistance index (HOMA) to Caucasian children with Type 2 diabetes mellitus.[11]

Differential Diagnosis of Type 2 Diabetes Mellitus in Children and Adolescents

Individuals with Type 2 diabetes may have clinical presentations indistinguishable from those of patients with other types of diabetes (see Table 3.5). This is relevant because as the number of children with Type 2 diabetes increases it becomes increasingly important to classify their diabetes correctly so that appropriate therapy may be instituted.

Typically, children with Type 1 diabetes are not overweight and have recent weight loss, polyuria, and poydipsia (see Table 3.6). They usually have a short duration of symptoms and frequently have ketosis; 30 per cent have ketoacidosis at presentation.[1] After metabolic stabilization, they may have an initial period of diminished insulin requirement, after which they require insulin for survival. Of children with Type 1 diabetes, five per cent have a first- or second-degree relative with the same disease.

TABLE 3.5 Classification of diabetes[1,13]

- Type 1 diabetes (absolute insulin deficiency):
  - immune mediated
  - idiopathic
- Type 2 diabetes (insulin resistance with relative insulin deficiency)
- Other specific types
  - Genetic defects of beta cell function (e.g. MODY)
  - Genetic defects in insulin action (e.g. lipoatrophic diabetes)
  - Diseases of the exocrine pancreas (e.g. cystis fibrosis)
  - Endocrinopathies (e.g. Cushing's syndrome)
  - Drug or chemical induced (e.g. glucorticoids)
  - Infections (e.g. congential rubella)
  - Uncommon forms of immune-mediated diabetes
  - Other genetic syndromes sometimes associated with diabetes (e.g. Prader-Willi syndrome)
- Gestational diabetes mellitus (GDM)

Children with idiopathic Type 1 diabetes may be difficult to distinguish from those with Type 2 diabetes. The majority of those described with idiopathic Type 1 diabetes have what has been termed atypical diabetes mellitus and are African-American.[1] Their family history is positive for early-onset diabetes in many relatives in multiple generations. Insulin may not be required for survival after the resolution of the acute metabolic deterioration. Metabolic control, however, is poor without insulin therapy, and ketoacidosis may occur.

TABLE 3.6 Clinical characteristics of Type 1, Type 2 and MODY diabetes mellitus

Clinical characteristic	Type 1 diabetes m.	Type 2 diabetes m.	MODY diabetes
Age when diagnosis is established	preschool–adolescents	>10 years	MODY 2: youth MODY 3: adolescents
Obesity	uncommon	common	uncommon
Gender	male = female	female > male	male = female
Relatives	5% Type 1 d.m.	75–100% Type 2 d.m.	100% MODY
Population	predominantly Caucasian	predominantly Americans of African, Hispanic, Asian and American Indian origin	
Beta cell autoantibodies	85–98%	uncommon	uncommon
Insulin, C-peptide	low	high	low
Ketoacidosis	frequently	<33%	uncommon
Associated disorders	autoimmune disorders (thyroid, adrenal, vitiligo), coeliac disease	Acanthosis nigricans PCOS Metabolic syndrome	

Maturity-onset diabetes of the young (MODY) is another rare form of diabetes in children, which includes several disorders caused by monogenic defects in beta cell function.[14] MODY 2 (defect in glucokinase) and MODY 3 (defect in HNF1α) are the most frequent types of MODY. Patients with MODY have a dominant genetic trait, usually are nonobese and have low fasting insulin levels. Recent studies suggest that the clinical presentation of MODY is broad, ranging from asymptomatic hyperglycaemia to a severe acute presentation. MODY has been reported in all races/ethnicities. These gene abnormalities are thought to be rare, and molecular diagnostic testing, currently only available in research laboratories, is required for specific classification. Until such testing becomes commonplace, children with MODY should be classified as having the type of diabetes that best fits their clinical picture.

Diagnostic Criteria of Type 2 Diabetes Mellitus in Children and Adolescents

The criteria for diagnosis of diabetes and impaired glucose metabolism in children and adolescents are presented in Tables 3.7 and 3.8. In the absence of unequivocal hyperglycaemia with acute metabolic decompensation, these criteria should be confirmed by repeat testing on a different day.

In most patients with diabetes, classification can be made reliably on the basis of clinical presentation and course.[1] In the unusual circumstance that requires a

TABLE 3.7 Criteria for the diagnosis of diabetes[1,3]

- Symptoms of diabetes plus casual glucose concentration:
  - ≥200 mg/dl (11.1 mmol/l) in venous plasma or capillary whole blood samples
  - ≥180 mg/dl (10.0 mmol/l) in venous whole blood samples
  - ≥220 mg/dl (12.2. mmol/l) in capillary plasma

  Casual is defined as any time of day without regard to time since last meal. The classic symptoms of diabetes include polyuria, polydipsia, and unexplained weight loss

or

- Fasting glucose:
  - ≥126 mg/dl (7.0 mmol/l) in venous or capillary plasma
  - ≥110 mg/dl (6.1 mmol/l) in venous or capillary whole blood samples

  Fasting is defined as no caloric intake for at least 8 hours

or

- Two-hours glucose during oral glucose tolerance test:
  - ≥200 mg/dl (11.1 mmol/l) in venous plasma or capillary whole blood sample
  - ≥180 mg/dl (10.0 mmol/l) in venous whole blood samples
  - ≥220 mg/dl (12.2. mmol/l) in capillary plasma

  The test should be performed using an oral glucose load containing the equivalent of 1.75 g/kg body weight (maximum 75 g) anhydrous glucose dissolved in water.

TABLE 3.8 Criteria for the diagnosis of impaired glucose metabolism in oral glucose tolerance test

	Time point	Venous plasma	Venous whole blood sample	Capillary plasma	Capillary whole blood sample
Normal	0 min	<100 mg/dl	<100 mg/dl	<100 mg/dl	<100 mg/dl
	2 hours	<140 mg/dl	<120 mg/dl	<160 mg/dl	<140 mg/dl
Impaired glucose tolerance	0 min	<126 mg/dl	<110 mg/dl	<126 mg/dl	<110 mg/dl
	2 hours	140–199 mg/dl	120–179 mg/dl	160–219 mg/dl	140–199 mg/dl
Impaired fasting glucose	0 min	100–125 mg/dl	100–109 mg/dl	100–125 mg/dl	100–109 mg/dl
	2 hours	<140 mg/dl	<120 mg/dl	<160 mg/dl	<140 mg/dl
Diabetes mellitus	0 min	>125 mg/dl	>109 mg/dl	>125 mg/dl	>109 mg/dl
	2 hours	>199 > mg/dl	>180 mg/dl	>219 mg/dl	>199 mg/dl

specific classification to be made, another test may be necessary, such as fasting insulin or C-peptide determination and, occasionally, beta cell autoantibody measurements (see Figure 3.1). To achieve a high degree of sensitivity, a combination of tests is required, which greatly increases the cost of classification. In the future, these tests may be standardized, more reliable and less expensive.

Individuals with Type 2 diabetes usually do not have autoantibodies to beta cell proteins; fasting insulin and C-peptide levels are elevated, although not as elevated as might be excepted for the degree of hyperglycaemia. Specific autoantibodies to

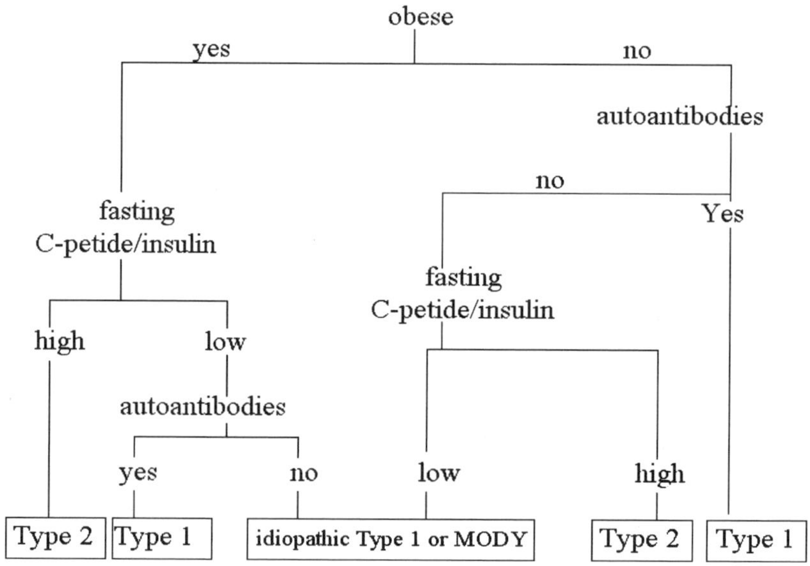

FIGURE 3.1 Flowsheet for classification of diabetes in children and adolescents[1]

insulin, to GAD-II or to tyrosine phosphatase insulin antibodies (IA)-2 and IA-2b are found at presentation in 85–98 per cent of individuals with immune-mediated Type 1 diabetes.[1] Type 1 diabetes mellitus also has a strong HLA association; however, HLA typing is not a useful diagnostic tool. Endogenous fasting insulin and C-peptide is low in Type 2 diabetes, with little or no increase after oral or intravenous glucose administration. Specific laboratory evaluation to classify diabetes in children should only be used by diabetologists with paediatric expertise and only when a definitive classification is clinically required.

Complications of Type 2 Diabetes Mellitus in Children and Adolescents

The chronic complications of diabetes in adults include macrovascular diseases such as accelerated development of cardiovascular disease leading to stroke and myocardial infarction, and microvascular diseases such as retinopathy, nephropathy and neuropathy leading to end-stage renal disease, loss of visual acuity and limb amputations. All of these complications contribute to the excess morbidity and mortality in individuals with diabetes.

They are only a few data concerning complications of Type 2 diabetes mellitus in childhood. Assessing trial data from adults and extrapolating to outcomes in children is fraught with difficulties. The largest follow-up study of Type 2 diabetes mellitus in adults was the UK Prospective Diabetes Study (UKPDS), which followed 5012 patients for a median of 10 years.[15] Clearly outcomes in terms of absolute numbers are non informative in children. One would not expect myocardial infarction rates to be similar in teenagers to those of median age 65 years, even if their glycaemic control were similar. On the other hand, the relative rates of events across quintiles of glycaemia are likely to be informative. The pathological process caused by hyperglycaemia is likely to be similar. The UKPDS observational analysis showed clear logarithmic association of risk with increasing glycaemia (see Figure 3.2). It would be perverse to suggest that these relative risks did not apply to children, and the conclusion must therefore be that diagnosis and aggressive control of glycaemia is a mandatory requirement if we are to reduce the burden of endpoints. Moreover, since the risk is logarithmic we should be especially assiduous in reducing glycaemia in those in the upper ranges of HbA_{1c}.

One notable outcome of the UKPDS analysis was the observation that the accrual of endpoints was a time-dependent process (see Figure 3.3). At higher levels of HbA_{1c} the effects become even more marked. Such observations have particular implications for onset of diabetes in childhood.

We know little about the onset and progress of macrovascualar disease in children with Type 2 diabetes mellitus. Arteriosclerosis is a time-dependent phenomenon, and thus the absolute time from diagnosis to developing pathological

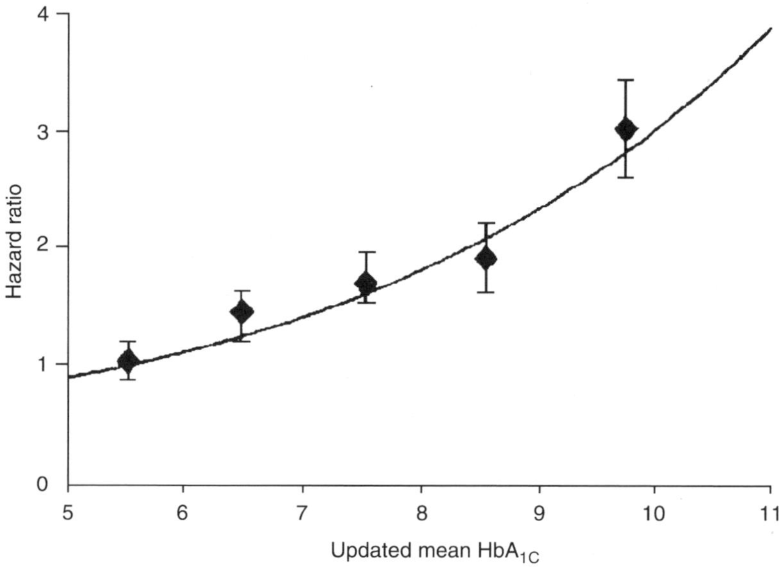

FIGURE 3.2 Data from the UKPDS showing logarithmic association of hazard ratio for all diabetes end-points against HbA_{1c}, showing a 21 per cent decrease in endpoints per one per cent lowering in HbA_{1c}[15]

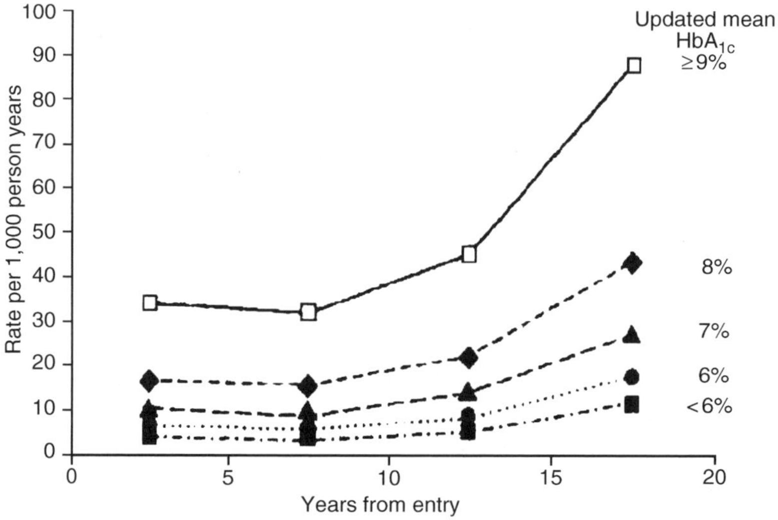

FIGURE 3.3 The absolute rate of accrual of microvascular endpoints in the UKPDS as a function of time (horizontal axis) and updated mean HbA_{1c}[15]

cardiovascular lesions may be many years—in that sense these children may be protected by age since they do not have pre-existing age-related cardiovascular disease. However, it is almost certain that they will develop an excess cardiovascular morbidity early in life.

Microvascular disease is the hallmark of hyperglycaemia diagnosed at a young age. Data from Japanese, Pima Indian children show the presence of microvascular diabetic complications already at diagnosis and follow-up.[10] In Japanese children, incipient retinopathy was detected in 36 per cent of the cases at the time of diagnosis, and in 39 per cent of the cases at 2 years' follow-up. Among Pima Indian children, 22 per cent had microalbuminuria, and at follow-up between 20 and 29 years of age 60 per cent had microalbuminuria and 17 per cent had already macroalbuminuria.

Screening for Type 2 Diabetes Mellitus in Children and Adolescents

Most of the European Caucasian children and adolescents with Type 2 diabetes and one-third of the American children were asymptomatic at diagnosis. According to this, the prevalence in a screening study in Germany of obese children was much higher than the prevalence rate reported in the standardized documentation system of diabetes in Germany.[5] Type 2 diabetes mellitus is characterized by absence of symptoms early in the disease. It is likely that, as with adults, undiagnosed Type 2 diabetes mellitus is a common condition in childhood. Screening of diabetes in high-risk populations is necessary since unrecognized hyperglycaemia would undoubtedly contribute to both microvascular and macrovascular risk in later life.[16] Screening studies demonstrated Type 2 diabetes mellitus in approximately one per cent of obese Caucasian children in Germany[5] and in four per cent of screened obese adolescents in particular ethnic groups in the USA.[11]

Consistent with the recommendations for screening in adults, only children at substantial risk for the presence or the development of Type 2 diabetes mellitus should be tested. Acknowledging the clinical presentation of Type 2 diabetes mellitus and that there are insufficient data to make definite recommendations, testing seems meaningful in overweight children and adolescents at onset of puberty in high-risk patients who display (1) a family history of Type 2 diabetes mellitus in first- and second-degree relatives or (2) signs of insulin resistance (acanthosis nigricans) or (3) conditions associated with insulin resistance (hypertension, dyslipidaemia, polycystic ovary syndrome) or (4) belong to a particular ethnic group (American Indians, African-Americans, Hispanics, Asians) and (5) in extremely obese children (see Table 3.9). Testing should be performed every two years starting at the age of 10 years or at onset of puberty if it occurs at a younger age.[1]

TABLE 3.9 Criteria for testing of Type 2 diabetes in children and adolescents (adapted from reference 1)

- overweight (BMI > 90th percentile)

plus

- one of the following risk factors:
  - family history of Type 2 diabetes in first- or second-degree relative
  - race/ethnicity (Asian, American Indian, Africa-American, Hispanic)
  - signs of insulin resistance or conditions associated with insulin resistance (acanthosis nigricans, hypertension, dyslipidaemia, PCOS)
  - extreme obesity (BMI > 99.5 percentile)

Requirements for testing an asymptomatic group include the availability of a test that is sensitive (few false negatives) and accurate with acceptable specificity (minimal number of false positives). HbA_{1c} is not a useful screening tool, since one-third of the asymptomatic children with Type 2 diabetes mellitus demonstrated normal values. Since fasting blood glucose failed to diagnose diabetes in one-quarter of children with Type 2 diabetes in the European cohort, the oral glucose tolerance test seems to be a better screening tool even if fasting glucose is preferred because of its lower costs and greater convenience.

Treatment of Type 2 Diabetes Mellitus in Children and Adolescents

The ideal goal of treatment is normalization of blood glucose values and HbA_{1c}. Successful control of the associated comorbidities, such as hypertension and dyslipidaemia, is also important. The ultimate goal of treatment is to decrease the risk of acute and chronic complications associated with diabetes.

Most of the recommended guidelines for treatment in children with Type 2 diabetes mellitus are extrapolated from experience gained in adults. Despite the severe manifestation, initial management of obese children and adolescents with Type 2 diabetes should consist of medical nutrition therapy with behaviour modification strategies for lifestyle change aiming at increasing physical activity. Weight loss and weight control are essential for reaching treatment goals. An improvement of the insulin resistance is not to be suspected before a reduction of SDS-BMI of at least 0.5[16] or a significant increase in physical activity. Since only a few youths with Type 2 diabetes mellitus can be treated with diet and exercise alone,[1] pharmacological intervention is frequently required to achieve a normoglycaemic state. Although insulin is the only drug approved for treatment in children, most paediatric diabetologists use oral agents for children with Type 2 diabetes mellitus. Advantages of oral agents include potentially greater compliance and convenience for the patient.

Clinical features suggesting initial treatment with insulin include dehydratation, presence of ketosis and acidosis.

All children with Type 2 diabetes mellitus should receive comprehensive self-management education. Self-management education should include teaching self-monitoring of blood glucose (SMBG). SMBG should be performed as needed and during periods of acute illness or when symptoms of hyper- or hypoglycaemia occur. Patients on insulin or sulfonylureas should also monitor periodically for asymptomatic hypoglycaemia. Routine blood glucose monitoring should be tailored to individual needs but should probably include a combination of fasting and postprandial glucose measurements. HbA_{1c} should be assayed to monitor glycaemic control and the results and their significance shared with the patient and the family.

Behaviour modification strategies for changing lifestyle, sedentary behaviour and decreasing high-calorie high-fat food choice should be implemented. Lifestyle changes cannot be imposed. They need to be accepted and indeed come from self-motivation. This self-motivation depends on education about glycaemia, blood pressure, lipids and the reasons for attention to good metabolic control. Adherence may be difficult, but the gains are immense. The families of those with the condition should be counselled, and siblings engaged in the education programmes.

Referral to a dietician with knowledge and experience in nutritional management of children with diabetes is necessary. Dietary recommendations should be culturally appropriate, sensitive to the family resources and provided to all caregivers. Encouraging healthy eating habits by the entire family is important.

Obesity has its own psychosocial consequences in children, sometimes leading to a positive feedback into comfort eating. Breaking such a cycle can be a huge challenge, and may need repeated reinforcement, much educational input to the children and their parents and the provision of exercise facilities and training courses in appropriate eating patterns.

Pharmacological Treatment of Type 2 Diabetes Mellitus in Children and Adolescents

If treatment goals with nutrition education and exercise are not met, pharmacological therapy is indicated. Currently, there are five types of glucose-lowering oral agent available (see Table 3.10).

Metformin, a biguanide, is undoubtedly the most appropriate starting point for pharmacological treatment in children with Type 2 diabetes mellitus. It does not, however, have a license for use in children. Metformin decreases hepatic glucose output and enhances primarily hepatic and also muscle insulin sensitivity without a direct effect on beta cell function. Metformin has the advantage of weight reduction and decrease in lipids without the risk of hypoglycaemia. Because of

TABLE 3.10 Treatment options of Type 2 diabetes mellitus in children and adolescents[18] (FDA, Federal Drug Administration (USA); EMEA, European Medicine Evaluation Agency (European))

Modality	Glycaemia reduction	Beta enhancing	Insulin resistance lowering	Use	FDA/EMEA approved	Notes
Diet and exercise	Yes	No	Yes	Yes	Yes	First-line approach Efficacy depends on successful lifestyle change
Insulin	Yes	No	No	Yes	Yes	Weight gain?
Metformin	Yes	No	Yes	Yes	No	Good safety record
Sulfonylureas	Yes	Yes	No	Yes	No	Good safety record in adults
Meglitinide analogues	Yes	Yes	No	?	No	Sparse data on their use
Thiazolidinediones	Yes	?	Yes	No	No	Weight gain, lack of long-term data
Acarbose	?	No	No	??	No	Side-effects may be unacceptable
Orlistat	?	No	No	??	No	Side-effects may be unacceptable
Surgical treatment of obesity	Yes	No	Yes	???		Some anecdotal evidence

concerns about lactate acidosis metformin is contraindicated in patients with impaired renal function and should be discontinued with the administration of radiocontrast material or hypocaloric diet. Metformin should not be used in patients with known hepatic disease, hypoxaemic conditions, severe infection or alcohol abuse. The most common side effects of metformin are gastrointestinal disturbances. The dose of metformin should be increased up to 2 g in split doses, unless there are gastrointestinal side-effects. Metformin has a good safety record, but should not be given if there is any doubt at all about the nature of the diagnosis—Type 1 diabetes in children is much more common worldwide than Type 2.

If monotherapy with metformin is not successful over a reasonable period of time (3–6 months), several alternatives can be considered. Some clinicians would add a sulfonylurea, which promotes insulin secretion. Other insulin secretogogues are acceptable as well as glucosidase inhibitor, but these have been less frequently used in children. All these agents have hypoglycaemia as potential side-effects, and the incidence of this is certainly greater in those with high beta cell functional reserve. In clinical practice this would be found in those with only minimal hyperglycaemia. No oral agent should be used during pregnancy.

Insulin treatment will often be the only feasible way of controlling hyperglycaemia. There is no specific contraindication in children. The UKPDS showed beyond any reasonable doubt that, even if patients are likely to put on weight, it is better to have improved glycaemic control than adopt a nihilistic view about the inevitability of the outcome. Insulin regimes should be adopted that are carefully tailored to lifestyle (bedtime insulin alone, twice-a-day insulin or multidose insulin regimes).

Monitoring and Treatment of Complications of Type 2 Diabetes Mellitus in Children and Adolescents

Since microvasuclar complications of Type 2 diabetes mellitus such as retinopathy and nephropathy already occur in children, dilated eye examinations should be performed. Screening for microalbuminuria should also be performed yearly. It is unclear whether foot examinations are important in children. Other than testing for and treating elevated blood pressure and lipid abnormalities, studies to detect macrovascular disease are probably not indicated, although there are no data in this age group.

Careful control of hypertension in children is critical. ACE inhibitors are the agents of choice in children with microalbuminuria. If normotension is not achieved, combination therapy with a-blockers, calcium antagonists or low-dose diuretics may be needed.

Prevention of Type 2 Diabetes Mellitus in Children and Adolescents

The financial and societal consequences of the emerging epidemic of Type 2 diabetes are substantial and demand an urgent public health response. Emphasis must be placed upon preventive behaviours and early detection. Prevention of Type 2 diabetes means prevention of obesity in childhood. The effect of weight loss on comorbid conditions and, most importantly, on the development of Type 2 diabetes has been unequivocally proven.[16,19] As prevention should start very early in life, perhaps even before birth, a population and community approach for prevention of obesity in childhood and hence Type 2 diabetes mellitus in childhood and adolescence seems to be the most promising and reasonable treatment strategy available at present.

However, primary prevention has proven to be difficult or impossible in most societies. A multidisciplinary team approach is needed to develop and secure preventive strategies. Good nutrition and modest exercise for pregnant women as well as monitoring of intrauterine growth of the foetus are mandatory. After birth, rapid weight gain should be avoided and the principles of good nutrition and physical activity be taught at all ages. Breast-feeding should be strongly recommended. Children's food choice can be influenced by early intervention and guidance. In fact, teacher training, modification of school meals and physical education are effective in reducing risk factors for obesity.[7]

The cost-effectiveness of group and mixed family-based treatments for childhood obesity has been tested and proven for motivated families. Therefore, family-based, behavioural treatment for obesity is also effective in preventing Type 2 diabetes mellitus and is also extremely cost effective. In unmotivated families, treatment remains difficult and frustrating for the patient and family, as well as for the multidisciplinary team caring for the obese child.

To prevent the development of Type 2 diabetes and its life-shortening sequelae, early detection of impaired glucose regulation may represent an appropriate strategy, as subjects with impaired glucose tolerance are at increased risk of developing this disease.[22] Recent intervention studies have convincingly demonstrated that adoption of a healthy lifestyle characterized by healthy eating, regular physical activity and subsequent modest weight loss can prevent the progression of impaired glucose tolerance to clinical diabetes.[23,24]

Conclusions

Type 2 diabetes mellitus is rare in childhood and adolescence, but recent reports indicate an increasing prevalence around the world, possibly due to increasing prevalence of obesity in children and adolescents. This is particularly the case in the USA but has also been reported in other countries in Asia and Europe. It is becoming increasingly clear that overweight children with clinical signs of insulin resistance (acanthosis nigricans, dyslipidaemia, hypertension, PCOS) or relatives with Type 2 diabetes mellitus or of particular ethnic populations (Asian, American Indian, African-Americans, Hispanics) above the age of 10 years should be screened for the presence of impaired glucose tolerance or overt Type 2 diabetes. Prevention and treatment of Type 2 diabetes mellitus should become one of the prime targets of public health intervention programmes. Much more attention should be given to the prevention and development of preventive strategies early in life. Finally, and most importantly, public awareness of the increasing health burden and economic dimension of the childhood obesity epidemic is of importance. Physicians should make the public aware of both the childhood obesity epidemic and its serious consequences, not least Type 2 diabetes mellitus.

References

1. American Diabetes Association. Type 2 diabetes in children and adolescents. *Diabetes Care* 2000; **23**: 381–389.
2. Fagot-Campagna A, Pettitt DJ, Engelgau MM, Burrows NR, Geiss LS, Valdez R, Beckles GL, Saaddine J, Gregg EW, Williamson DF and Narayan KM. Type 2 diabetes among North American children and adolescents: an epidemiologic review and a public health perspective. *J Pediatr* 2000; **136**: 664–672.

3. Drake AJ, Smith A, Betts PR, Crowne EC and Shield JPH. Type 2 diabetes in obese white children. *Arch Dis Child* 2002; **86**: 207–208.
4. Rami B, Schober E, Nachbauer E and Waldhör T. Type 2 diabetes mellitus is rare but not absent in children under 15 years of age in Austria. *Eur J Ped* 2003; **162**: 850–852.
5. Wabitsch M, Hauner H, Hertrampf M, Muche R, Hay B, Mayer H, Kratzer W, Debatin KM and Heinze E. Type 2 diabetes mellitus and impaired glucose regulation in Caucasian children and adolescents with obesity living in Germany. *Int J Obes* 2004; **28** (2): 307–313.
6. Ebbeling CA, Pawlak DB and Ludwig DS. Childhood obesity: public-health crisis, common sense cure. *Lancet* 2002; **360**: 473–482.
7. Kiess W, Böttner A, Raile K, Kapellen T, Müller G, Galler A, Paschke R and Wabitsch M. Type 2 diabetes mellitus in children and adolescents: a review from a European perspective. *Horm Res* 2003; **59** (Suppl. 1): 77–84.
8. Edelstein SL, Knowler WC, Bain RP, Andres R, Barrett-Connor EL, Dowse GK, Haffner SM, Pettitt DJ, Sorkin JD, Muller DC, Collins VR and Hamman RF. Predictors of progression from impaired glucose tolerance to NIDDM: an analysis of six prospective studies. *Diabetes* 1997; **46** (4): 701–710.
9. Haffner SM, Stern MP, Mitchell BD, Hazuda HP and Patterson JK. Incidence of type II diabetes in Mexican Americans predicted by fasting insulin and glucose levels, obesity, and body-fat distribution. *Diabetes* 1990; **39** (3): 283–288.
10. Arslanian SA. Type 2 diabetes in children: clinical aspects and risk factors. *Horm Res* 2002; **57** (Suppl. 1): 19–28.
11. Sinha R, Fisch G, Teague B, Tamborlane WV, Banyas B, Allen K, Savoye M, Rieger V, Taksali S, Barbetta G, Sherwin RS and Caprio S. Prevalence of impaired glucose tolerance among children and adolescents with marked obesity. *N Engl J Med* 2002; **346**: 802–810.
12. Arslanian SA. Metabolic differences between Caucasian and African-American children and the relationship to Type 2 diabetes mellitus. *J Pediatr Endocrinol Metab* 2002; **15** (Suppl. 1): 509–517.
13. Genuth S, Alberti KG, Bennett P, Buse J, Defronzo R, Kahn R, Kitzmiller J, Knowler WC, Lebovitz H, Lernmark A, Nathan D, Palmer J, Rizza R, Saudek C, Shaw J, Steffes M, Stern M, Tuomilehto J and Zimmet P. Expert committee on the diagnosis and classification of diabetes mellitus. Follow-up report on the diagnosis of diabetes mellitus. *Diabetes Care* 2003; **26**: 3160–3167.
14. Velho G and Froguel P. Genetic metabolic and clinical characteristics of maturity onset diabetes of the young. *Eur J Endocrinol* 1998; **138**: 233–239.
15. Stratton IM, Adler AI, Neil HA, Matthews DR, Manley SE and Cull CA *et al.* Association of glycaemia with macrovascular and microvascular complications of Type 2 diabetes (UKPDS 35): prospective observational study. *BMJ* 2000; **321**: 405–412.
16. DCCT Research Group. The effect of intensive treatment of diabetes on the development and progression of long-term complications in insulin-dependent diabetes mellitus. *N Engl J Med* 1993; **329**: 977–986.
17. Reinehr T and Andler W. Changes in the atherogenic risk-factor profile according to degree of weight loss. *Arch Dis Child* 2004; **89** (5): 419–422.
18. Matthew DR and Wallace TM. Children with Type 2 diabetes: the risks of complications. *Horm Res* 2002; **57** (Suppl. 1): 34–39.
19. Reinehr T, Kersting M, Alexy U and Andler W. Long-term follow-up of overweight children: after training, after a single consultation session and without treatment. *J Pediatr Gastroenterol Nutr* 2003; **37**: 72–74.
20. Campbell K, Waters E, O'Meara S and Summerbell C. Interventions for preventing obesity in childhood. *Obes Rev* 2001; **2**: 149–157.
21. Reinehr T, Brylak K, Alexy U, Kersting M and Andler W. Predictors to success in outpatient training in obese children and adolescents. *Int J Obes* 2003; **27** (9): 1087–1092.

22. The DECODE Study Group. Glucose tolerance and mortality: comparison of WHO and American Diabetes Association diagnostic criteria. *Lancet* 1999; **354**: 617–621.
23. Tuomilehto J, Lindstrom J, Eriksson JG, Valle TT, Hamalainen H, Ilanne-Parikka P, Keinanen-Kiukaanniemi S, Laakso M, Louheranta A, Rastas M, Salminen V and Uusitupa M. Finnish diabetes prevention study group. Prevention of Type 2 diabetes mellitus by changes in lifestyle among subjects with impaired glucose tolerance. *N Engl J Med* 2001; **344**: 1343–1350.
24. Diabetes Prevention Program Research Group. Reduction in the incidence of Type 2 diabetes with lifestyle intervention or metformin. *N Engl J Med* 2002; **346**: 393–403.

2 Screening for Type 2 Diabetes

4

Screening for Undiagnosed Diabetes: Whom, Where, When and How

Tim Kenealy, Bruce Arroll and **Peter Müller**

Undiagnosed Diabetes and Its Harms

Most people with diabetes go through an intermediary phase (IGT and/or IFG) before developing diabetes. Diabetes may be present 4–7 years before diagnosis and some degree of impaired glucose metabolism may be present for up to 12 years before diabetes is diagnosed.[1]

Macrovascular risk rises with blood glucose even within the normal range.[2] Studies of acute myocardial infarction have shown four per cent[3] to 5.3 per cent[4] of patients had undiagnosed diabetes. (In the study by Tenerez *et al.* an additional 21 per cent of patients had known diabetes.)[3] Microvascular disease has a higher glucose threshold, developing when an individual's glucose metabolism deteriorates further and they become diabetic. Nevertheless, in the UKPDS trial 36 per cent of patients with newly diagnosed diabetes already had retinopathy.[5] Because people with diabetes typically have no or minimal symptoms prior to developing permanent damage, the only effective method for early detection is screening asymptomatic people.

The Rate of Undiagnosed Diabetes in New Zealand

Simmons and colleagues collected data on people with known (self-identified) diabetes in South Auckland suburbs by a door-to-door survey from 1992 to 1995

Prevention of Type 2 Diabetes Edited by Manfred Ganz
 ISBN: 0-470-85733-1

TABLE 4.1 Prevalence (per cent) of self-reported diabetes by ethnic and age groups, from a door-to-door survey in South Auckland (1985 WHO criteria)[8]

Age	European	Maori*	Pacific	Other**
<10	0.2	0	0.1	0.1
10–19	0.2	0.1	0.1	0.3
20–29	0.5	0.4	0.2	0.3
30–39	0.7	2.2	1.1	1.0
40–49	1.5	6.7	4.7	4.1
50–59	3.8	13.2	12.1	8.0
60+	5.9	15.4	11.7	12.8

*Includes some people of mixed Maori/Pacific ethnicity.
**Mostly Asian.

and published a series of articles as this work progressed.[6–8] They reported diabetes in 1881 of 90 447 residents of all ages, a crude rate of 2.1 per cent. Table 4.1 shows their estimates of diabetes prevalence by age and ethnicity, after adjustment for age and under-ascertainment (which was estimated by comparing the door-to-door survey results with local general practice diabetes registers). No adjustment was made for socio-economic status of respondents compared with national figures. Therefore, if these figures are extrapolated to the New Zealand population they may overestimate diabetes prevalence, which is known to be inversely related to income,[9,10] because average South Auckland incomes are lower than the New Zealand average.[11]

To identify both known and previously unknown diabetes and impaired glucose tolerance, in 1988–1990 Scragg and colleagues surveyed people working in large companies in Auckland and Tokoroa. They administered an OGTT to 5677 people between the ages of 40 and 64. Table 4.2 shows a summary of the diabetes prevalence they reported, by age and ethnicity. If extrapolated to the whole population, these figures are likely to underestimate the number with

TABLE 4.2 Prevalence (per cent) of known and newly diagnosed diabetes by ethnic and age groups, in a working population in Tokoroa and Auckland, using OGTT (1985 WHO criteria)[10]

Age		European	Maori	Pacific	Asian
40–44	new	0.4	2.1	3.6	4.8
	known	0.4	3.6	0.8	4.8
45–49	new	1.0	7.3	1.0	0.0
	known	0.8	4.0	4.8	0.0
50–54	new	1.0	3.1	3.7	6.3
	known	1.0	4.1	11.9	6.3
≥55	new	1.0	6.6	6.7	9.1
	known	2.4	10.5	5.4	0.0

TABLE 4.3 Estimated prevalence (per cent) of undiagnosed diabetes in New Zealand, by age and ethnicity (1999 WHO criteria)[12]

Age	European	Maori	Pacific	Asian
30–39	1.2	3.5	1.8	1.6
40–49	2.3	10.8	7.5	6.6
50–59	6.0	21.1	19.3	12.9
≥60	9.4	24.6	18.7	20.5

diabetes, as they did not include people who were not working. Even within the working population, the authors reported that the rate of diabetes was inversely related to income.

When Scragg re-analysed his data, using 1999 WHO criteria, he found a ratio of undiagnosed (1999 WHO) to diagnosed (1985 WHO) of 1.6:1, which did not vary by age or ethnic group.[12] This ratio can be applied to Simmons' prevalence of known diabetes,[8] shown in Table 4.1, to estimate prevalence of undiagnosed diabetes, shown in Table 4.3. That prevalence is over five per cent for all people from age 50 and for all non-European ethnic groups from age 40.

Should We Screen for Diabetes?

In a 1968 WHO report, Wilson and Jungner proposed ten criteria to assess whether a screening programme is appropriate.[13]

1. The condition should be an important health problem.
2. There should be an accepted treatment for patients with recognized disease.
3. Facilities for diagnosis and treatment should be available.
4. There should be a recognizable latent or early symptomatic stage.
5. There should be a suitable test or examination.
6. The test should be acceptable to the population.
7. The natural history of the condition... should be understood.
8. There should be an agreed policy on whom to treat as patients.
9. The cost of case finding... should be economically balanced in relation to possible expenditure on medical care as a whole.
10. Case finding should be a continuing process and not a 'once and for all' project.

More recently, Gray added criteria to meet the requirements of evidence-based medicine, particularly the need for good randomized controlled trial evidence that a screening programme reduced mortality (cited by the New Zealand National Health Committee).[14] The UK National Screening Committee, of which Gray is a member, has set out current screening criteria,[15]and there are other lists with similar messages.[14,16]

The key issues raised will be addressed. First, there has been no randomized controlled trial measuring survival and morbidity amongst people who are screened compared with those who are not. (An interesting small-cohort study from Germany compared 32 pairs of people with Type 1 or Type 2 diabetes, matched for age and sex, and showed no difference in survival between those presenting spontaneously with symptoms and those detected by screening for glycosuria.[17]) It should be noted here that the most relevant comparison for a randomized controlled trial is between screening, followed by 'usual practice' care, and not screening, with 'usual practice' care. An Anglo–Danish–Dutch study to address these issues is currently in the early stages.[18]

Nevertheless, it seems that a strong case can still be made for screening high-risk people. The high relative and absolute risks of premature death and morbidity from microvascular and macrovascular disease are well known. Effective treatments are readily available. A precursor phase is present and detectable and the rate of progression to diabetes has been documented in many populations.[19] Diagnostic criteria are agreed.

It is unlikely that people with diagnosed diabetes are importantly different from those with undiagnosed diabetes. The DECODE group pointed to similar mortality hazard ratios for both known diabetic and screen-diagnosed diabetic people compared with those without diabetes.[20] NHANES II data indicated that those with undiagnosed diabetes had higher total cholesterol and triglycerides than those whose diabetes was diagnosed, and their rates of uncontrolled hypertension were similar (and nearly double the rate of those without diabetes).[21] High rates of diabetes damage are found to be already present when diabetes if first diagnosed; as mentioned earlier, 36 per cent already had retinopathy at the start of the UKPDS trial.[6] Another report from the same trial noted that people with diabetes symptoms (who might therefore seek medical attention) had similar rates of macrovascular and microvascular disease as did those without symptoms.[22]

It is worth noting that all discussions of the duration of diabetes prior to diagnosis under 'usual care' cite a single important paper from M Harris *et al.*[2] These authors considered the close relationship between duration of known diabetes and prevalence of retinopathy. Given the high incidence at diagnosis, they extrapolated back to a time of zero incidence (4–7 years), then added a further 5 years based on a paper by Jarret.[23] He had reported on a small cohort of 30 patients from the Whitehall study on impaired glucose tolerance who had subsequently developed diabetes. Of these 30, followed for minimum of 3 years after diagnosis of diabetes, eight developed retinopathy, none in less than 5 years from developing diabetes. (Harris *et al.* misquoted the number of patients in Jarrett's report. Their argument remains sound if more tenuous.)

Facilities for screening and diagnosis are available in primary care. The availability of facilities for treatment, and their capacity to expand to meet demand, varies across disciplines and around the country. It is common to recommend that screening not go ahead in the absence of adequate facilities.[24] However, delaying screening until the system is fully staffed in all disciplines in all areas is unrealistic. It seems reasonable to encourage increased screening combined with monitoring and remedial action to increase services as and where needed. On the other hand, case finding is not, currently, a continuous process. This is probably best achieved with the aid of computerized reminder systems. Such systems, albeit incomplete, are currently available in New Zealand only within general practice.

The only study of patients' perception of Type 2 diabetes screening reported that patients considered it useful and not burdensome.[25] Shaw *et al.* reviewed the psychological impact of screening tests in general, including tests for Type 1 diabetes, cancer, Huntington's chorea and AIDS.[26] They concluded that in the short term anxiety and depression were more common amongst those who test positive than amongst those who test negative, but that this effect did not persist. They made the interesting observation that the effect of positive tests was often more marked on family members than on the individual concerned.

The only economic study of diabetes screening in New Zealand is in a loose model constructed by PricewaterhouseCoopers on commission from Diabetes New Zealand.[27] The model took three policy scenarios for expending public health money on diabetes – current expenditure ongoing, increased expenditure and major up-front investment including more screening – and predicted an overall saving to the taxpayer over 20 years if major expenditure is committed now. A cost-effectiveness study from the US Centers for Disease control suggested that screening was cost effective, particularly for younger people, down to age 25 (who might gain more quality of life years than older people), and ethnic minorities (who have a higher prevalence of diabetes).[28] A UK group was less convinced by the US group findings, pointing to their sensitivity to assumptions made.[29] Both groups principally assumed that treatment of diabetes improved microvascular but not macrovascular disease.

The payment that New Zealand community laboratories receive for a glucose test is NZ$2.22 (about £0.80) and that for HbA_{1c} is NZ$10.36 (about £3.80), although this does not represent the full costs of identifying candidates for screening, blood collection, testing and follow-up of results. Nearly all the cost of diabetes comes from treating people with diabetes, which should be compared with the costs of failure to diagnose and failed treatment. There is limited information about the cost of treatment and control. However, tight blood pressure control has been shown to be cost effective[30,31] and modelling studies of costs and benefits of best-practice treatment suggest benefits comparable with other commonly accepted treatments.[28,32,33]

It is inappropriate to restrict consideration of the value to screening solely to a discussion of whether control of glucose benefits microvascular disease (which it clearly does) and macrovascular disease (which is subject to more debate). Appropriate management of diabetes includes managing all the associated cardiovascular risk factors, including smoking, blood pressure and lipids. Treatment for each of these individually is clearly beneficial, as is a multi-factorial approach to combined risk management,[34] and structured care processes to ensure this happens in routine practice.[35–40] One might suggest that risk factors other than glucose can be managed without knowing that a patient has diabetes, but Harris *et al.* pointed to the benefits of lower blood pressure and lipid targets in those with diabetes compared with those without diabetes.[41] This indicates improved patient outcomes when a person with diabetes is known to have the condition.

While the value of screening for Type 2 diabetes may not have been sufficiently proven for those who are responsible for using public funds to develop formal public health screening programmes,[42] nevertheless practicing clinicians must make decisions based on the evidence currently available. Screening, at least in 'high-risk' groups, is firmly supported by reasonable extrapolation from strong evidence. Treatment of people with known diabetes is beneficial. It seems unlikely that those with undiagnosed diabetes are importantly different from those with diagnosed diabetes. Screening can detect diabetes earlier than would be found by 'usual care'. Primary care seems the only viable venue for screening. The biggest question is, can general practice provide what is needed – systematic opportunistic screening? This question is currently being addressed by the Diabetes, Heart Disease and Stroke Prevention Project in the UK.[43]

Theory of Screening

Please note that this section is primarily theoretical. The reader may wish to skip this section and continue with the following section, 'Screening theories are difficult to apply to diabetes: implications of the diagnostic criteria for screening decisions'.

Screening means doing a simple test to see whether it is worth doing further, more definitive, diagnostic tests on a patient. A screening test is used to divide people into two or more groups at different risks of having diabetes: either high (needing further testing) and low (not needing further testing), or high (needing further testing), medium (different testing) and low (no further testing). Cut-off test values are chosen as dividing lines among the groups.

The results of screening tests can be compared with the results of a 'gold standard' test. In the case of diabetes, the gold standard is the OGTT. Other examples

TABLE 4.4 An example of screening using fasting plasma glucose (FPG) in 44 592 people in Queensland, Australia; overall diabetes prevalence 20.0 per cent[44]

Screening using fasting glucose, cut-off $\geq$ 6 mmol/l		Classification after OGTT	
		Diabetes	No diabetes
	Test +ve	$a = 7567$	$b = 9824$
	Test −ve	$c = 1351$	$d = 25\,851$
Totals		8918	35 675

a = true positive, b = false positive, c = false negative, d = true negative.

of gold standard tests include breast histology compared with screening mammography or an angiogram compared with a screening exercise electrocardiogram.

Let us use the example of some real numbers from Australia, shown in Table 4.4.[44]

For completeness, Table 4.5 below explains the commonly used measures of screening effectiveness, using the same notation and numbers as Table 4.4.

The aim of all screening is to go from a pre-test probability to a post-test probability. We can calculate a post-test probability using a 2×2 table or a nomogram. The pre-test probability for the data used in Table 4.4 is the prevalence of diabetes, 20 per cent. The post-test likelihood of a positive test (in this case a fasting glucose >6 mmol/l) is $a/(a + b) = 44$ per cent chance of diabetes. This result would definitely require us to go on and do an OGTT. The post-test likelihood of a negative test works out at 4.9 per cent. This is below our five per cent threshold for screening, so no further testing is required for this patient.

We could arrive at the same conclusion using a nomogram, which is quicker than creating a new 2×2 table when using it for a range of pre-test probabilities. Figures 4.1–4.3 show nomograms using the same likelihood ratios as used in our 2×2 table. The first vertical line represents the pre-test probability. The middle line is the likelihood ratio and the third line is the post-test probability. The post-test probabilities are obtained by running a rule from one side (pre-test probability) through the likelihood ratio to the far side. The line for a positive test crosses the post-test probability line at about 44 per cent. The line for a negative test crosses the line at about five per cent.

The pre-test likelihood in Figure 4.1 is five per cent. The post-test likelihood is about 14 per cent, which suggests we should do a ‘gold standard’ test. The likelihood ratio used in Figure 4.1 comes from Table 4.5 and is 3 for a positive test and 0.21 for a negative test. A negative test gives about a 1.1 per cent likelihood of disease, requiring no further testing. When the pre-test likelihood is

TABLE 4.5 Measures of screening effectiveness, using notation and numbers from Table 4.4. These formulae apply only to 2 × 2 tables – they do not work for 2 × *n* tables

Term	Formula	Description	Worked example
Prevalence, also known as the pre-test likelihood and pre-test probability	$a + c/(a + b + c + d)$	proportion who have the disease	8918/44 593 = 0.20 = 20%
		Fixed properties of a test	
Sensitivity	$a/a + c$	proportion of those with the disease who have a positive test	7567/8918 = 0.85
Specificity	$d/d + b$	proportion of those without the disease who have a negative test	25 851/35 675 = 0.72
Likelihood ratio for a positive test	sensitivity/(1 – specificity)		0.85/(1 – 0.72) = 3.0
Likelihood ratio for a negative test	(1 – sensitivity)/specificity		(1 – 0.85)/0.15 = 0.21
		Vary with prevalence	
Positive predictive value, also known as the post-test likelihood of a positive test (PTL +ve)	$a/a + b$	proportion of those with a positive test who have the disease	7567/17 391 = 0.44 = 44%
Post-test likelihood of a negative test (PTL –ve)*	$c/c + d$	proportion of those with a negative test who have the disease	1351/27 202 = 0.049 = 4.9%
Negative predictive value*	$d/d + c$	proportion of those with a negative test who do not have the disease	25 851/27 202 = 95%
False positive/true positive	b/a		9824/7567 = 1.3
False negative/true negative	c/d		1351/25 851 = 0.05

*PTL –ve is clinically more useful than negative predictive value, as we wish to know the likelihood of a patient having diabetes despite a negative screening test.

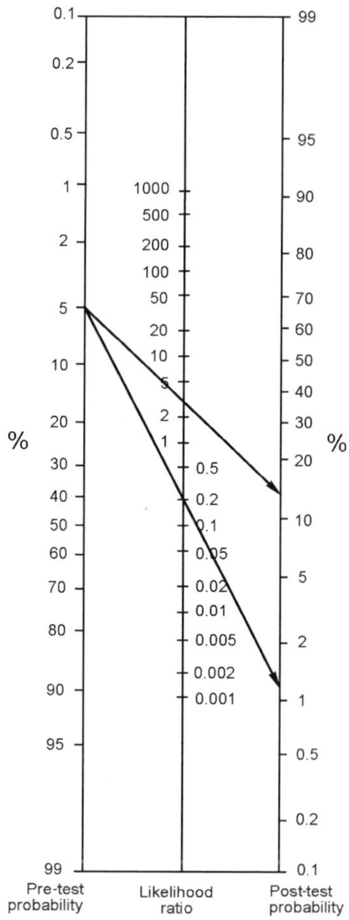

FIGURE 4.1 Prevalence (pre-test probability) of five per cent. Likelihood ratio of a positive test = 3. Likelihood ratio of a negative test = 0.21 (from Table 4.5). A positive test has a post-test likelihood of 14 per cent for having diabetes. A negative test means the person has a 1.1 per cent chance of having diabetes

about 20 per cent, as shown in Figure 4.2, a positive test has a post-test likelihood of 43 per cent and a negative test means the person has about a five per cent chance of having diabetes. At 20 per cent prevalence it could be argued that a 'gold standard' glucose tolerance test is indicated as the initial test rather than a fasting glucose. In Figure 4.3, where the pre-test probability is 60 per cent, a positive test gives an 82 per cent chance of diabetes and a negative test gives about a 24 per cent chance of diabetes. This shows the danger of performing a screening test in a high-prevalence setting and we should perhaps go to a glucose tolerance test immediately rather than risk a false negative test.

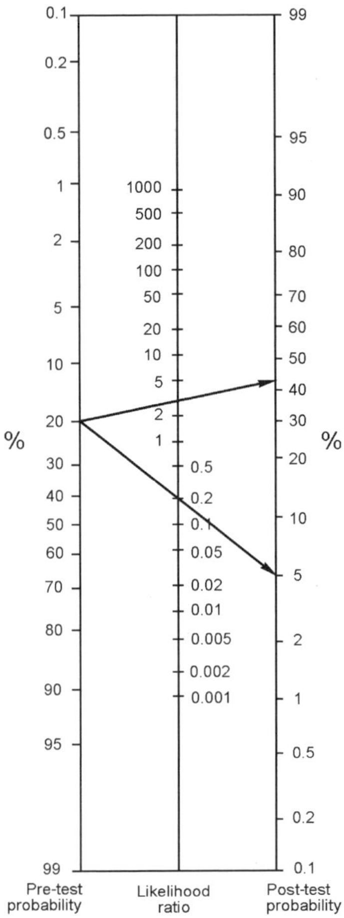

FIGURE 4.2 Prevalence (pre-test probability) 20 per cent. Likelihood ratio of a positive test = 3. Likelihood ratio of a negative test = 0.21 (from Table 4.5). A positive test has a post-test likelihood of 43 per cent for diabetes. A negative test has a post-test likelihood of about five per cent for having diabetes

We can choose an approximate pre-test probability from data we already know about a patient. Table 4.3 gives the proportion of people in New Zealand with undiagnosed diabetes in groups defined by age and ethnicity. It is equally possible to define such groups by other or additional characteristics including weight, family history or cardiovascular disease status when the increased diabetes risk associated with these factors is known. Table 4.3 shows a prevalence of 24.6 per cent of undiagnosed diabetes for Maori aged over 60 years. If the individual was more than 20 per cent above ideal body weight (Table 4.7) then the pre-test probability could be $2.7 \times 24.6 = 66.42$ per cent. There are other ways of estimating a pre-test probability. One could measure the prevalence in one's own clinical

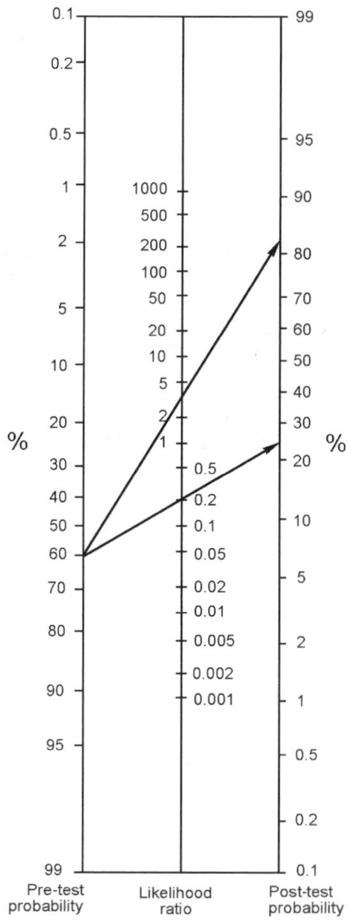

FIGURE 4.3 Prevalence (pre-test probability) 60 per cent. Likelihood ratio of a positive test = 3. Likelihood ratio of a negative test = 0.21 (from Table 4.5). The post-test likelihood of a positive test is 82 per cent. The post-test likelihood of a negative test is still 24 per cent for having diabetes. In this situation a screening test may be misleading and a 'gold standard' test is appropriate

setting based on past experience or measurement. It could be a guess. So long as the guess was based on reasonable grounds then it would not matter if one clinician suggested a pre-test probability of five per cent while another said 15 per cent. Such differences are unlikely to change management.

The post-test likelihoods of a positive and a negative test clearly vary markedly with diabetes prevalence. It is interesting to consider a general approach to using screening, diagnostic and gold standard tests, as suggested for breast cancer and other conditions where the prevalence is generally below five per cent, such as shown in Table 4.6. The table is expanded from ideas published by Sackett *et al.*[45]

TABLE 4.6 Test performance depends on prevalence. General schematic diagram concerning screening, not specific to diabetes. The figures are for a fasting glucose with sensitivity 0.85 and specificity 0.72, from Table 4.4

Prevalence	99%	60%	20%	5%	1%	0.1%
PTL +ve	99.9%	82%	43%	14%	3%	0.3%
PTL −ve	95%	24%	5%	1.1%	<0.1%	0.02%
False +ve/true +ve	0.003	0.21	1.3	6	32	329
False −ve/True −ve	21	0.31	0.05	0.011	0.002	0.0002

<- - - - - - screen* - - - - - ->

<- - - - - - - diagnostic test* - - - - - ->

<- - - treat or - - - ->
perform gold standard**

false +ve the problem

tests 'works well'

false −ve the problem

*The one test, a fasting glucose, could be called a 'screening test' in the prevalence range of 0.1 to about five per cent and a 'diagnostic test' in the mid-prevalence range.
**In the high-prevalence range we could ideally use a gold standard, i.e. a glucose tolerance test.

False positives are a problem when the prevalence is low. Each false positive needs to be investigated, thereby creating anxiety and physical danger (from unnecessary surgery and investigation) for those who do not have the disease. Alternatively, false negatives are a problem in high-prevalence settings, when treatment and/or gold standard testing are needed.

Sensitivity ('true positive' rate) and specificity ('true negative' rate) will vary as the cut-off point is varied; when one goes up, the other goes down. Once the cut-off is chosen, sensitivity and specificity are regarded, in principle, as constant properties of that test. Nevertheless, a wide range of sensitivity and specificity may be found unless they are established in populations with a sufficient range of both diabetes prevalence and any other factors that may affect test performance;[46] i.e. they should include people like those we intend to test in New Zealand.

Because sensitivity will always increase at the expense of specificity, and because the PPV depends on the population being tested, there is no single 'best' cut-off value to use. Given the value of treating diabetes, it is reasonable to choose tests with a high sensitivity to minimize the number of people with diabetes who are missed in the screening process. This inevitably means screening more people, most of whom will not have diabetes. Nevertheless, many of those without diabetes may prove to have lesser degrees of impaired glucose metabolism, including IGT. Recent studies have shown that treating IGT with lifestyle changes or drugs reduces the numbers of people going on to develop frank diabetes.[47–49] Finally, screening for diabetes is likely to detect other associated and modifiable health risks including obesity, dyslipidaemia, high blood pressure, smoking and sedentary lifestyles.

Screening Theories are Difficult to Apply to Diabetes: Implications of the Diagnostic Criteria for Screening Decisions

The formal diagnostic criteria for diabetes create two overlapping groups of people with diabetes. Some people with diabetes will have only a raised fasting glucose, some will have only a raised random or 2 hour value on the OGTT and some may have both, as shown schematically in Figure 4.4. It is worth noting that IGT lies between normal and diabetes by the 2 hour criterion. IFG lies between normal and diabetes by the fasting criterion. Some people have both IGT and IFG.

Actual numbers in each category vary with the population tested. However, in an elderly European population, one-third of people with diabetes had a fasting value <7 mmol/l but a 2 hour value ≥ 11.1 mmol/l on an OGGT.[20] Isolated elevation of the 2 hour glucose seems to be more common in the elderly, the less obese and some Asian populations.[50] Analysis of the New Zealand workforce data from a younger age group suggests this group includes about four per cent undiagnosed diabetes.[51] Furthermore, because the OGTT uses a larger glucose test meal than most people ever normally consume, a person's random glucose will rarely be as high as their 2 hour OGTT test value. There is also concern that people with an elevated 2 hour glucose value may be more at risk of cardiovascular disease than those with only an elevated fasting glucose,[52,53] although this finding was not confirmed in the NHANES III study,[54] in which subjects were younger and heavier. These factors have important implications for choice of screening tests to use and how to interpret them.

We have six conditions to diagnose (diabetes on fasting criteria, 2 hour criteria or both, IGT, IFG and normal), yet we seek a single screening test. It is clear why the OGTT is the 'gold standard' test, as it definitely classifies each of these conditions. A fasting glucose is a logical screening test to detect IFG and diabetes

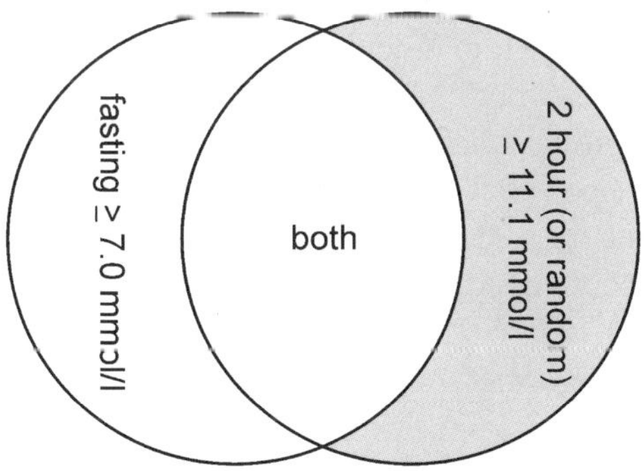

FIGURE 4.4 The diagnostic criteria for diabetes create two overlapping groups of people, who have diabetes on the fasting criterion, the 2 hour criterion or both. IGT lies between normal and diabetes by the 2 hour criterion. IFG lies between normal and diabetes by the fasting criterion. Some people have both IGT and IFG. The diagram is schematic only

according to the fasting criteria or those meeting both fasting and 2 hour criteria. It is clearly not such a good test to identify IGT or those with diabetes on the 2 hour criteria alone. Furthermore, in screening terminology, a fasting test is not only a 'screening' test but is also part of a 'gold standard' test for IFG and for some people with diabetes.

Decisions about which screening test to use, and which cut-offs to use, are hampered by lack of clear decisions about how many people with diabetes we are prepared to miss (false negatives), and how many people with IGT we are determined to find (sensitivity).

Current Recommendations, New Zealand and International

No major international organization recommends mass population screening for diabetes, though they accept or promote screening of individual patients at increased risk of diabetes or cardiovascular disease.[19,42,55,56] All the international organizations recommend screening using some form of glucose test. None recommend using HbA_{1c} for screening. Screening criteria have necessarily been revised since recent consensus agreement on new diagnostic criteria for the diagnosis of type 2 diabetes.[50,57,58]

The ADA 2003 guidelines recommend screening every patient at age 45, then three-yearly, using a fasting plasma glucose.[56] If the result is <7.0 mmol/l an OGTT should be performed on those at high risk of diabetes. If the result is ≥ 7.0 mmol/l, the person should be retested on another day to confirm the diagnosis of diabetes. Capillary glucose testing is discouraged.

Recent Australian guidelines recommend testing groups with a five per cent or higher prevalence of undiagnosed diabetes, with re-testing of high-risk groups yearly and lower-risk groups three-yearly.[19] In Australia, the five per cent risk includes everyone over age 55 and others according to additional risk factors (over an above age). For example, they recommend screening Aboriginals, Torres Strait Islanders and Pacific, Indian and Chinese people from age 35. They prefer a fasting venous glucose, where >7.0 mmol/l suggests diabetes is likely but to be confirmed, 5.5–6.9 mmol/l indicates the need for an OGTT and <5.5 is normal.

The New Zealand Society for the Study of Diabetes (NZSSD) first published a consensus statement on screening for diabetes in 1995.[59] This was revised in 2002, with current recommended screening cut-offs for fasting glucose of <5.5 (re-screen in 3 years), 6.0–6.9 (OGTT for high-risk people) and >6.9 mmol/l indicating diabetes if confirmed on another day.[12]

Current Practice in New Zealand

There is considerable variation in the tests GPs say they use most often to screen for diabetes. In 1999 in South Auckland, 37 per cent used a random glucose,

28 per cent a fasting glucose and 16 per cent used a capillary sample and self-monitoring meter; the remainder mostly use combinations of these same methods.[60]

Sporadic screening using capillary blood with a self-monitoring meter has been happening for many years in a variety of settings including many pharmacies, school galas, community clinics, from Public Health Nurse caravans and on marae (communal meeting places of the indigenous Maori population).

Many laboratories report so many low HbA_{1c} results that it seems that many GPs are now using HbA_{1c} as part of their screening process for diabetes. One-third of HbA_{1c} results in Auckland in 2002 were under 5.5 per cent (personal communication, G Braatvedt, 2002).

Private laboratories around the country report a variety of 'reference ranges' for fasting glucose, random glucose and HbA_{1c}, with a variety of interpretive comments. For example, in the year 2000, the upper end of the normal random glucose reference range varied around the country from 7.5 to 9.5 mmol/l.[51] Similarly, the normal reference range for HbA_{1c} varied from 3.5 to 4.0 at the lower end, and from 6.2 to 6.4 per cent at the upper end, partly depending on the method used to measure HbA_{1c}. Even if glucose is tested when patients are in hospital, elevated levels are often not followed up and are usually not even noted on discharge documents.[61,62] Hospital laboratories typically present glucose results with a reference range (which may vary around the country), but no interpretive comments. In practice this leaves the most junior doctors and those in a range of non-medical specialties without potentially helpful interpretive advice. None of the community or hospital 'reference ranges' in the year 2000 corresponded to the 'decision points' of screening recommendations current then or now.[12]

Studies of Practical Screening in New Zealand

There are only two published studies of attempts at practical diabetes screening in New Zealand. In 1989–90 Bourn and Mann[63] invited all the 39–70-year-old patients registered with two GPs in one practice in Dunedin to have a random laboratory blood glucose test. The population was largely New Zealand European, some 67 per cent responded and nine people were newly diagnosed with diabetes, all over age 50.

In 1993 Lawrenson *et al.*[64] undertook an extensive community campaign visiting halls, marae, shops and other venues throughout the Waikato. They targeted Maori over age 20, Europeans over age 40, the obese and those with a family history of diabetes. They used BM stix and a Reflolux meter for the initial non-fasting screening test. They chose cut-offs of less than 6.5 mmol/l as normal (88 per cent of those tested), greater than 8 mmol/l as screen positive for diabetes (3.6 per cent) and a value between 6.5 and 8.0 mmol/l as an indication to re-test in three months (8.8 per cent). (The percentages do not quite add to 100 and there appears to be a minor addition error in the relevant published table.) Of the 162 with a value $\geq$8.0 mmol/l, 141 had an OGTT; of these 79 were normal, 56 had Type 2 diabetes (using 1985 WHO criteria), five had IGT and one woman had gestational diabetes. This gives a positive predictive value for diabetes of 0.42. The data are not available to calculate sensitivity and specificity, nor to determine whether different cut-off values for screen positive and screen negative would have resulted in detection of a greater proportion of people with undiagnosed diabetes. Despite testing 5589 people they found only 56 people with previously undetected diabetes (mostly over age 50). They therefore recommended future screening of all New Zealanders over 50 and younger Maori with a body mass index $\geq$30 kg/m^2. The subsequent regression model by Johnson and Baker indicated that, with this meter, if the 'true' plasma glucose were 8.0 mmol/l the mean meter reading would be 8.3, with 95 per cent of readings falling between 6.2 and 10.4.[65]

Systematic Opportunistic Screening in General Practice

'Opportunistic screening' for diabetes means that a patient is screened for diabetes while seeking medical attention for an unrelated issue. According to the 1996/97 Health Survey, GPs are the most widely used health professionals, with 80 per cent of adults in New Zealand visiting a GP at least once in a year.[66] The proportion increases to over 90 per cent for people aged over 65. Similar proportions visit at least once a year across all income brackets and all ethnic groups – 81 per cent for European, 77 per cent for Maori, 79 per cent for Pacific – apart from 62 per cent for 'other' ethnic groups. In principle, the opportunity exists for most of the population to be screened for diabetes, including most of those who might be considered at 'high risk' of diabetes. An increasing number of specialized primary care services are being established to provide services more specifically aimed at Maori and Pacific people. Nevertheless, these services typically employ GPs and practice nurses and use the same practice systems and computer software as 'mainstream' general practices.

Several studies have invited all people registered at a particular practice to attend for diabetes screening. Bourn and Mann had a response rate of 67 per cent, as mentioned above.[63] Lawrence *et al.* had a response rate of 35 per cent.[67] These efforts, however, were one-time events that would need to be repeated indefinitely. The opportunity exists to establish 'systematic opportunistic screening' for diabetes, that is, to organize systems of care that assist GPs and practice nurses to appropriately screen people when they consult for some other purpose. However, the effectiveness of 'systematic opportunistic screening' as a means to reach the national population needs to be evaluated.

We recently conducted a randomized controlled trial to test two strategies designed to increase opportunistic screening for diabetes in routine general practice in New Zealand. The trial compared screening rates in four intervention arms: patient reminders, computer reminders, both reminders and usual care. The trial lasted two months. The computer reminder was an icon that flashed only for patients considered eligible for screening. The patient reminder was a diabetes risk self-assessment sheet, based on an ADA form,[68,69] filled in by patients and given to the GP during the consultation. Patients were considered eligible if they were age 50 or more, had no diabetes code in their computer record and no laboratory glucose test in their record for the previous three years. The participants were 107 GPs in 66 practices, who saw 19 187 individuals age 50+. Of these people, 5628 were eligible for screening for diabetes. The primary outcome was whether each eligible patient who attended during the trial was or was not tested for blood glucose. Analysis was by intention to treat and allowed for clustering by GP.

Computer reminders were more effective (OR 2.55, 95 per cent CI 1.68–3.88) than patient reminders (OR 1.72, 1.21–2.43) and both reminders (OR 1.69, 1.11–2.59) compared with usual care. Patients were more likely to be screened if they visited the GP repeatedly, if they were non-European patients, if they were 'regular' patients of the practice and if their GP had a higher screening rate prior to the study. GP gender, age, tenths worked, consultation rate, practice size, patient charges and GP attitudes to guidelines, preventive care, diabetes care and screening for diabetes were not significant in the final model.

Let us briefly consider the potential of systematic opportunistic screening for diabetes in general practice in terms of the impact on the total New Zealand population of people with undiagnosed diabetes. We want to find the cumulative probability of these people being diagnosed per year. For our purposes some simple estimates will suffice. (A fuller model would include the compounding effect of the increased screening rate stimulated by computer reminders and include the incidence of new diabetes.) Let us assume that diabetes is present for 5 years before diagnosis under 'usual care',[2] that there are 70 000 people with undiagnosed diabetes,[51] that 60 per cent of these will visit a GP once in a year and 25 per cent will visit a GP twice in a year (an approximation based on Ministry of Health figures[66]), that the probability of them being screened for diabetes currently is 0.14 for one visit and 0.16 for two visits and that with computer reminders the probability would be 0.27 for one visit and 0.31 for two visits (taken from our study). It works out that in one year some 8600 people would have their diabetes diagnosed under the current system compared with some 16 765 people if all GPs in New Zealand were using computer reminders. Systematic opportunistic screening for one year may lead to the benefit of treating diabetes for more than 8000 people for 5 years.

Who to Test: Which Groups are at Relatively High Risk?

Table 4.7 shows recognizable groups of people who are at substantially increased risk of developing diabetes. The list is not exhaustive and the risk factors are cumulative.

TABLE 4.7 Groups of people who are at substantially increased risk of developing diabetes. The list is not exhaustive and the risk factors are cumulative

Major risk factors for Type 2 diabetes[19,69]	Approximate increased risk of diabetes
1. A parent, brother or sister with Type 2 diabetes	40–50% lifetime risk[70]
2. Obesity (i.e. $\geq$20% over desired body weight or BMI $\geq$27 kg/m^2)	exponential, e.g. 2.7 × risk with gain 8–11 kg[71]
3. Race/ethnicity (e.g. Polynesian, Asian, African, Hispanic)	Maori and Pacific 2–3 × European[11,72]
4. Age $\geq$45 years	progressive; age 60 2–3 × age 40[11,72]
5. Previously identified IFG or IGT	IFG 25 per cent, IGT 50% lifetime risk[73]
6. Hypertension ($\geq$140/90 mm Hg in adults)	twofold[74,75]
7. HDL cholesterol level $\leq$0.90 mmol/l and/or triglyceride level $\geq$2.8 mmol/l	twofold[74]
8. History of gestational diabetes mellitus	40–70% lifetime risk[7]
9. Polycystic ovaries	twofold[76]

Based on similar information, the ADA published a screening questionnaire, which attempted to select high-risk asymptomatic people for screening.[69] The questionnaire has been validated only in a white American population and the current ADA guidelines do not encourage its use.[56] Although Welborn *et al.*[75] used a questionnaire to pre-select people in a large Australian screening trial, they did not publish the questionnaire details.

Using known risk factors, it is possible to estimate the risk of an individual for having current undiagnosed diabetes. Such risk estimation would need to be simple for patient or practice staff use, though could be much more complex if calculated by a computer algorithm. In practice, a computer algorithm is limited to using the data available within the computer (or supplied at the time by the user). The overall population prevalence of known and unknown diabetes in New Zealand is 4–5 per cent.[77] It therefore seems appropriate to pick a risk figure of not less than five per cent, a figure also nominated in the recent Australian guidelines.[19]

Various groups with a risk of five per cent or more of undiagnosed diabetes can be recognized, depending on the information available. If patient age is the only information available, then all patients age 50 or over (without known diabetes) should be screened. If ethnicity data are also available, screening would be appropriate for all non-Europeans $\geq$age 40 and Europeans $\geq$age 50. If additional risk factors are known, as in Table 4.7, one can identify those patients with approximately a twofold increased risk of undiagnosed diabetes. Thus it would be appropriate to screen non-Europeans $\geq$age 30 and Europeans $\geq$age 40 if they have any combination of BMI $>$ 30, a first-degree relative with Type 2 diabetes, hypertension, obesity, raised triglycerides, lowered HDL or polycystic ovaries. A

TABLE 4.8 Age–ethnic subgroups ranked in descending order of relative yield for undiagnosed diabetes (1999 WHO criteria). Relative yield is the proportion of the total number of people with undiagnosed diabetes, relative to that subgroup proportion of the total population (≥age 30). Results except relative yield are percentages[51] (With thanks to R Scragg)

Ethnic–age group	Undiagnosed diabetes prevalence	Proportion of NZ population		Proportion of NZ total undiagnosed diabetes		Relative yield
			Cumulative		Cumulative	
M: 60+	24.6	1.2	1.2	5.2	5.2	4.5
M: 50–59	21.1	1.4	2.5	5.2	10.4	3.8
A: 60+	20.5	0.4	2.9	1.3	11.7	3.7
P: 50–59	19.3	0.5	3.3	1.6	13.4	3.5
P: 60+	18.7	0.4	3.8	1.4	14.8	3.4
A: 50–59	12.9	0.5	4.2	1.1	15.8	2.3
M: 40–49	10.8	2.5	6.7	4.8	20.6	2.0
E: 60+	9.4	25.4	32.1	43.2	63.8	1.7
P: 40–49	7.5	0.9	33.0	1.2	65.0	1.4
A: 40–49	6.6	1.2	34.2	1.4	66.5	1.2
E: 50–59	6.0	14.9	49.1	16.4	82.8	1.1
Groups above have higher yield than total NZ population (relative yield = 1) Cut-point based on the recommendation to screen groups with prevalence >5%						
M: 30–39	3.5	4.0	53.1	2.6	85.4	0.6
E: 40–49	2.3	20.9	74.0	8.9	94.3	0.4
P: 30–39	1.8	1.4	75.4	0.5	94.7	0.3
A: 30–39	1.6	1.7	77.1	0.5	95.2	0.3
E: 30–39	1.2	22.9	100	4.8	100	0.2

M = Maori; P = Pacific; A = Asian; E = European.

final group consists of those with a past history of IFG or IGT, previous gestational diabetes, or known cardiovascular disease (MI, IHD, angina, CVA, TIA), who should be screened regardless of age. This group has a relatively high rate of progression from nondiabetes to diabetes and/or an increased risk of micro- or macrovascular damage if they do have diabetes.

The rates of undiagnosed diabetes in New Zealand by age and ethnic subgroups (shown previously in Table 4.3) are repeated in the first two columns of Table 4.8. The proportion of the total New Zealand population ≥age 30 is given for each subgroup. The proportion of undiagnosed diabetes in the New Zealand population ≥age 30 is then calculated for each subgroup. This proportion of undiagnosed diabetes is divided by the proportion of the population for each subgroup to give the relative yield.

A comparison of cumulative undiagnosed diabetes with cumulative New Zealand population shows the proportion of all undiagnosed cases, along with the proportion of the general population ≥30 years, covered by alternative targeted screening strategies. For example, a policy to screen subgroups with a relative yield >2.0 would cover about 20.6 per cent of undiagnosed diabetes cases, coming from about 6.7 per cent of the general population. Extending the screening programme to subgroups with a relative yield >1.0 would cover 82.8 per cent of undiagnosed cases coming from 49.1 per cent of the general population (a marginal gain of 62.2 per cent extra diabetes cases by screening an extra 42.4 per cent of the population).

How to Test: Specific Screening Tests and Cut-off Values?

General caveats

Test results vary, so there can be – usually small – differences between results of the same test on the same person on different occasions. This happens partly because of variations in the testing procedures, especially with capillary meters, but mostly because of genuine variation within individual people. For example, one study performed two OGTTs 2–6 weeks apart on the same subjects.[78] The percentages classified both times as normal, IGT and diabetes were only 91, 48 and 78 per cent respectively. It is also worth noting that blood glucose may be raised under conditions of acute infective, traumatic or circulatory stress, but normal when tested later.

There are two general difficulties affecting most studies of sensitivity and specificity of specific tests for diabetes. The first is the changes of diagnostic criteria. The 1999 WHO criteria classify more people as having diabetes than do either the 1985 WHO criteria or the 1997 ADA criteria.[20,52,73] The sensitivity of any given test and cut-off value is therefore lower under the 1999 WHO criteria than under the previous criteria. Any publication before 1999 needs to be interpreted in this light.

Second, few studies have performed both screening and OGTT tests on all subjects. Most studies perform an initial screen followed by an OGTT only on the 'screen positive' people. Hence they are unable to comment on the false-negative rate of their initial screen. Many published studies report on results of people already referred for an OGTT. The group tested is therefore pre-selected, but we do not know the selection criteria, i.e. they are not a group we can confidently recognize clinically. The groups may therefore have already excluded a disproportionate number of people who would otherwise test as false positive, false negative or true negative. The published results may therefore give unrealistically high sensitivities, high or low specificities and high positive predictive values.

It should also be clear that the subsequent comments apply to screening for diabetes in people who are asymptomatic. People with symptoms of possible diabetes should have a fasting or random glucose. If the levels are ≥7.0 or ≥11.1 mmol/l, respectively, that person has diabetes by definition. If the levels are lower, then interpretation is the same as for an asymptomatic person.

Some people with a combination of the risk factors shown in Table 4.7 are at sufficiently high risk of diabetes that screening is not necessary and one can reasonably proceed directly with diagnostic testing.

Fasting venous plasma glucose

The fasting glucose is usually the lowest glucose level for an individual over a 24 hour period and is relatively constant for that individual. The normal population range is small compared with that for a non-fasting glucose. The ADA defines 'fasting' as having no food or drink, apart from water, for 8 hours before the test.[69] However, a fasting glucose should be done in the morning, as a test in the afternoon can be as much as 1 mmol/l lower than in the morning.[79]

According to the diagnostic criteria, people with a fasting glucose $\geq$7.0 mmol/l have diabetes by definition as long as it is confirmed on another day. It is less clear how to interpret lower levels of fasting glucose.

In a European study of people aged 60–80, half the people with a fasting glucose of 6.1–6.9 mmol/l had diabetes according to their 2 hour glucose in an OGTT, and constituted one-third of all people with diabetes.[20] In a high-risk US population one-quarter of those with diabetes had a fasting glucose $\leq$6.0 mmol/l.[80] Data from an Australian laboratory series of OGGTs are shown in Table 4.4. One can calculate a sensitivity and specificity of 95 and 37 per cent respectively for a cut-off value of $\geq$5.5 mmol/l. An OGTT is appropriate for the 53 per cent of this group with a fasting glucose of 5.5–6.9 mmol/l.

On the other hand, most populations tested will not have an overall prevalence of 20.0 per cent, so fewer people in each of the glucose categories of Table 4.9 will have diabetes. For example, in 2002 a laboratory in Taranaki, New Zealand, performed 1249 OGTTs. Of these 335 people had a fasting glucose of 5.5–6.0 mmol/l. Of these, 13 (3.9 per cent) proved to have diabetes on the 2 hour criterion and 66 had IGT (personal communication, J Shuker, 2003).

TABLE 4.9 Test performance of fasting plasma glucose (FPG) in 44 592 people having an OGTT in Queensland, Australia, overall diabetes prevalence 20.0 per cent. The 16 per cent not listed had an FPG $\geq$7.0 mmol/l[44]

FPG <5.5 mmol/l 31% of population			FPG 5.5–6.0 mmol/l 30% of population			FPG 6.1–6.9 mmol/l 23% of population		
NGT	IGT	DM	NGT	IGT	DM	NGT	IGT	DM
77%	19%	3%	67%	26%	7%	39%	39%	22%

NGT = normal glucose tolerance, IGT = impaired glucose tolerance, DM = diabetes mellitus.

There is general agreement that those with a fasting glucose <5.5 mmol/l are highly unlikely to have current diabetes.[19,50,59]

For some patients a fasting sample will be less convenient than a nonfasting sample. Fasting samples, however, also provide the opportunity for testing of serum lipids, although fasting makes little difference to any lipid except triglycerides.[81] Lawrence and Robinson have an interesting variation.[82] They suggested that if a fasting glucose is >5.5 mmol/l a person be further tested for hypertension and dyslipidaemia, even if they are not further tested for diabetes.

Conclusion

Fasting glucose is the most commonly recommended screening test for diabetes. A cut-off value of ≥5.5 mmol/l has a high sensitivity but a low specificity for diabetes. Large numbers of people will still need an OGTT because the fasting test does not detect those who would have diabetes only according to a raised 2 hour test on OGTT.

Random (nonfasting) venous plasma glucose

A random (nonfasting) glucose test has been taken at an unknown (or nonstandard) time after an unknown (or nonstandard) amount of food. Random values are more biologically variable than fasting glucose and are therefore more difficult to interpret.

In 2000 the ADA recommended that if a random glucose is >8.9 mmol/l then two fasting tests be performed as a diagnostic test.[69] The most recent ADA recommendations mention no specific random glucose figure to use in deciding when to follow a random glucose with an OGTT.[56] Recalculation of the data from Welborn *et al.*[75] gives a positive predictive value of 0.12 for a random glucose >5.5 mmol/l to diagnose diabetes under 1985 WHO criteria. As people with a negative screen did not have further testing, sensitivity and specificity cannot be calculated.

Simmons and Williams collected a random glucose during a door-to-door survey in Coventry, UK.[83] The glucose was later measured by a laboratory auto-analyser. They offered an OGTT to subjects with a raised capillary glucose and a random selection of 10 per cent of the remaining subjects. A capillary glucose of 7.0 mmol/l had 52 per cent sensitivity in Europeans and 68 per cent sensitivity in South Asians, for diabetes according to 1985 WHO criteria. (Whole blood glucose can be 15 per cent lower than the plasma glucose values used throughout this thesis, but the relationship is variable.)[50] Other surveys[64,84] have measured random glucose using capillary blood and home test meters, which introduce an additional level of imprecision, as described next.

Conclusion

When using venous plasma glucose, the same cut-off should apply as for a fasting glucose, i.e. an OGTT should be performed if the test is $\geq$5.5 mmol/l. However, if the test was clearly post-prandial then realistic interpretation is less clear.

Capillary glucose measured on meters for self-testing

Sample types, calibration and cut-offs

Although the specimen applied to the test strip is of course capillary blood, preferably from a finger, the result displayed on a given device depends on several factors. Manufacturers may calibrate their system to indicate the glucose level in capillary whole blood, capillary plasma, venous whole blood or venous plasma. The type of calibration can vary in different regions of the world and should be mentioned in the enclosed labelling documents. The final step of the calibration has to be performed by the end-user when inserting a lot-specific code number or a code key into the meter.

For the purpose of screening, it is important to know the relationships between the different sample types, as these clearly show the need for different cut-offs. As seen in Figure 4.5, a cut-off for plasma-calibrated systems of 7.0 mmol/l corresponds to 6.1 mmol/l for blood.

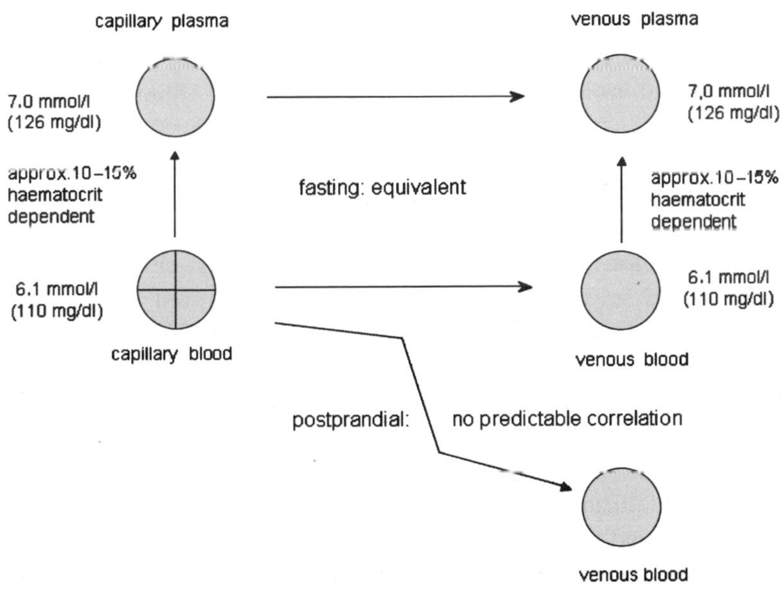

FIGURE 4.5 Blood/plasma & arterial/venous differences: The relationship between glucose levels in capillary blood and venous blood is relatively predictable in the fasting state but not in the nonfasting state

The conversion of glucose values from capillary whole blood to venous whole blood is determined by the arterio-venous difference. In the fasting state the glucose concentrations in arterial, capillary and venous blood are supposed to be almost equivalent. However, large differences can be observed in the post-prandial state.[85,86] Conversion factors cannot be given or lead to unpredictable errors.

The conversion from blood to plasma (e.g. capillary blood to capillary plasma) seems to have a similar complexity. The blood–plasma difference is mainly influenced by the cellular constituents of blood, with a smaller influence from the concentration of proteins. Our own comparison studies indicate a venous blood/venous plasma correction of 1.11–1.12,[87] which is consistent with the factor of 1.11 recommended by the International Federation of Clinical Chemistry and Laboratory Medicine (IFCC).[88]

Clinical requirements and analytical performance of self-monitoring of blood glucose (SMBG)

The analytical performance of blood glucose monitoring systems for self-testing mirrored to the requirements from a clinical point of view have been a matter of discussion for the past 20 years. Clarke[89] in 1987 and Koschinsky[90] in 1988 provided early technical reports, and the American Diabetes Association (ADA) first published consensus recommendations in 1987.[91,92] The International Standardization Organization (ISO) has provided more recent standards for criteria for the accuracy of SMBGs.[93]

Mostly these authors have suggested that 95 per cent of all results of the glucose readings on a SMBG system should fall within a certain range (e.g. ±15 per cent) in comparison to an established laboratory reference procedure. 'Inaccuracy', or deviation of the SMBG system from the reference consists of two components, bias and imprecision. Bias is the deviation of the mean of the system readings from the mean of the reference readings. Imprecision is the range of deviation around the system mean, measured as coefficient of variation (cv) which is standard deviation as a per cent of system mean.[65,94] During the last decade it seems that there has been more improvement in performance of SMBG systems regarding imprecision than in bias. It has to be emphasized that, for clinical use in screening or diabetes management, imprecision and bias can be equally important. Table 4.10 shows the readings to be expected on meters used in New Zealand, based on trials with a minimum of 50 tests per meter.

Bühling has stated that when used by well trained personnel the accuracy of the analysed systems was acceptable for use in gestational diabetes screening,[95] and Haeckel asserted that SMBG systems properly calibrated by the manufacturers could be used for diagnosis as well as laboratory procedures.[96] Nevertheless, our interpretation of the information above is that the meters are suitable for 'on the

TABLE 4.10 Predicted reading of monitors at a 'true' whole blood glucose of 6.1 mmol/l (equivalent to a venous plasma glucose of 7.0 mmol/l). Based on equations from Johnson and Baker[65]

Monitor name in published data	95% limits of expected readings	Rank market share*	Comment
Companion 2	4.9–8.2	1	now Precision Plus
Advantage	4.6–7.4	2	replaced with Advantage II
Glucocard	6.1–8.6	3	now Glucocard Super
Glucometer Elite	6.2–8.2	4	replaced with Glucometer Esprit

*Based on PHARMAC data Jan–May 2000; these four account for approximately 95% of test strip sales.

spot' testing of symptomatic people, with a subsequent laboratory test; they are too inaccurate for screening asymptomatic people, as most people with asymptomatic diabetes will have only modestly elevated blood glucose.

HbA_{1c}

Glucose reacts non-enzymatically and irreversibly with adult haemoglobin to form HbA_{1c}, which persists for the life of the red blood cell – about 3–4 months. It is not affected by fasting. Unfortunately, many studies of HbA_{1c} have used a variety of methods that have poor precision compared with modern HbA_{1c} ion exchange high-performance liquid chromatography methods. Kilpatrick *et al.*[97] suggested that HbA_{1c} could never be an adequate screening test for diabetes because of significant biological variability within and especially between people. Nevertheless, a 1993 meta-analysis of 10 studies indicated that HbA_{1c} has a sensitivity of 80 per cent and specificity >90 per cent for detection of diabetes by 1985 WHO criteria.[98] A 1996 meta-analysis of 34 studies even suggested that an $HbA_{1c} \geq 7$ per cent could be the best option available to identify 'treatment-requiring' diabetes.[99]

Ko *et al.* used 1985 WHO criteria to examine a group of Chinese referred for OGTT.[100] Recalculating their data for an $HbA_{1c} \geq 5.5$ per cent gives a sensitivity of 92 per cent and specificity of 44 per cent. Rohlfing *et al.* assessed HbA_{1c} as a screening test for undiagnosed diabetes according to 1997 ADA criteria in 6559 asymptomatic people over age 20 in the US.[101] Forty-three per cent of their subjects were non-Hispanic white, 27 per cent non-Hispanic black and 30 per cent Mexican-American. They state that an HbA_{1c} of 5.6 per cent had a sensitivity of 83 per cent and specificity of 84 per cent. However, they also noted that at 6.1 per cent the sensitivity ranged from 57 to 84 per cent and specificity ranged from 93 to 98 per cent according to subject ethnicity.

No international body currently recommends screening using HbA_{1c}. Ethnic differences in HbA_{1c} may be relevant in New Zealand. There are no published data applying to Maori and Pacific people. New Zealand laboratories still use more than one assay technique and the results are not fully comparable between methods. Finally, HbA_{1c} cannot be used to formally diagnose diabetes, so glucose testing is needed regardless.

Conclusion

Test characteristics are at least as good as for random glucose. An $HbA_{1c} \geq 5.5$ per cent indicates the need for further testing, either a fasting glucose or OGTT, and an $HbA_{1c} \geq 7$ per cent probably indicates 'treatment-requiring' diabetes. Nevertheless, this still needs to be confirmed by glucose testing, so HbA_{1c} is not recommended as a sole test.

Fructosamine

In a similar way to its reaction with haemoglobin, glucose also reacts non-enzymatically and irreversibly with albumin (protein) in blood. The test is relatively cheap, is automated and has excellent measurement precision. Results are not affected by fasting. Albumin has a short half-life in the circulation and thus fructosamine reflects mean glucose over the preceding 2–3 weeks. Whilst fructosamine concentration is closely correlated with HbA_{1c}, fructosamine concentration alone cannot predict HbA_{1c} values and vice versa due to multiple mechanisms including fructosamine being lower in those who are obese or have albuminuria.[102]

Some studies[103,104] found fructosamine wanting as a screening test in populations with a high prevalence of diabetes, but a Japanese group[105] reported a sensitivity of 96.7 per cent for diabetes using 1985 WHO criteria and a cut-off of $\geq$290 µmol/l. Another Japanese group rated fructosamine as the most cost-effective screening method, at least in Japan.[106] Baker *et al.*[107] tested a New Zealand group of workers and found a sensitivity of 81.1 per cent and a specificity of 97.6 per cent for diabetes under the 1985 WHO criteria, at a cut-off of 296 µmol/l.

Because HbA_{1c} has been used for long-term diabetes outcome studies, whereas fructosamine has not, fructosamine has become decreasingly used to monitor diabetes and therefore decreasingly available for screening purposes. Many laboratories in New Zealand no longer offer the test.

Conclusion

It may have appealing test characteristics but fructosamine is not recommended as a screening test in New Zealand.

Combining fasting glucose with HbA_{1c} or fructosamine

The potential advantage of combination testing with a fasting glucose and either HbA_{1c} or fructosamine is reducing the number of false negative tests from a fasting glucose alone, i.e. detecting some of those people with a fasting glucose $\leq$7.0 mmol/l but who would have diabetes on the 2 hours test of an OGTT.[100,101,108]

Ko *et al.* examined the combined use of a fasting plasma glucose and HbA_{1c} or fructosamine for the screening of diabetes in 2877 Hong Kong Chinese patients at high risk for diabetes undergoing OGTT; the prevalence of diabetes in the population tested was 22 per cent.[100] All patients had a family history of diabetes or past GDM or IGT or were obese. Eighty per cent were female and they were relatively young, with a mean age of 37 years. Diabetes and IGT were diagnosed using the 1985 WHO criteria; however, only a further 1.2 per cent of their patients had a glucose 7.0–7.7, i.e. had diabetes by 1999 WHO criteria. Table 4.11 shows the likelihood ratio of having diabetes when a positive screen consists of both a fasting glucose $\geq$ 5.6 mmol/l and an $HbA_{1c} \geq 5.5$ per cent.

Combination tests are not well established internationally and there are no published figures for the performance of these tests in a New Zealand population. Additional laboratory glucose tests would still be required to confirm diabetes in asymptomatic people.

Conclusion

Screening using combinations of fasting glucose and either HbA_{1c} or fructosamine is promising, but not yet well established.

Urine testing

Blood glucose levels above the renal threshold for the reabsorption of glucose from the nephron result in glucose in the urine. This threshold is variable and

TABLE 4.11 2877 Chinese subjects classified as normal, IGT or diabetes by paired values of fasting plasma glucose (FPG) and HbA_{1c} (1985 WHO criteria).[100] Likelihood ratio of having diabetes with both FPG $\geq$ 5.6 and $HbA_{1c} \geq$ 5.5 compared to having one or both tests below these cut-off values

FPG (mmol/l)	HbA_{1c} (%)	Normal	IGT	Diabetes	Likelihood ratio
$\geq$5.6	$\geq$5.5	132	221	527	5.36
$\geq$5.6	<5.5	64	52	27	0.84
<5.6	$\geq$5.5	683	234	48	0.19
<5.6	<5.5	714	150	25	0.10

increases with age. Murray *et al.* undertook a community study of European New Zealanders in Rangiora in 1967.[109] Their numbers have been re-calculated here. People provided urine 90 minutes and blood two hours after taking 50 g oral glucose (nonfasting). The authors noted that 99 per cent of people gave a urine specimen, suggesting this method was acceptable. Those with a blood glucose $\geq$7.22 mmol/l were requested to obtain an OGTT (using 1985 WHO criteria). 'Moderate' or 'heavy' glycosuria on Ames Uristix was present 1 hour after a 50 g glucose load in 35 of 60 people with diabetes and in 201 of 2426 without diabetes. This gives a sensitivity of 58 per cent and specificity of 92 per cent against OGTT. Davies *et al.* proposed that patients self-test for glycosuria, stating a sensitivity of 43 per cent and specificity of 98 per cent.[110] On the other hand, urinalysis of all medical admissions to Auckland hospital over one year did not result in detection of a single new case of diabetes.[111]

The performance of the test is unknown for a non-European population, for current test strips and against 1999 WHO diagnostic criteria. Current patient acceptability is unknown.

Conclusion

Urine testing is not recommended, though it may be more effective than commonly thought.

Questionnaires as an initial screen

A small number of questionnaires have been developed to use as an initial screening tool for diabetes.[68,112,113] A related approach used routinely collected data to assign a diabetes risk score to individual patients.[114,115] These methods collect known risk factors for diabetes and apply weightings to produce a score that can be used to decide whether or not to screen for diabetes. Ruige *et al.*,[112] Herman *et al.*[68] and Baan *et al.*[113] assessed their questionnaires against 1985 WHO diabetes criteria. Park *et al.* predicted raised HbA_{1c} rather than formally diagnosed diabetes.[114] Scragg re-analysed his New Zealand data[11] assessing risk factors against newly diagnosed diabetes using 1999 WHO criteria (personal communication, R Scragg, 2002). He noted that after logistic regression only age and ethnicity were significantly associated with diabetes. Questions about family history performed poorly as many people did not know whether they had a relative with diabetes. Regardless of the results of a questionnaire, a blood glucose test is still required for the formal diagnosis of diabetes.

Conclusion

Questionnaires formalize the process that GPs probably currently undertake informally. There is currently no questionnaire available that has been validated for a New Zealand population. In the meantime, GPs can only use simple age and ethnicity data plus the known factors that increase diabetes risk.

Screening Intervals

An individual who has a negative or normal screening test needs re-testing after an interval. There are no direct trial data to guide us on ideal intervals. The ideal interval between screens is a function of the chance of missing diabetes on the screening test (false negative), the rate of people newly developing diabetes over a particular interval and the risk of diabetes causing damage to either of these groups in the interval between the screening tests.

The rate of newly developing diabetes over a given interval is lower for those at low risk and higher for those at high risk, and can be estimated by examining the risk between consecutive age groups in Tables 4.1–4.3. The risk of any person developing microvascular or macrovascular damage per year was relatively small when estimated in a modelling study.[116] Overall, some five per cent of those people without diabetes at initial screening will progress to diabetes within 3 years. All those with a negative screening test should be recalled for re-screening 3 yearly. In contrast, people with previous IGT, IFG and gestational diabetes have a higher rate of progression to diabetes, of the order of five per cent per year.[19] It is reasonable to screen this sub-group yearly.

Difficulty Applying Recommendations to Individual Patients

Determining cut-off values according to test sensitivity and sensitivity in population groups is one thing. Applying these figures to individual patients may be more difficult. For example, consider the Australian figures in Table 4.4. The pre-test probability of any member of the population tested having diabetes was 20.0 per cent. After the test 16 per cent have a glucose of $\geq$7.0 mmol/l. They probably have diabetes, although this needs to be confirmed on a repeat test. A further 31 per cent have a glucose $<$5.5 mmol/l and need no further testing. However, after the test neither doctor nor patient is sure whether the remaining 53 per cent have diabetes. Furthermore, this remaining group now has probabilities of having diabetes of 22 per cent (for those with a fasting test 6.1–6.9 mmol/l) and six per cent for those with a fasting test 5.5–6.0 mmol/l. Yet, somewhat counter-intuitively, it is now suggested that these people with a lower risk than the original whole group nevertheless need a more onerous test, the OGTT. In practice in New Zealand the pre- and post-test probabilities will be smaller, as it is recommended to test groups with a total prevalence of undiagnosed diabetes of five per cent or more (rather than 20.0 per cent as in the example). It is not known how many GPs, others health-care providers and patients opt not to follow up a screening test with an

OGTT, especially for those with a screening test 5.5–6.0 mmol/l. Research is needed into the decisions and the decision-making processes involved.

Screening Algorithms for Asymptomatic People

The above discussion about use and interpretation of specific screening tests is summarized in the algorithms below. It is recommended to screen those at five per cent or more risk of undiagnosed diabetes. By age and ethnicity in New Zealand this means Europeans at age 50 or more and all others at age 40 or more. Screening at earlier ages is appropriate for those with the risk factors listed in Table 4.7.

Option 1: fasting glucose (mmol/l)

- glucose ≥ 7.0 — re-test another day; diabetes if ≥ 7.0
- glucose 5.5–6.9 — consider OGTT
- glucose < 5.5 — re-test in 1–3 years; see screening intervals

Option 2: fasting glucose + HbA_{1c}

- glucose ≥ 7.0 — re-test another day; diabetes if ≥ 7.0
- glucose $\geq$ 5.5–6.9 or $HbA_{1c} \geq 5.5\%$ — consider OGTT
- glucose < 5.5 + $HbA_{1c} \geq 5.5\%$ — consider OGTT
- FG < 5.5 + $HbA_{1c} < 5.5\%$ — re-test in 1–3 years; see screening intervals

Option 3: nonfasting (random) glucose

- glucose ≥ 11.1 — re-test another day (preferably fasting); diabetes if fasting ≥ 7.0
- glucose 5.5–11.0 — consider OGTT (see discussion)
- glucose < 5.5 — re-test in 1–3 years; see screening intervals

Summary

While we await randomized controlled trial data to more precisely define the value of screening for Type 2 diabetes, it seems reasonable to extrapolate from available data. To provide the following advice for practicing clinicians. Undiagnosed diabetes causes similar harms to those caused by diagnosed diabetes. For every person with diagnosed diabetes there may be another with undiagnosed diabetes. Screening of high-risk individuals is justified against standard criteria and is widely recommended by international bodies.

We recommend screening people at five per cent risk or more of undiagnosed diabetes. (In New Zealand this means Europeans age 50 or more and all others at age 40 or more.) Groups at higher risk include those with hypertension, dyslipidaemia, the obese and those with a family history of diabetes or with previous IGT, IFG or gestational diabetes. The formal criteria for diagnosing diabetes create two overlapping groups of people, those with a fasting glucose ≥ 7.0 mmol/l and those with a glucose ≥ 11.1 mmol/l on a random glucose or a 2 hours test in the OGTT. Only an OGTT can identify both groups. The recommended process is therefore to start with a fasting glucose and follow with an OGTT only for those with a glucose 5.5–6.9 mmol/l. A random glucose may be used, although it is more difficult to interpret. Capillary glucose, HbA_{1c}, fructosamine and urinary glucose testing are not recommended as screening tests. Those with a negative screening test should be re-screened in 3 years. Those with previous IGT, IFG or gestational diabetes should be re-screened yearly. There are unanswered questions about how individual GPs and patients do or should follow up a fasting glucose of 5.5–6.0 mmol/l. The answers ideally depend on more accurate assessment than is usually available of an individual's risk factors and associated pre-test probability of diabetes.

The biggest challenge will be to screen the large number of at-risk people. The best opportunity for screening appears to be systematic opportunistic screening, i.e. systematically screening people who attend a primary health-care provider for some other reason.

References

1. Harris M, Klein R, Welborn T and Knuiman M. Onset of NIDDM occurs at least 4–7 years before clinical diagnosis. *Diabetes Care* 1992; **15** (7): 815–819.
2. Khaw K, Wareham N, Luben R, Bingham S, Oakes S and Welch A *et al.* Glycated haemoglobin, diabetes, and mortality in men in Norfolk cohort of European Prospective Investigation of Cancer and Nutrition (EPIC-Norfolk). *BMJ* 2001; **322**: 15–18.
3. Tenerez A, Lonnberg I, Berne C, Nilsson G and Leppert J. Myocardial infarction and prevalence of diabetes mellitus. Is increased glucose at admission a reliable criterion for the diagnosis of diabetes? *Eur Heart J* 2001; **22** (13): 1102–1110.
4. Oswald G, Corcoran S and Yudkin J. Prevalence and risks of hyperglycaemia and undiagnosed diabetes in pateints with acute myocardial infarction. *Lancet* 1984; **1** (8389): 1264–1267.
5. UK Prospective Diabetes Study (UKPDS) Group. Intensive blood-glucose control with sulphonylureas or insulin compared with conventional treatment and risk of complications in patients with Type 2 diabetes (UKPDS 33). *Lancet* 1998; **352** (9131): 837–853.
6. Simmons D, Gatland B, Leakehe L and Fleming C. Frequency of diabetes in family members of probands with non-insulin dependent diabetes. *J Int Med* 1995; **237** (3): 315–321.
7. Simmons D, Gatland B, Fleming C, Leakehe L and Scragg R. Prevalence of known diabetes in a multiethnic community. *New Zealand Med J* 1994; **107**: 219–222.
8. Simmons D, Harry T and Gatland B. Prevalence of known diabetes in different ethnic groups in inner urban South Auckland. *New Zealand Med J* 1999; **112**: 316–319.

9. Simmons D, Shaw L, Kenealy T and Scragg R. Ethnic differences in diabetes knowledge and education: the South Auckland diabetes survey. *New Zealand Med J* 1994; **107**: 197–200.
10. Scragg R, Baker J, Mecalf P and Dryson E. Prevalence of diabetes mellitus and impaired glucose tolerance in a New Zealand multiracial workforce. *New Zealand Med J* 1991; **104**: 395–397.
11. Statistics New Zealand. Auckland Region, standard regional tables, by Territorial Local Authority: Statistics New Zealand, http://www.stats.govt.nz/domino/external/web/ExtraPages.nsf/htmldocs/Standard+Regional+Tables+-+Auckland+Region accessed 23 May 2003. 2001.
12. Kenealy T, Braatvedt G and Scragg R. Screening for type 2 diabetes in non-pregnant adults in New Zealand: practical recommendations. *New Zealand Med J* 2002; **115** (1152): 194–196.
13. Wilson J and Jungner G. *Principles and Practice of Screening for Disease*. 1968. Geneva: World Health Organization.
14. National Advisory Committee on Health and Disability. *Screening to Improve Health in New Zealand*. 2003. Wellington: National Advisory Committee on Health and Disability.
15. The UK National Screening Committee. *The UK National Screening Committee's Criteria for Appraising the Viability, Effectiveness and Appropriateness of a Screening Programme*. 2003. London: UK National Screening Committee.
16. Barratt A, Irwig L, Glasziou P, Cumming R, Raffle A and Hicks N *et al*. Users' guides to the medical literature XVII. How to use guidelines and recommendations about screening. *JAMA* 1999; **281** (21): 2029–2034.
17. Schneider H, Lischinski M and Jutzi E. Survival time after onset of diabetes: 29-year follow-up mortality study in a diabetes cohort from a rural district. *Diabete Metabolisme* 1993; **19**: 152–158.
18. Lauritzen T, Griffin S, Borch-Johnsen K, Wareham N, Wolffenbuttel B and Rutten G. Anglo–Danish–Dutch study of intensive treatment in people with screen detected diabetes in primary care. The ADDITION study: proposed trial of the cost-effectiveness of an intensive multifactorial intervention on morbidity and mortality among people with Type 2 diabetes detected by screening. *Int J Obesity Relat Metab Disorders* 2000; **24** (Suppl. 3): S6–S11.
19. Australian centre for diabetes strategies. *National Evidence Based Guidelines for the Management of Type 2 Diabetes Mellitus*. 2001. Sydney: Australian Centre for Diabetes Strategies.
20. DECODE Study Group on behalf of the European diabetes epidemiology group. Consequences of the new diagnostic criteria for diabetes in older men and women. *Diabetes Care* 1999; **22** (10): 1667–1671.
21. Harris M. Undiagnosed NIDDM: clinical and public health issues. *Diabetes Care* 1993; **16** (4): 642–652.
22. Colagiuri S, Cull CA and Holman RR, Group ftUPDSU. Are lower fasting plasma glucose levels at diagnosis of Type 2 diabetes associated with improved outcomes? UK Prospective Diabetes Study 61. *Diabetes Care* 2002; **25** (8): 1418–1424.
23. Jarrett R. Duration of non-insulin-dependent diabetes and development of retinopathy: analysis of possible risk factors. *Diabet Med* 1986; **3**: 261–263.
24. New Zealand society for the study of diabetes. Core components of a diabetic service. *New Zealand Med J* 1995; **108** (1010): 434–435.
25. Adriaanse M, Snoek F, Dekker J, van der Ploeg H and Heine R. Screening for Type 2 diabetes: an exploration of subjects' perceptions regarding diagnosis and procedure. *Diabet Med* 2002; **19** (5): 406–411.
26. Shaw C, Abrams K and Marteau TM. Psychological impact of predicting individuals' risks of illness: a systematic review. *Soc Sci Med* 1999; **49**: 1571–1598.

27. Diabetes New Zealand, PricewaterhouseCoopers. *Type 2 Diabetes: Managing for Better Health Outcomes.* 2001. Wellington: Diabetes New Zealand.
28. CDC Diabetes Cost-Effectiveness Study Group. The cost-effectiveness of screening for Type 2 diabetes. *JAMA* 1998; **280**: 1757–1763.
29. Raikou M and McGuire A. The economics of screening and treatment in Type 2 diabetes mellitus. *Pharmacoeconomics* 2003; **21** (8): 543–564.
30. Gray A, Raikou M, McGuire A, Fenn P, Stevens R and Cull C *et al.* Cost effectiveness of an intensive blood glucose control policy in patients with Type 2 diabetes: economic analysis alongside randomised controlled trial (UKPDS 41). *BMJ* 2000; **320**: 1373–1378.
31. UK prospective diabetes study group. Cost effectiveness analysis of improved blood pressure control in hypertensive patients with Type 2 diabetes: UKPDS 40. *BMJ* 1998; **317** (7160): 720–726.
32. Elliott W, Weir D and HR B. Cost-effectiveness of the lower treatment goal (of JNC VI) for diabetic hypertensive patients. *Arch Intern Med* 2000; **160**: 1277–1283.
33. Eastman R, Javitt J, Herman W, Dasbach E, Copley-Merriman C and Maier W *et al.* Model of complications of NIDDM: II. Analysis of the health benefits and cost-effectiveness of treating NIDDM with the goal of normoglycaemia. *Diabetes Care* 1997; **20** (5): 735–744.
34. Gaede P, Vedel P, Larsen N, Jensen G, Parving H and Pedersen O. Multifactorial intervention and cardiovascular disease in patients with Type 2 diabetes. *N Engl J Med* 2003; **348** (5): 383–393.
35. Griffin S and Kinmonth A. Diabetes care: the effectiveness of systems for routine surveillance for people with diabetes. *The Cochrane Library of Systematic Reviews* 1998(1).
36. Olivarius ND, Beck-Nielsen H, Andreasen A, Horder M and Pedersen P. Randomised controlled trial of structured personal care of Type 2 diabetes mellitus. *BMJ* 2001; **323**: 1–9.
37. Foulkes A, Kinmonth A, Frost S and Macdonald D. Organised personal care – an effective choice for managing diabetes in general practice. *J R Coll Gen Practitioners* 1989; **39**: 444–447.
38. Singh B, Holland MR and Thorn PA. Metabolic control of diabetes in general practice clinics: comparison with a hospital clinic. *BMJ* 1984; **289**: 726–728.
39. Pringle M, Stewart-Evans C, Coupland C, Williams I, Allison S and Sterland J. Influences on control in diabetes mellitus: patient, doctor, practice, or delivery of care? *BMJ* 1993; **306**: 630–634.
40. Norris SL, Nichols PJ, Caspersen CJ, Glasgow RE, Engelgau MM and Leonard J Jr *et al.* The effectiveness of disease and case management for people with diabetes. A systematic review. *Am J Prevent Med* 2002; **22** (4, S1): 15–38.
41. Harris R, Donahue K, Rathore SS, Frame P, Woolf S and Lohr K. Screening adults for Type 2 diabetes: a review of the evidence for the U.S. Preventive Services Task Force. *Ann Intern Med* 2003; **138** (3): 215–229.
42. Wareham N and Griffin S. Should we screen for Type 2 diabetes? Evaluation against National Screening Committee criteria. *BMJ* 2001; **322**: 986–988.
43. Diabetes, Heart Disease and Stroke Prevention Project. http://www.nelh.nhs.uk/screening/diabetesproject/home.htm.
44. Appleton C. Problems with new criteria for diagnosis of diabetes mellitus [letter]. *Med J Australia* 1999; **171**: 107–108.
45. Sackett DL, Haynes RB, Guyatt GH and Tugwell P. *Clinical Epidemiology. A Basic Science for Clinical Medicine*, 2nd edn. Boston, MA: Lippincott Williams and Wilkins.
46. Feinstein A. *Clinical Epidemiology: the Architecture of Clinical Research.* 1985. Philadelphia, PA: Saunders.

47. Swinburn B, Metcalf P and Ley S. Long-term (5-year) effect of a reduced-fat diet intervention in individuals with glucose intolerance. *Diabetes Care* 2001; **24**: 619–624.
48. Pan X-R, Li G and Hu Y *et al.* Effects of diet and exercise in preventing NIDDM in people with impaired glucose tolerance: The Da Qing IGT and diabetes study. *Diabetes Care* 1997; **20** (4): 537–544.
49. Tuomilehto J, Lindstrom J, Eriksson J, Valle T, Hamalainen H and Ilanne-Parikka P *et al.* Prevention of Type 2 diabetes mellitus by changes in lifestyle among subjects with impaired glucose tolerance. *N Engl J Med* 2001; **344** (18): 1343–1350.
50. Alberti K and Zimmet P, on behalf of a WHO Consultation. *Definition, Diagnosis and Classification of Diabetes Mellitus and its Complications.* 1999. Geneva: department of noncommunicable disease surveillance. World Health Organization.
51. Kenealy T, Scragg R and Braatvedt G. *Screening for Diabetes in Asymptomatic Non-Pregnant Adults in New Zealand.* 2000. Wellington: Health Funding Authority.
52. DECODE Study Group. Glucose tolerance and mortality: comparison of WHO and American Diabetes Association diagnostic criteria. *Lancet* 1999; **354**: 617–621.
53. Bastyr E, Graf C, Stuart C, Zagar A, Brodows R and Robertson K *et al.* Therapy focused on lowering postprandial glucose, not fasting glucose, may be superior for lowering HbA_{1c}. *Diabetes Care* 2000; **23** (9): 1236–1241.
54. Resnick H, Harris M and Brock D *et al.* American Diabetes Association diabetes diagnostic criteria, advancing age and cardiovascular risk profiles. Results from the 3rd National Health and Nutrition Examination Survey (NHANES III). *Diabetes Care* 2000; **23**: 176–180.
55. US Preventive Services Task Force. Screening for Type 2 diabetes mellitus in adults: recommendations and rationale. *Ann Intern Med* 2003; **138** (3): 212–214.
56. American Diabetes Association. Screening for Type 2 diabetes. *Diabetes Care* 2003; **26** (Suppl.): S21–S24.
57. Colman P, Thomas D, Zimmet P, Welborn T, Garcia-Webb P and Moore M. New classification and criteria for diagnosis of diabetes mellitus. *New Zealand Med J* 1999; **112**: 139–141.
58. Expert Committee of the American Diabetes Association. Report of the expert committee on the diagnosis and classification of diabetes mellitus. *Diabetes Care* 1997; **20**: 1–15.
59. New Zealand Society for the Study of Diabetes. Screening for diabetes in asymptomatic individuals. *New Zealand Med J* 1995; **108** (1011): 464–465.
60. Kenealy T, Kenealy H, Arroll B, Scott D, Scragg R and Simmons D. Diabetes care by General Practitioners in South Auckland: changes from 1990 to 1999. *New Zealand Med J* 2002; **115** (1164):U219, Oct 25.
61. Krebs J. Diabetes is still unrecognised in the 1990's: a report of a hospital audit [letter]. *New Zealand Med J* 2000; **113** (1103): 42.
62. Simmons D and Laughton S. Diabetes on the surgical wards in an area with a high prevalence of diabetes. *New Zealand Med J* 1993; **106**: 156–157.
63. Bourn D and Mann J. Screening for non-insulin dependent diabetes mellitus and impaired glucose tolerance in a Dunedin general practice – is it worth it? *New Zealand Med J* 1992; **105** (935): 207–210.
64. Lawrenson R, Dunn P, Jury D and Sceats J. Discover diabetes: screening for diabetes mellitus in the Waikato. *New Zealand Med J* 1993; **106**: 522–524.
65. Johnson R and Baker J. Accuracy of devices used for self-monitoring of blood glucose. *Ann Clin Biochem* 1998; **35**: 68–74.
66. Ministry of Health. *Taking the Pulse: The 1996/97 New Zealand Health Survey.* 1999. Wellington: Ministry of Health.

67. Lawrence J, Bennett P, Young A and Robinson A. Screening for diabetes in general practice: cross sectional population study. *BMJ* 2001; **323**: 548–551.
68. Herman W, Smith P, Thompson T, Engelgau M and Aubert R. A new and simple questionnaire to identify people at increased risk for undiagnosed diabetes. *Diabetes Care* 1995; **18** (3): 382–387.
69. American Diabetes Association. Screening for Type 2 diabetes. *Diabetes Care* 2000; **23** (Suppl. 1): S20–S23.
70. Yki-Jarvinen H. Pathogenesis of non-insulin dependent diabetes mellitus. *Lancet* 1994; **343**: 91–95.
71. Colditz G, Willett W, Rotnitzky A and Manson J. Weight gain as a risk factor for clinical diabetes mellitus. *Ann Intern Med* 1995; **122**: 481–87.
72. Simmons D. Diabetes and its complications in New Zealand: an epidemiological perspective. *New Zealand Med J* 1996; **109** (1025): 245–247.
73. Davies M. New diagnostic criteria for diabetes – are they doing what they should? *Lancet* 1999; **354**: 610–611.
74. Schmidt M, Watson R, Duncan B, Metcalf P, Brancati F and Sharrett A *et al.* Clustering of dyslipidaemia, hyperuricaemia, diabetes, and hypertension and its association with fasting insulin and central and overall obesity in a general population. *Metabolism* 1996; **45** (6): 699–706.
75. Welborn T, Reid C and Marriott G. Australian diabetes screening study: impaired glucose tolerance and non-insulin-dependent diabetes mellitus. *Metabolism* 1997; **46** (12 Suppl. 1): 35–39.
76. Legro R, Kunselman A, Dodson W and Dunaif A. Prevalence and predictors of risk for Type 2 diabetes mellitus and impaired glucose tolerance in polycystic ovary syndrome: a prospective, controlled study of 254 affected women. *J Clin Endocrinol Metab* 1999; **84**: 165–169.
77. Health Funding Authority. *Diabetes 2000*. 2000. Wellington: Health Funding Authority.
78. Mooy J, Grootehuis P, de Vries H, Kostense P, Poop-Snijders C and Bouter L *et al.* Intra-individual variation of glucose, specific insulin and pro-insulin concentrations measured by two oral glucose tolerance tests in a general Caucasian population: the Hoorn Study. *Diabetologia* 1996; **39**: 298–305.
79. Troisi R, Cowie C and Harris M. Diurnal variation in fasting plasma glucose: implications for diagnosis of diabetes in patients examined in the afternoon. *JAMA* 2000; **284** (24): 3157–3159.
80. Perry R, Shankar R, Fineberg N, McGill J and Baron A. HbA_{1c} measurement improves the detection of Type 2 diabetes in high risk individuals with nondiagnostic levels of fasting plasma glucose. *Diabetes Care* 2001; **24**: 465–471.
81. Booth S and Lacey R. Effect of food on estimation of high-density lipoprotein and total cholesterol in normal subjects. *Ann Clin Biochem* 1982; **19**: 176–181.
82. Lawrence J and Robinson A. Screening for diabetes in general practice. *Preventive Cardiology* 2003; **6** (2): 78–84.
83. Simmons D and Williams D. Random blood glucose as a screening test for diabetes in a biethnic population. *Diabet Med* 1994; **11**: 830–835.
84. Engelgau M, Thompson T, Smith P, Herman W, Aubert R and Gunter E *et al.* Screening for diabetes mellitus in adults. The utility of random capillary blood glucose measurements. *Diabetes Care* 1995; **18** (4): 463–466.
85. Colagiuri S, Sandbæk A, Carstensen B, Christensen J, Glumer C and Lauritzen T *et al.* Comparability of venous and capillary glucose measurements in blood. *Diabet Med* 2003; **20** (11): 953–956.

86. Haeckel R, Brinck U, Colic D, Janka H-U, Püntmann I and Schneider J *et al.* Comparability of blood glucose concentrations measured in different sample systems for detecting glucose intolerance. *Clin Chem* 2002; **48** (6): 936–939.
87. Mueller P and Sauter H. Accutrend Glucose Venenblutmessungen mit Code für venöses Blut. *Boehringer Mannheim Evaluation Report.* 1994. Mannheim: Boehringer Mannheim.
88. Burnett R, D'Orazio P, Fogh-Andersen N, Kuwa K, Kulpmann W and Larsson L *et al.* IFCC Recommendation on reporting results for blood glucose. *Clinica Chimica Acta; international journal of clincal chemistry* 2001; **307**: 205–209.
89. Clarke W, Cox D, Gonder-Frederick L, Carter W and Pohl S. Evaluating clinical accuracy of systems for self-monitoring of blood glucose. *Diabetes Care* 1987; **10** (5): 622–628.
90. Koschinsky T, Dannehl K and Gries F. New approach to technical and clinical evaluation of devices for self-monitoring of blood glucose. *Diabetes Care* 1988; **11**: 619–629.
91. American Diabetes Association. Consensus statement on self-monitoring of blood glucose. *Diabetes Care* 1994; **17**: 81–86.
92. American Diabetes Association. Consensus statement on self-monitoring of blood glucose. *Diabetes Care* 1987; **10**: 95–99.
93. International Organization for Standardization. *In Vitro Diagnostic Test Systems – Requirements for Blood-Glucose Monitoring Systems for Self-Testing in Managing Diabetes Mellitus.* 2003. Geneva: International Organization for Standardization (ISO).
94. Johnson R and Baker J. Analytical error of home glucose monitors: a comparison of 18 systems. *Ann Clin Biochem* 1999; **36**: 72–79.
95. Buehling K, Henrich W, Kjos S, Siebert G, Starr E and Dreweck C *et al.* Comparison of point-of-care-testing glucose meters with standard laboratory measurement of the 50g-glucose-challenge test (GCT) during pregnancy. *Clin Biochem* 2003; **36**: 333–337.
96. Puentmann I, Wosniok W and Haeckel R. Comparison of several Point-of-Care Testing (POCT) glucometers with an established laboratory procedure for the diagnosis of Type 2 diabetes using the discordance rate. A new statistical approach. *Clin Chem Lab Med* 2003; **41** (6): 809–820.
97. Kilpatrick E, Maylor P and Keevil B. Biological variation of glycated haemoglobin. *Diabetes Care* 1998; **21**: 261–264.
98. Hanson R, Nelson R and McCance D *et al.* Comparison of screening tests for non-insulin dependent diabetes mellitus. *Arch Intern Med* 1993; **153**: 2133–2140.
99. Peters A, Davidson M, Schringer D and Hasselblad V. A clinical approach to the diagnosis of diabetes mellitus: an analysis using glycosylated haemoglobin levels. *JAMA* 1996; **276**: 1246–1252.
100. Ko G, Chan J, Yeung V, Chow C, Tsang L and Li J *et al.* Combined use of a fasting plasma glucose concentration and HbA_{1c} or fructosamine predicts the likelihood of having diabetes in high risk subjects. *Diabetes Care* 1998; **21**: 1221–1225.
101. Rohlfing C, Little R, Wiedmeyer H, England J, Madsen R and Harris M *et al.* Use of GHb (HbA_{1c}) in screening for undiagnosed diabetes in the U.S. population. *Diabetes Care* 2000; **23** (2): 187–191.
102. Braatvedt G, Drury P and Cundy T. Assessing glycaemic control in diabetes: relationships between fructosamine and HbA_{1c}. *New Zealand Med J* 1997; **110**: 459–462.
103. Guillausseau P, Charles M, Paolaggi F, Timsit J, Chanson P and Peynet J *et al.* Comparison of HbA_{1c} and fructosamine in diagnosis of glucose tolerance abnormalities. *Diabetes Care* 1990; **13**: 898–900.
104. Swai A, Harrison K, Chuwa L, Makene W, McLarty D and Alberti K. Screening for diabetes: does measurement of serum fructosamine help? *Diabet Med* 1988; **5**: 648–652.
105. Kasezawa N, Kiyose H, Ito K, Iwatsuka T, Kawai H and Goto Y *et al.* Criteria for screening diabetes mellitus using serum fructosamine level and fasting plasma glucose level. The

Japanese Society of Multiphasic Health Testing and Services (JMHT) Fructosamine Working Committee. *Methods Information Med* 1993; **32** (3): 237–240.

106. Shirasaya K, Miyakawa M, Yoshida K, Takahashi E, Shimada N and Kondo T. Economic evaluation of alternative indicators for screening for diabetes. *Preventive Med* 1999; **29** (2): 79–86.
107. Baker J, Metcalf P, Scragg R and Johnson R. Fructosamine Test-Plus, a modified fructosamine assay evaluated. *Clin Chem* 1991; **37**: 552–556.
108. Wiener K and Roberts N. The relative merits of HbA_{1c} and fasting plasma glucose as first line diagnostic tests for diabetes mellitus in non-pregnant subjects. *Diabe Med* 1998; **15**: 558–563.
109. Murray J, Laing J, Cotter A, Lovell-Smith H, Jepson L and Beaven D. Diabetes mellitus in European New Zealanders. *New Zealand Med J* 1969; **69** (444): 271–275.
110. Davies MJ, Williams DRR, Metcalfe J and Day JL. Community screening for non-insulin-dependent diabetes mellitus: self-testing for post-prandial glycosuria. *Q J Med* 1993; **86** (10): 677–684.
111. Issacs R. A prospective study of routine dipstick urinalysis in acute medical admissions to Middlemore Hospital [letter]. *New Zealand Med J* 1986: 467.
112. Ruige J, de Neeling J, Kostense P, Bouter L and Heine R. Performance of an NIDDM screening questionnaire based on symptoms and risk factors. *Diabetes Care* 1997; **20** (4): 491–496.
113. Baan C, Ruige J, Stolk R, Witteman J, Dekker J and Heine R *et al.* Performance of a predictive model to identify undiagnosed diabetes in a health care setting. *Diabetes Care* 1999; **22** (2): 213–219.
114. Park PJ, Griffin SJ, Sargeant L and Wareham NJ. The performance of a risk score in predicting undiagnosed hyperglycemia. *Diabetes Care* 2002; **25** (6): 984–988.
115. Griffin SJ, Little PS, Hales CN, Kinmonth AL and Wareham NJ. Diabetes risk score: towards earlier detection of Type 2 diabetes in general practice. *Diabetes/Metab Res Rev* 2000; **16** (3): 164–171.
116. Eastman R, Javitt J, Herman W, Dasbach E, Abrozck A and Dong F *et al.* Model of complications of NIDDM: I. Model construction and assumptions. *Diabetes Care* 1997; **20** (5): 725–734.

5

Genetic Screening and Prevention of Type 2 Diabetes

Paolo Pozzilli

Introduction

Type 2 diabetes is probably the best example of a multifactorial disease (Figure 5.1). This condition is the result of the interaction between genetic and environmental factors where the latter play a major role in the clinical expression of the disease. Although evidence for a genetic component in Type 2 is high, only 10 per cent of the genetic risk factors for this type of diabetes have been identified, compared with approximately 65 per cent in the case of Type 1 diabetes. The clinical heterogeneity observed in Type 2 diabetes, which, with all probability reflects the different forms of inheritance, offers the most probable explanation of this fact. Hence, Type 2 diabetes may be considered a syndrome linked to several genetic variants with clinically defined sub-types, which are, however, dependent upon environmental factors. To determine the genetic factors involved in this disease, a model approach was that of differentiating the potential monogenic forms of the disease. To this end, this strategy has offered interesting results in families with early-onset Type 2 diabetes, such as maturity-onset diabetes of the young (MODY) or severe types of insulin resistance, which has led to the identification of genetic mutations in several genes including glucokinase, insulin and insulin receptor genes.

Most of the genes identified as likely contributors to the more common forms of Type 2 diabetes have been characterized by means of a candidate gene approach. Using this approach, various genes have been identified, including the insulin receptor substrate 1 (IRS 1), fatty acid binding protein (FABP 2) and glycogen synthase genes. However, it has been suggested that these genes are putative

Prevention of Type 2 Diabetes Edited by Manfred Ganz
 ISBN: 0-470-85733-1

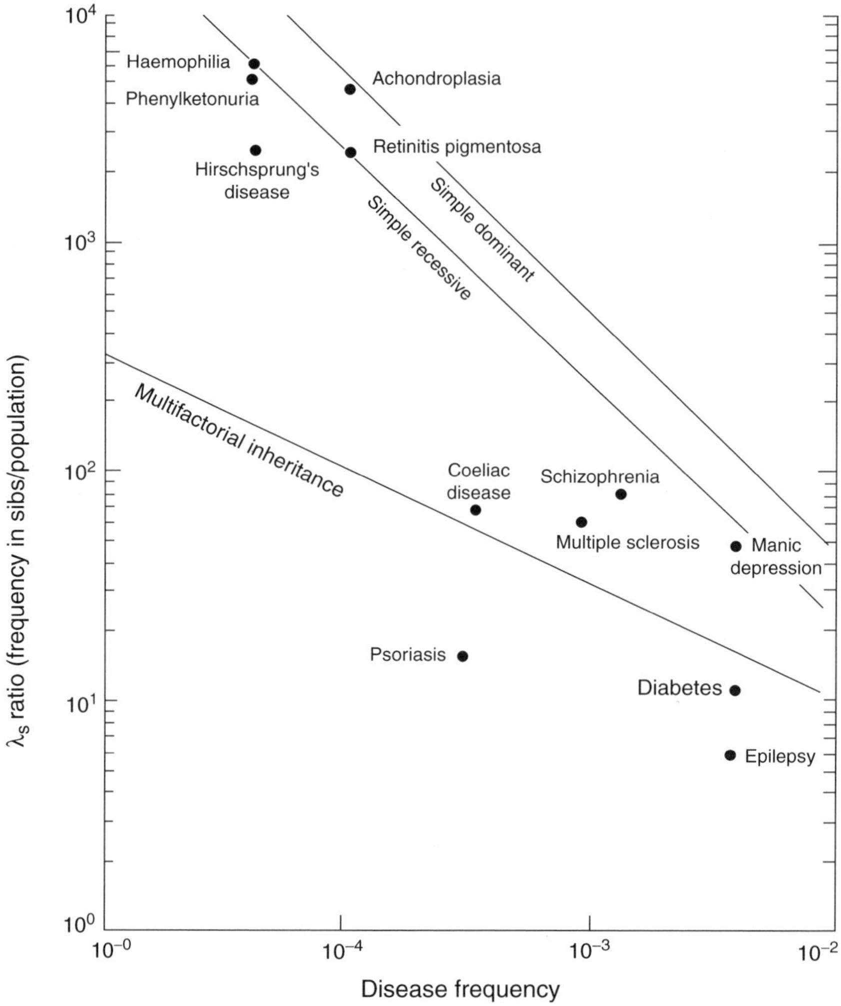

FIGURE 5.1 The relationship between genetics (expressed as λ_s ratio) and frequency of different multifactorial diseases. Note that diabetes falls below the line of the multifactorial inheritance. Modified from *An Introduction to the Genetics of Diabetes: a Practical Guide*, Pozzilli P. (ed.), Medpress Ltd., Kent

factors responsible for insulin resistance associated with diabetes rather than with the disease itself. Currently, many other cDNA and genomic clones that contain genes with a known function are at present being studied with an aim to identify polymorphic regions within or near these genes that can be used as genetic markers with microsatellite regions, as they are ideal tools for studies of this type.

The great advances made in the area of molecular genetics have led to the use of genetic markers to identify subjects at risk for both Type 1 and Type 2 diabetes.

For the former, where fewer genes are likely to be involved in the disease pathogenesis and the contribution of genetic factors is probably higher than in Type 2 diabetes, a number of relevant observations have been made, which have brought about the beginning of the era of genetic screening at birth for disease prevention.

Lessons from Type 1 Diabetes for Genetic Screening

Type 1 diabetes is an autoimmune disease that destroys insulin-producing pancreatic beta cells and some of the major genes predisposing to Type 1 diabetes have been identified. This autoimmune process targets several islet beta cell components, many of which have been identified. The characterization of autoantibodies against beta cell antigens, markers of the autoimmune response, are being used as a predictor of disease development during the long phase of prediabetes.

Most importantly, the identification of genes that predispose to Type 1 diabetes has been a major achievement over the past few years.[1] Although multiple genes may contribute to the development of Type 1 diabetes, research has shown that the principal genes predisposing to this disease are alleles of the major histocompatibility complex (MHC).[2] This complex (also known as human leukocyte antigens (HLA)) is closely involved in the activation of T-cells and regulation of the immune response.[3] The HLA types most closely associated with Type 1 diabetes are the alleles DR3 and DR4.[4] Between 80 and 90 per cent of patients with Type 1 diabetes are positive for one or both of these high-risk alleles. However, about 30–40 per cent of individuals without diabetes also have these HLA alleles. Thus, the HLA type of an individual is a necessary but not a determinant factor to signal a predisposition to Type 1 diabetes. Although the role of HLA polymorphism in Type 1 diabetes and other autoimmune diseases is well known, polymorphisms in other immune-related regions have also been implicated in disease susceptibility. In addition to HLA alleles (IDDM susceptibility genes), the insulin gene on Chr 11q15 (IDDM2) and CTLA-4 on 2q33 (IDDM12) are other loci specifically identified as potentially contributing to Type 1 diabetes susceptibility.[5] Variation in CTLA-4 has been reported to contribute to Type 1 diabetes susceptibility in several populations, although some studies have found no association between the two.[6] The interaction of CTLA-4 and B-7 (CD80) is responsible for the co-stimulation of T cells during antigen presentation. Experimental and murine studies have demonstrated a central role for CTLA-4 in promoting apoptosis in CD4+ and CD8+ lymphocytes in order to down-regulate activated T lymphocytes.[7]

Current studies also seek to identify additional genes (especially non-HLA genes) that predispose individuals to Type 1 diabetes as well as arriving at a better understanding of beta cell biology with the ultimate goal of replacing beta cell function, including pancreatic islet transplantation.

Methods for Early Prediction of Type 1 Diabetes and Prevention Strategies

One of the most important observations made over the past 20 years has been that of recognising in which that Type 1 diabetes as a slow, progressive autoimmune disease antibody markers can be detected several years prior to development of clinical disease. The ability to detect and predict this form of diabetes is important for identifying strategies of intervention and prevention of the autoimmune response towards beta cells. Prevention is ultimately the most effective cure of any disease and early attempts at preventing Type 1 diabetes based on combining genetic and immunological markers are now ongoing.

Over the past few years, a number of studies have been implemented in Europe and the United States to identify subjects at risk of developing Type 1 diabetes based upon genetic screening. The first study, the DAISY study (Diabetes AutoImmunity Study in the Young) started in the mid-1990s. Up to now more than 20 000 newborns from the general population have been identified with the high risk HLA DR3/DR4 haplotype.[8] These newborns are being followed up for the presence of antibodies to glutamic acid decarboxylase (GAD), a tyrosine phosphate-like molecule (IA-2) and insulin autoantibodies (IAA), the main aim being to identify the generation of islet-cell-related antibodies. This is the first study to have used a genetic marker within the general population to identify those who are at high risk of developing diabetes based on positivity for islet cell autoimmunity.

In Europe, the TRIGR project (Trial to Reduce Insulin dependent diabetes in Genetically at Risk individuals) has recently been set up.[9] This study is based on the identification of newborns considered to be at high diabetic risk, being offspring of a diabetic (Type 1) parent or having a sibling in the family with the disease. High-diabetic-risk newborns also identified as possessing the high-risk HLA-associated genetic markers are then followed up for the development of islet cell autoimmunity. Most important, a cow's milk hydrolysate or normal cow's milk formula (as control) is administered to these newborns up to 8 months of age to find out whether the avoidance of this protein in the first months of life could prevent islet cell autoimmunity and, ultimately, the emergence of Type 1 diabetes.

Two studies have been set up in Italy; DIABFIN and PREVEFIN. The first, like DAISY, identifies individuals who carry the high-risk HLA genotype from within the general population.[10] Up to now more than 10 000 individuals have been HLA typed at birth and positive markers for Type 1 diabetes were found in only 0.9 per cent of the population. These newborns are being followed up, as in the DAISY study, to define the natural history of autoimmunity to islet cell antigens.

In the other study, PREVEFIN, an ongoing trial in Italy, similar entry criteria have been adopted (high-risk individuals identified with the genetic markers DR3/DR4 in the general population), but in this case the newborns are randomized to vitamin D supplementation and, similarly to the TRIGR study, one group receives a cow's milk hydrolysate and the other a normal cow's milk formula.[11] The above study designs are the best examples of how genetic screening performed both in the general population at high risk for the disease and in selected groups (first-degree relatives of Type 1 diabetic probands) can be applied to identify those who could benefit from preventative therapy. We are still in the early phases, but nevertheless the model is promising and can be applied to other disease conditions.

Type 2 Diabetes: Where do We Stand as regards Genetic Screening?

Type 2 diabetes is a complicated, multifactorial disease in which interaction between multiple genes and multiple environmental factors ultimately results in the development of hyperglycaemia. Type 2 diabetes is characterized by resistance to insulin action in different tissues coupled with an inability of the pancreas to deliver insulin in a precisely regulated amount and fashion to control glucose homeostasis. Such defects, insulin resistance and relative beta cell failure, ultimately lead to high blood glucose levels and clinically overt Type 2 diabetes.

The disease is extraordinarily common, and affects about 6 per cent of the US population and 3–5 per cent of the population in Western Europe, and is therefore the most significant form of diabetes from a public health perspective. Obesity and reduced physical activity, major problems both in the US and Western Europe, are important risk factors for Type 2 diabetes and more than 80 per cent of subjects with Type 2 diabetes are obese. Evidence suggests that controlling these risk factors can help prevent the development of diabetes in many genetically susceptible individuals.[12]

The major obstacles that prevent a full understanding of the genetics of Type 2 diabetes are firstly that Type 2 diabetes is a highly heterogenous disease and not a single disease, secondly, that most Type 2 cases probably need to manifest more than one genetic defect to become clinically evident, and lastly, the variability of age at the time of clinical onset of Type 2 diabetes may lead to false negatives if an individual is screened too early in life.

Recently, there have been several major research advances in the understanding of Type 2 diabetes. Several genes involved in some subtypes of Type 2 diabetes have been identified,[13] although their role in the disease process is far from being elucidated. Recent data has shown that obesity, physical inactivity and other lifestyle factors are crucial environmental risk factors in genetically susceptible individuals for disease development.[14] To help in understanding how these environmental factors, particularly obesity, are involved in the progression to Type 2 diabetes, the genes involved in the development of obesity in animal models,[15] as well as the genes regulating neurohormones and other proteins involved in the control of appetite and energy balance[16] have been identified and studied. Since insulin resistance is one of the most important features of this multifactorial disease,[17] the various genetically controlled steps involved in peripheral insulin action in diverse cell types as well as the genes controlling insulin secretion from pancreatic beta cells are being investigated – with the aim of defining a genetic profile of the high risk individual. Lastly, new noninvasive technologies are being used to study metabolic derangements in affected patients and animals, which include nuclear magnetic resonance (NMR) and positron emission tomography (PET) to correlate the genetic susceptibility to a pathophysiological trait.[18]

Currently, several challenges still remain in order to have a clearer understanding of how and why individuals develop Type 2 diabetes and to design preventative measures. It will be necessary to identify the genes that confer disease susceptibility to common forms of Type 2 diabetes and obesity and to use good animal model systems to assist in this process. It will also be necessary to define the molecular mechanisms responsible for insulin resistance and defects in insulin secretion. In relation to this, a better definition of the genetic traits regulating appetite, energy expenditure and control of body weight and their involvement with insulin action and secretion will help clarify the role of obesity in Type 2 diabetes. It will also be important to identify other environmental factors that transform a predisposition to Type 2 diabetes into overt clinical disease and the mechanisms involved. It looks as if we are still far from using genetic screening to identify subjects and risks for Type 2 diabetes. Nevertheless, we need to pursue this approach if we would like to intervene successfully for disease prevention in genetically predisposed individuals.

Genes that are Identified with a Predisposition to Type 2 Diabetes: The New Scene

Genetic association analysis that uses thousands of single-nucleotide polymorphism (SNP) markers has become a promising alternative to a genome-wide linkage scan. Therefore, in the past three years a new scenario has been created thanks to the availability of SNP markers and wide genome screening in the search for genes predisposing to Type 2 diabetes.

Genome scans in families with Type 2 diabetes have identified a putative locus on chromosome 20q. For this study, linkage disequilibrium mapping was used in an effort to narrow a 7.3 Mb region in an Ashkenazi Type 2 diabetic population. The region encompassed a 1-logarithm of odds (LOD) interval around the SNP microsatellite marker D20S107, which gave a LOD score of >3 in linkage analysis of a combined Caucasian population. It was found that this 7.3 Mb region contained 25 known and 99 predicted genes.[19]

The Pro12Ala polymorphism in the PPARgamma2 gene has been associated with a reduced risk of Type 2 diabetes and insulin resistance. Recently, an association between dizygotic twinning and PPARgamma gene polymorphisms was put forward. The phenotypic appearance of the two polymorphisms (Pro12Ala and exon 6C $\rightarrow$ T) in PPARgamma was investigated among elderly twins (207 monozygotic (MZ) and 342 diaygotic (DZ)) and studied to see whether they could explain previously reported differences in plasma glucose and insulin profiles among MZ and DZ twins. A significant impact of the Prof12 Ala and polymorphism on glucose tolerance, diabetic status, homeostasis model assessment for insulin resistance, and plasma insulin profiles in twins was demonstrated. Thus, this study supports a role for both the intrauterine environment (thrifty phenotype) and for genetics (thrifty genotype) in the aetiology of insulin resistance and perhaps glucose intolerance in twins.[20]

An autosomal genome scan for genes contributing to the development of Type 2 diabetes and which affect the body mass index (BMI) in the Japanese population (164 families, 256 affected sib-pairs) was recently carried out. It was found that 12 regions showed nominally significant multipoint evidence of linkage with Type 2 diabetes.[21]

The genes ABCC8 and KCNJ11, which encode the subunits sulfonylurea receptor 1 (SUR1) and inwardly rectifying potassium channel (Kir6.2) of the beta cell ATP-sensitive potassium (K(ATP)) channel, control insulin secretion. Common polymorphisms in these genes (ABCC8 exon 16-3t/c exon 18 T/C, KCNJ11 E23K) have been variably associated with Type 2 diabetes, but no large (approximately 2000 subjects) case–control studies have been performed. The role of these three variants was evaluated by studying 2486 British subjects: 854 with Type 2 diabetes, 1182 population control subjects and 150 parent–offspring Type 2 diabetes trios.[22] The E23K allele was associated with diabetes in the case–control study (odds ratio (OR) 1.18 (95 per cent CI 1.04–1.34), $P = 0.01$) but did not show familial association with diabetes. Neither exon 16 nor exon 18ABCC8 variants were associated with the disease. Meta-analysis of all case–control data showed that the E23K allele was associated with Type 2 diabetes, but the ABCC8 variants were not associated. These results confirm that E23K increases risk of Type 2 diabetes and show that large-scale association studies are important for the identification of disease susceptibility alleles.

Despite these fascinating and enlightening studies, we are not yet ready to use this information in the clinical setting.

How Can we Track the Prediabetes Period Using Genetic Markers?

A sedentary life-style and caloric abundance have created new physiological conditions capable of changing the level of expression of a number of genes involved in fuel metabolism and body weight regulation. In the past, it is likely that the genetic variants or alleles of these genes were important in the adaptation of human physiology to evolutionary constraints. The nature and prevalence of polymorphisms responsible for quantitative variations of complex metabolic traits may have been different among human populations, depending on their environmental and ancestral genetic background. These polymorphisms could probably explain differences observed today in disease susceptibility and prevalence among various groups or populations of humans. From complex traits to potentially complex alleles, understanding the molecular genetic basis underlying quantitative variation will continue to be a growing concern among geneticists dealing with obesity and Type 2 diabetes, two main disorders of the modern era. Genomics and genetic epidemiology now allow high-level linkage and association studies to be designed. The pooling of large trans–geographic cohorts may in fact increase the genetic heterogeneity of studied traits and dilute genotype–phenotype associations. Type 2 diabetes as well as obesity can be subjected to a pregenetic dissection of complexity into simpler quantitative traits (QTs). This dissection is based on pathogenic mechanisms, the time course of the traits and the individual's age within the predisease period, rather than on descriptive parameters after disease diagnosis. Such an approach to phenotypes may ease the way for future associations to be established between QTs of intermediate complexity and genetic polymorphisms.

Genetic Screening for MODY and Potential Preventive Strategy

Maturity-onset diabetes of the young (MODY) is a clinically heterogeneous group of disorders characterized by nonketotic diabetes mellitus, an autosomal dominant mode of inheritance, onset usually before the age of 25, (frequently in childhood or adolescence), and a primary defect in the function of the beta cells of the pancreas. MODY can result from mutations in any one of at least six different genes (Table 5.1). One of these genes encodes the glycolytic enzyme glucokinase (associated with MODY 2) and the other five encode transcription factors including hepatocytic nuclear factor (HNF-) 4α (associated with MODY 1), HNF-1α (MODY 3) insulin promoter factor 1 (IPF-1 (MODY 4)), HNF-1β (MODY 5) and neurogenic differentiation factor 1 (NeuroD1), also known as beta cell E-box transactivator 2 (BETA2 (MODY 6)). All these genes are expressed in beta cells, and mutation of any of them leads to beta cell dysfunction and onset of diabetes. These genes are also expressed in other tissues, and abnormalities in liver and kidney function may also be evident in some forms of MODY. Factors that affect insulin sensitivity, such as infection, puberty, pregnancy and (in rare cases) obesity, may trigger the onset of diabetes and increase the severity of hyperglycaemia in patients with MODY, but otherwise nongenetic factors have no relevant role in the development of this form of genetically determined diabetes.

Genetic testing for MODY has now reached the clinical stage in a few centres equipped for this type of investigation. Diagnostic genetic testing can confirm the definite MODY subtype and allows specific advice regarding management of the disease. In families where a MODY gene is identified, it may be advisable to offer

TABLE 5.1 MODY-related genes and the clinical phenotypes associated with mutations in the genes

MODY type	Gene	Clinical features	Most common treatment	Molecular bases	Clinical features of homozygous states
MODY 1	HNF-4α	Diabetes, microvascular complications (in many cases), reduction in serum concentrations of triglycerides, apolipoproteins, AII and CIII and Lp(a) lipoprotein	Oral hypoglycaemic agent, insulin	Abnormal regulation of gene transcription in beta cells, leading to a defect in metabolic signalling of insulin secretion, beta cell mass, or both	
MODY 2	Glucokinase	Impaired fasting glucose, impaired glucose tolerance, diabetes, normal proinsulin-to-insulin ration in serum	Diet and exercise	Defect in sensitivity of beta cells to glucose due to reduced glucose phosphorylation, defect in hepatic storage of glucose as glycogen	Permanent neonatal diabetes, requiring insulin treatment
MODY 3	HNF-1 α	Diabetes, microvascular compilations (in many cases), renal glycosuria, increased sensitivity to sulfonylurea drugs, increased proinsulin-to-insulin ration in serum	Oral hypoglycaemic agents, insulin	Abnormal regulation of gene transcription in beta cells leading to a defect in metabolic signalling of insulin secretion, beta cell mass, or both	
MODY 4	IPF-1	Diabetes	Oral hypoglycaemic agents, insulin	Abnormal transcriptional regulation of beta cell development and function	Pancreatic agenesis and neonatal diabetes requiring insulin treatment
MODY 5	HNF-1β	Diabetes, renal cysts and other abnormalities of renal development, progressive nondiabetic renal dysfunction, leading to chronic renal insufficiency and failure, internal genital abnormalities (in female carriers)	Insulin	Abnormal regulation of gene transcription in beta cells, leading to a defect in metabolic signalling of insulin secretion, beta cell mass, or both	
MODY 6	NeuroD1, or BETA2	Diabetes	Insulin	Abnormal transcriptional regulation of beta cell development and function	

genetic tests to other family members with signs of hyperglycaemia. As regards therapy for hyperglycaemia, the identification of a mutation allows a more defined therapeutic strategy. For instance, families with glucokinase diagnosed MODY can be reassured that it is unlikely they will need therapy except in cases of pregnancy.[23] In those families where HNF-1a is identified, progression of the disease is likely; however, patients can be well managed with sulfonylureas for years, only much later switching to insulin therapy. Unfortunately, as of yet, with the more recently defined MODY types, specific therapeutic guidance is not possible.

In all cases, after appropriate counselling, families should decide whether or not predictive testing is necessary. In the case of adults the issue is less problematic; in the case of children, parents have to balance their wishes with the rights of the child. It is advisable that the diabetes team discuss the possibility of genetic testing together with a clinical geneticist who presents the dominant inheritance of MODY in a simple, way using a pictorial family tree. Topics to be considered include the following: (a) difficulty in identifying the age at which diabetes will develop, although it will occur in 99 per cent of cases; (b) implications of identifying a child as a future diabetic, a finding that will involve frequent blood testing to identify a child with diabetes in the future; (c) insurance and job prospects; (d) the concept that when test results are positive, there is no return to the status of 'not knowing'; (e) a child when reaching adult age might be disappointed with the decision that a genetic test of this type was performed on him/her. These concepts are common to all genetic disorders, but in this case the advantage is that the early treatment of hyperglycaemia in MODY can result in good metabolic control of the disease, which certainly contributes to prevent long-term diabetic complications. So our recommendations are that, in the appropriate clinical settings, testing for MODY be performed in families where the disease is likely to occur.

Conclusion

Genetic screening for Type 2 diabetes aimed at identifying subjects at disease risk for prevention studies is not yet a reality and is limited to research settings only. The case is different for MODY families, where genetic screening is feasible. For clinical Type 2 diabetes, we are still in a phase where we need to clarify how susceptibility genes interact and how the environment exercises its effect on them.

For MODY, the fact that six genes that cause the disease have been identified has already paved the way to preventative approaches. This is particularly important since in this case young subjects are involved. At present, while we wait for more sensitive genetic markers to be discovered, we need to concentrate on regular screening for subjects at risk for Type 2 diabetes based on the identification of known environmental risk factors associated with this disease.

In conclusion, for future research strategies, the following should be taken into consideration:

(a) It is not feasible at present to extrapolate the role of a genetic defect in the pathogenesis of Type 2 diabetes based exclusively on the identification of an altered protein, even though the function of that protein may be relatively well understood.

(b) To identify the significance of a specific defect in the pathogenesis of this disease requires the combination of *in vivo* and *in vitro* studies.

(c) The analysis of genetic defects that occur in individual families with Type 2 diabetes may significantly contribute to the understanding of the mechanism causing this form of diabetes and must be pursued.

Acknowledgements

I would like to acknowledge the contribution of Andrea Stoler and Tanya Szendelly in preparing this chapter.

References

1. Bottino R, Lemarchand P, Trucco M and Giannoukakis N. Gene- and cell-based therapeutics for Type I diabetes mellitus. *Gene Ther* 2003; **10**: 875–889.
2. Tait BD, Colman PG, Morahan G, Marchinovska L, Dore E, Gellert S, Honeyman MC, Stephen K and Loth A. HLA genes associated with autoimmunity and progression to disease in Type 1 diabetes. *Tissue Antigens* 2003; **61**: 146–153.
3. Notkins AL. Immunologic and genetic factors in Type 1 diabetes. *J Biol Chem* 2002; **277**: 43545–43548.
4. Knip M, Kukko M, Kulmala P, Veijola R, Simell O, Akerblom HK and Ilonen J. Humoral beta-cell autoimmunity in relation to HLA-defined disease susceptibility in preclinical and clinical Type 1 diabetes. *Am J Med Genet* 2002; **115**: 48–54.
5. Ueda H, Howson JM, Esposito L and Heward J. Association of the T-cell regulatory gene CTLA4 with susceptibility to autoimmune disease. *Nature* 2003; **423**: 506–511.
6. Kristiansen OP, Pociot F, Bennett EP, Clausen H, Johannesen J, Nerup J and Mandrup-Poulsen T. IDDM7 links to insulin-dependent diabetes mellitus in Danish multiplex families but linkage is not explained by novel polymorphisms in the candidate gene GALNT3. The Danish Study Group of Diabetes in Childhood and The Danish IDDM Epidemiology and Genetics Group. *Hum Mutat* 2000; **15**: 295–296.
7. Kouki T, Sawai Y, Gardine CA, Fisfalen ME, Alegre ML and DeGroot LJ. CTLA-4 gene polymorphism at position 49 in exon 1 reduces the inhibitory function of CTLA-4 and contributes to the pathogenesis of Graves' disease. *J Immunol* 2000; **165**: 6606–6611.
8. Graves PM, Rotbart HA, Nix WA, Pallansch MA, Erlich HA, Norris JM, Hoffman M, Eisenbarth GS and Rewers M. Prospective study of enteroviral infections and development of beta-cell autoimmunity. Diabetes Autoimmunity Study in the Young (DAISY). *Diabetes Res Clin Pract* 2003; **59**: 51–61.

9. Hamalainen AM, Ronkainen MS, Akerblom HK and Knip M. Postnatal elimination of transplacentally acquired disease-associated antibodies in infants born to families with Type 1 diabetes. The Finnish TRIGR Study Group. Trial to reduce IDDM in the genetically at risk. *J Clin Endocrinol Metab* 2000; **8511**: 4249–4253.
10. Napoli F, Minicucci L, Cotellessa M, Padovani P, Pezzolo F, Giannattasio A, Di Siena RP, Bazzigaluppi E, Buzzetti R, Falorni A, Cherubini V, Multari G, Crinò A, Pozzilli P and Lorini R. Screening for Type 1 diabetes genetic risk in newborns of continental Italy. Primary prevention (PREVEFIN study). *Horm Res* 2002; **58** (Suppl. 2), 77.
11. Buzzetti R, Galgani A, Petrone A *et al.* Newborn screening for prediction of Type 1 diabetes genetic risk in continental Italy (Diabfin Study). *Diabetologia* 2002; **45** (Suppl. 2): A49.
12. Gloyn AL. The search for Type 2 diabetes genes. *Ageing Res Rev* 2003; **2**: 111–127.
13. Shih DQ and Stoffel M. Molecular etiologies of MODY and other early-onset forms of diabetes. *Curr Diab Rep* 2002; **2**: 125–134.
14. Mayer-Davis EJ and Costacou T. Obesity and sedentary lifestyle: modifiable risk factors for prevention of Type 2 diabetes. *Curr Diab Rep* 2001; **1**: 170–176.
15. Mauvais-Jarvis F, Kulkarni RN and Kahn CR. Knockout models are useful tools to dissect the pathophysiology and genetics of insulin resistance. *Clin Endocrinol* 2002; **57**: 1–9.
16. Air EL, Strowski MZ, Benoit SC, Conarello SL, Salituro GM, Guan XM, Liu K, Woods SC and Zhang BB. Small molecule insulin mimetics reduce food intake and body weight and prevent development of obesity. *Nat Med* 2002; **8**: 179–183.
17. Gerich JE. Contributions of insulin-resistance and insulin-secretory defects to the pathogenesis of Type 2 diabetes mellitus. *Mayo Clin Proc* 2003; **78**: 447–456.
18. Garvey WT, Kwon S, Zheng D, Shaughnessy S, Wallace P, Hutto A, Pugh K, Jenkins AJ, Klein RL and Liao Y. Effects of insulin resistance and Type 2 diabetes on lipoprotein subclass particle size and concentration determined by nuclear magnetic resonance. *Diabetes* 2003; **52**: 453–462.
19. Permutt MA, Wasson J, Love-Gregory L, Ma J, Skolnick G, Suarez B, Lin J and Glaser B. Searching for Type 2 diabetes genes on chromosome 20. *Diabetes* 2002; **51** (Suppl. 3): S308–S315.
20. Poulsen P, Andersen G, Fenger M, Hansen T, Echwald SM, Volund A, Beck-Nielsen H, Pedersen O and Vaag A. Impact of two common polymorphisms in the PPARgamma gene on glucose tolerance and plasma insulin profiles in monozygotic and dizygotic twins: thrifty genotype, thrifty phenotype, or both? *Diabetes* 2003; **52**: 194–198.
21. Iwasaki N, Cox NJ, Wang YQ, Schwarz PE, Bell GI, Honda M, Imura M, Ogata M, Saito M, Kamatani N and Iwamoto Y. Mapping genes influencing Type 2 diabetes risk and BMI in Japanese subjects. *Diabetes* 2003; **52**: 209–213.
22. Gloyn AL, Weedon MN, Owen KR, Turner MJ, Knight BA, Hitman G, Walker M, Levy JC, Sampson M, Halford S, McCarthy MI, Hattersley AT and Frayling TM. Large-scale association studies of variants in genes encoding the pancreatic beta-cell KATP channel subunits Kir6.2 (KCNJ11) and SUR1 (ABCC8) confirm that the KCNJ11 E23K variant is associated with Type 2 diabetes. *Diabetes* 2003; **52**: 568–572.
23. Froguel P, Vaxillaire M, Sun F and Velho G *et al.* Close linkage of the glucokinase locus on chromosome 7p to early onset non insulin dependent diabetes mellitus. *Nature* 1992; **356**: 152–164.

6

Screening Parameters and Techniques: Limitations and Opportunities

Knut Borch-Johnsen and **Charlotte Glümer**

Type 2 diabetes is a common, chronic disorder associated with a high risk of developing late diabetic complications. Population-based surveys have consistently shown that many individuals have undiagnosed Type 2 diabetes and this, combined with the poor prognosis and the beneficial effect of treatment, has led to the suggestion to screen for Type 2 diabetes. The focus of this chapter is a review of techniques and strategies used for screening for diabetes, while the issue of 'whether to screen or not' is covered in the following chapter.

Screening for Type 2 diabetes is a complicated issue for several reasons. The first question is how to screen – what screening tests should be used. The second question is whom to screen (population based screening or targeted screening). The third question is how to organize the screening. This chapter will discuss these topics by reviewing

1. the epidemiology of type 2 diabetes with a focus on the prevalence of undiagnosed diabetes
2. what screening is and how to evaluate the screening test
3. screening strategies
    a. screening instruments and methods
    b. stepwise screening strategies

Prevention of Type 2 Diabetes Edited by Manfred Ganz
 ISBN: 0-470-85733-1

4. who should be screened (targeted screening strategies)
5. recommendations.

The Epidemiology of Type 2 Diabetes

Over the last few decades the number of individuals with Type 2 diabetes has increased world wide, affecting industrialized as well as developing countries.[1] The most important reason for this is the demographic changes with increasing life expectancy and growth of the middle aged and old population world wide. The age-specific prevalence of diabetes is however also increasing[2] due to lifestyle changes, with decreasing physical activity and increasing prevalence of obesity. In the United States of America the prevalence of obesity (defined as a body mass index $>30\,kg/m^2$) has increased from 12 per cent in 1991 to 20.9 per cent in 2002.[3] The highest increase in the burden of diabetes, measured both as increase in number of individuals with diabetes and as increase in the age-specific prevalence of the disease, is seen in Asia, and in particular in India and China.[1]

Type 2 diabetes is a disease with a long asymptomatic period. This explains why a substantial proportion of patients (20–40 per cent) have one or more late diabetic complications diagnosed at the time of clinical diagnosis of diabetes.[4–8] The true length of this period is unknown for obvious reasons, but it has been estimated that the period from development of diabetes until clinical diagnosis on average is between 5 and 11 years.[4] It is this long latent period that creates the potential window for screening for diabetes. Population-based studies from several different parts of the world consistently show that approximately 50 per cent of all cases of diabetes are undiagnosed,[9–11] and this would be the target group for screening activities.

When evaluating screening strategies it is important to consider regional and ethnicity-driven differences in the clinical features characterizing the diabetic patient. In all countries and all ethnic groups the prevalence of diabetes increases with increasing age, but the age by which the prevalence of diabetes starts to increase is lower in Asia than in the white Caucasian populations in Europe and North America.[12] Ethnicity also modifies the effect of weight and body mass index (BMI) on the prevalence of diabetes. While the pattern is the same in all populations – increasing prevalence of diabetes with increasing BMI – the risk associated with a given BMI varies considerably between populations. In India the prevalence of diabetes starts to increase at a BMI of $21–23\,kg/m^2$ while in Europe the major increase only occurs at levels of BMI above $25–27\,kg/m^2$. Thus the epidemiology of diabetes shows considerable heterogeneity across the world, and this has implications for application of screening strategies across ethnic groups.

What is Screening and How do We Evaluate a Screening Test?

Screening is the first step in identifying individuals with undiagnosed disease and can be defined as 'an examination of asymptomatic persons to classify them as likely or unlikely to have the disease. Persons likely to have the disease should then undergo diagnostic testing and be treated if they are found to have the disease'.[13] This definition clearly separates the screening test from the diagnostic test and is applicable to most screening tests for cancer where cytological tests such as the vaginal smear for cervical cancer or radiological tests such as mammography for breast cancer are used to identify individuals at high risk of having previously undiagnosed cancer. In these situations *sensitivity* and *specificity* measure the ability of the test to correctly classify an individual as diseased (sensitivity) or nondiseased (specificity). The ideal screening test should have high sensitivity and high specificity, but increasing the sensitivity of a test inevitably leads to a loss of specificity. For a given test (e.g. a biological marker) the sensitivity can be estimated for a variety of values of the biological marker in question. For each value the specificity can also be calculated. Given these sets of combinations of sensitivity and specificity a so-called *receiver operating characteristic (ROC) plot* can be derived. The y-axis is the sensitivity (true positive fraction) and the x-axis is the false positive fraction (1 – specificity), and thus the ROC plot graphically exposes the association between sensitivity and specificity. The area under the curve (AUC) is a measure of diagnostic accuracy and describes the probability of a diseased person having a test result more abnormal than a nondiseased individual. A value of 0.5 means that the screening test is worthless (does not discriminate between diseased and nondiseased individuals), while a value of 0.8 means that in four out of five cases the diseased individual will have a more abnormal test result than the nondiseased.[14] The 'optimal' threshold or cut-off is often referred to as the point optimizing sensitivity and specificity. This will be defined by the 45° tangent of the ROC curve, but this assumes that sensitivity and specificity are equally important. This is rarely the case. If the disease screened for is very severe with an effective treatment if diagnosed, then sensitivity should be given very high priority. In contrast, if the disease in question is slowly developing with a relatively good prognosis and if the diagnostic test is associated with serious discomfort or even risk of complications or even death, then the diagnostic test should not be offered to individuals who are nondiseased, and thus specificity would be given high priority. In diabetes screening is typically done by some measure of blood glucose, and thus the screening tests could be identical to the diagnostic testing. This may cause confusion with respect to the evaluation of the characteristics (sensitivity and specificity) of the screening test as discussed later in relation to the individual tests. The screening tests for diabetes can be divided into two groups, the first involving measurement of biological markers such as blood glucose, HbA_{1c}, urinary glucose, genetic markers etc. measured individually or in combination as part of a stepwise screening strategy. These methods are dealt with in the next section of this chapter. The second group of tests involves the phenotypical characteristics of the individual used to develop risk scores/risk charts. These will be dealt with in the fourth section of this chapter.

Screening Strategies

Screening for diabetes can be done either by a single screening method or through a stepwise strategy. The screening instruments are partly the same using the two different strategies, and the theoretical advantage of using the stepwise strategy is that this may reduce the number of blood tests and oral glucose tolerance tests and thereby reduce the total cost of a screening programme. This section will first deal with the screening tests individually and then with the stepwise screening strategies.

Random capillary blood glucose is a blood glucose measurement taken at a random point of time independent of the duration since last meal. The advantage of the test is that there are very few requirements, the test can be made any time of the day, and – if based on bed-side equipment for measurement of blood glucose – gives an immediate answer to the individual screened. Only a few studies have systematically evaluated these screening strategies.[15,16] As shown in Table 6.1 the performance of random capillary glucose is far from optimal, and in the Finnish study the performance was particularly poor in women. The low sensitivity and specificity may be explained by the variability in the time from last meal until the blood test. Thus the performance of the test could be improved if a fixed period of time since the last meal were used, but then the major advantage of the random capillary blood glucose – the flexibility – would disappear. In conclusion, the usefulness of random blood glucose as an isolated screening test for diabetes is limited. However, a low random glucose (<4.5 mmol/l) is associated with a very low probability of having undiagnosed diabetes, and thus the test can be used to exclude diabetes in some individuals (30–40 per cent of the population).

Glycated haemoglobin (HbA_{1c}) is a measure of the stable, irreversible, non-enzymatic glycation of the haemoglobin molecule. HbA_{1c} is a good and stable marker of mean blood glucose in diabetic individuals, and is used to monitor the metabolic control in individuals with diabetes.[17] HbA_{1c} is stable over time, and represents an estimate of the mean blood glucose in the 4–8 weeks preceding the test. This stability of the measurement makes it a good candidate for a screening test for diabetes. Furthermore, the measurement is operationally simple as it requires capillary blood from the ear-lobe or a finger, it can be measured at any time of the day and the sample is stable during transportation to the laboratory.

Unfortunately, HbA_{1c} has been shown to be unable to separate individuals with normal glucose tolerance from individuals with previously undiagnosed diabetes. In USA, 60 per cent of individuals with screen-detected diabetes, based on the

TABLE 6.1 Sensitivity and specificity of screening tests for diabetes

Test	Metabolic state	Cut-point	Sensitivity (%)	Specificity (%)	Reference
Capillary glucose	Random	≥6.2	63	92	15
	Random	≥6.7	75	88	16
HbA_{1c}		≥5.6	35	100	30
		≥5.6	83	84	31
		≥5.8	92	89	32
		≥6.0	85	91	33
		≥6.0	60	91	34, 35
		≥6.1	77	79	36
		≥6.2	81	88	37
		≥6.3	66	98	38
Capillary glucose	Fasting	≥5.0	83	79	39
		≥6.7	75	93	40
Venous plasma glucose	Fasting	≥5.3	78	83	41
		≥5.5	73	90	30
		≥5.7	80	91	42
		≥5.8	76	89	43
		≥5.8	85	84	36
		≥6.0	68	93	44
		≥6.0	83	81	45
		≥6.0	90	66	46
		≥6.1	80	90	47
		≥6.1	88	87	48
		≥6.1	95	90	31
		≥7.8	52	99	35

measurement of fasting plasma glucose, have an HbA_{1c} in the normal range.[18] If a high cut-off value for HbA_{1c} were used, then that would lead to low sensitivity and high specificity as shown in Table 6.2.

TABLE 6.2 Diagnostic criteria for diabetes based on different blood samples by WHO in 1999[49]

		Glucose concentration (mmol/l)		
		Whole blood		Plasma venous
		Venous	Capillary	
Diabetes Mellitus	Fasting	≥6.1	≥6.1	≥7.0
	2 hours	≥10.0	≥11.1	≥11.1
Nedsat glukose tolerance (IGT)	Fasting	<6.1	<6.1	<7.0
	2 hours	6.7–9.9	7.8–11.0	7.8–11.0
Impaired fasting glycaemia (IFG)	Fasting	5.6–6.0	5.6–6.0	6.1–7.0
	2 hours (if measured)	<6.7	<7.8	<7.8

Another problem using HbA_{1c} as a screening test is the lack of standardization of the test between laboratories. Only very recently has an international standard been developed,[19] enabling standardization of assays across the world, but this standardization has only just begun.

Fasting blood or plasma glucose is the glucose value measured in the morning (prior to 10 am) after at least 8 hours of fasting. It can be measured on capillary blood or plasma, and these measurements give different results, with the diagnostic value for diabetes being 6.1 mmol/l if based on venous or capillary whole blood and 7.0 mmol/l if based on venous plasma (Table 6.2). The diagnosis of diabetes is based on fasting plasma glucose of 7.0 mmol/l or above, or 11.1 mmol/l or above 2 hours following a standardized 75 g oral glucose tolerance test. Fasting values below 7.0 mmol/l can, however, be found in individuals with a diabetic glucose tolerance test. In the DECODE study more than one-third of individuals with a diabetic 2 hour glucose had a nondiabetic fasting plasma glucose value,[20] and in Asian populations the proportion is even higher.[21] Thus, if fasting plasma glucose is to be used as a screening test for diabetes, a lower cut-off than the diagnostic value of 7.0 mmol/l must be used, and an oral glucose tolerance test must be performed in the remaining individuals. As shown in Table 6.1 the sensitivity and specificity of fasting plasma glucose will depend on the cut-off chosen for the screening test.

Combined screening strategies based on a combination of the above listed methods or combining a questionnaire with glucose measurements have been used. Four studies have combined measurement of HbA_{1c} and fasting plasma glucose and one has combined the American Diabetes Association (ADA) questionnaire with random capillary blood glucose. The results of these strategies are given in Table 6.3. Theoretically, these strategies should improve sensitivity and specificity, but this is generally not the case. The real advantage is that they will reduce the number of individuals requiring diagnostic testing.

TABLE 6.3 Sensitivity and specificity of combined screening strategies

Test	Sensitivity (%)	Specificity (%)	Reference
$HbA_{1c} \geq 5.5\%$ and fasting plasma glucose ≥ 5.6 mmol/l	84	84	36
$HbA_{1c} \geq 6.0\%$ and fasting plasma glucose ≥ 7.8 mmol/l	40	99	35
$HbA_{1c} \geq 6.1\%$ and fasting plasma glucose ≥ 6.1 mmol/l	69	96	50
$HbA_{1c} \geq 5.9\%$ and fasting plasma glucose ≥ 6.1 mmol/l	68	92	51
ADA questionnaire and random capillary blood glucose ≥ 6.7 mmol/l	58	94	16

Who Should be Screened – Targeted Screening Strategies Based on Phenotypical Characteristics

Type 2 diabetes does not hit individuals at random but occurs (predominantly) in individuals with one or more risk factors for developing Type 2 diabetes. The major risk factors for developing diabetes include age, gender, family history, obesity, ethnicity, previous gestational diabetes, presence of other components of the metabolic syndrome and physical inactivity. These features of diabetes have been used to develop screening instruments based on different combinations of the above listed features. At present six different risk scores have been published, of which five have been validated on independent populations. The risk scores are based either on *questionnaires* or on *routinely recorded data in medical records*. The questionnaires are all based on the major risk factors for Type 2 diabetes. They are self-administered and based on information known by the screened individual such as age, body mass index, family history of diabetes, physical activity, gestational diabetes and markers of the metabolic syndrome.[16,22–24] The last screening instruments are based on data already collected and gathered in the record of the general practitioner.[25,26]

These questionnaires have all been developed based on population-based surveys, and they perform almost equally well with respect to sensitivity, while the specificity differs between the questionnaires (Table 6.4). All questionnaires developed so far have been developed based on white Caucasian populations, and thus it is unknown how they will perform in nonwhite or non-Caucasian populations. Furthermore all these questionnaires have been developed and validated on the basis of prevalence screening studies. If used as part of a repeated screening programme where all prevalent cases are identified at baseline and only new (incident) cases are identified in the screening programme, the performance of the tests is likely to change, but it is rather unpredictable how they will change.

Limitations, Perspectives and Recommendation

Screening for diabetes should only be conducted if diabetes fulfils the criteria for screening outlined by the World Health Organisation in 1968,[27] and whether this is the case will vary between countries and regions. If, based on the total evidence provided, the health authorities decide to screen for diabetes, then two decisions must be made: first, who should be offered screening for diabetes, and second, how screening should be conducted (choice of test and organization for screening).

In most populations the prevalence of undiagnosed diabetes will be relatively low and of the order of 2–5 per cent depending on the age, ethnicity and level of obesity. This argues in favour of a high-risk screening strategy where screening for diabetes is offered to those considered at high risk of developing diabetes. The existing risk scores offer a rational and well validated strategy for this, but they

TABLE 6.4 Performance of validated risk scores for diabetes

		Population			Performance			
Type of data	Risk score	Number in validation population	Number of screen-detected case	Age	Sensitivity	Specification	Positive predictive value	Fraction needing diagnostic test(%)
Self-administered questionnaires	ADA risk score[23]	1471	157	$\geq$20	75	51	Not available	52
	Dutch risk score[22]	786	32	45–74	72	56	7	45
	Inter99[24]	2874	117	30–60	67	74	10	28
Routinely gathered data	Dutch risk score[25]	2484	110	50–74	78	44	Not available	Not available
	UK risk score[26]	528	23	40–64	77	72	11	30

have been developed for white Caucasians only. There is a need for modifications of the screening instruments for use in other ethnic groups. This work is in progress within the DETECT-2 project,[28] where centres from all over the world contribute with data.

The second question – how screening should be performed – has two elements. The first would be the organizational – how to identify the high-risk population. Having the risk score, the question then is how to distribute it. Using a high-risk approach seems to be simpler because the number of blood tests decreases. However, this implies stepwise screening. For each additional step the complexity of the strategy will increase. This will inevitably result in decreased compliance in the population as well at the general practitioner level. This element of screening has so far been neglected in the evaluation of screening strategies, but the ongoing ADDITION study[29] is also evaluating the organisational aspect of screening. Evaluation of this must be performed in other regions and with other screening instruments as well. Furthermore, to obtain an acceptable overall performance of the strategy, the sensitivity has to be reasonably high for the questionnaire without a too high test positive fraction.

For the choice of blood test the current recommendation would be to use a measure of fasting plasma or capillary whole blood as the next step in the screening strategy. Measurement of blood glucose instead of measurement of blood glucose markers (e.g. HbA_{1c}) in the second step leads to a less complex strategy; furthermore, blood glucose measurement is a part of the diagnostic testing. Measurement of fasting plasma glucose would allow classification of more than 50 per cent of the screen-detected diabetic individuals on the basis of fasting glucose alone, and the test would identify the additional 5–10 per cent who would have to undergo an oral glucose tolerance test, necessary to identify the (substantial) proportion of cases with screen-detected diabetes and nondiabetic fasting glucose values.

The performance of different measurements of hyperglycaemia has been evaluated and different risk scores have been developed and validated in white Caucasians. The overall performance of these tools is similar, although ethnic differences occur. No new screening tools are expected to be implemented in the near future.

The future challenge is to set up and evaluate the feasibility of regional high-risk screening strategies consisting of a population-specific risk assessment combined with a glucose measurement.

References

1. King H, Aubert RE and Herman WH. Global burden of diabetes 1995–2025: prevalence, numerical estimates and projections. *Diabetes Care* 1998; **21**: 1414–1431.

2. Drivsholm T, Ibsen H, Schroll M, Davidsen M and Borch-Johnsen K. Increasing prevalence of diabetes mellitus and impaired glucose tolerance among 60-year old Danes. *Diabet Med* 2001; **18**: 126–132.
3. Mohdad AH, Ford ES, Bowman BA, Dietz WH, Vinicor F, Bales VS and Marks JS. Prevalence of obesity, diabetes and obesity-related health risk factors. *JAMA* 2003; **289**: 76–79.
4. Harris MI, Klein R, Welborn TA and Knuiman MW. Onset of NIDDM occurs at least 4–7 years before clinical diagnosis. *Diabetes Care* 1992; **15**: 815–819.
5. Klein R, Klein BE, Moss SE, Davis MD and DeMets DL. The Wisconsin epidemiology study of diabetic retinopathy III. Prevalence and risk of diabetic retinopathy when age at diagnosis is 30 or more years. *Arch Opthalmol* 1984; **102**: 527–532.
6. Glatthaar C, Welborn TA, Stenhouse NS and Garcia-Webb P. Diabetes and impaired glucose tolerance. A prevalence estimate based on the Busselton 1981 survey. *Med J Aust* 1985; **143**: 436–440.
7. Gall MA. Albuminuria in non-insulin-dependent diabetes mellitus. Prevalence, causes and consequences. *Dan Med Bull* 1997; **44**: 465–485.
8. Rajala U, Laakso M, Qiao Q and Keinanen-Kiukaanniemi S. Prevalence of retinopathy in people with diabetes, impaired glucose tolerance and normal glucose tolerance. *Diabetes Care* 1998; **21**: 1664–1669.
9. Mooy JM, Grootenhuis PA, de Vries H, Valkenburg HA, Bouter LM, Kostence PJ and Heine RJ. Prevalence and determinants of glucose intolerance in a Dutch Caucasian population. The Hoorn Study. *Diabetes Care* 1995; **18**: 1270–1273.
10. Dunstan DW, Zimmet PZ, Welborn TA, Cameron AJ, Shaw D, de Court, Jolley D and McCarty DJ. The Australian Diabetes, Obesity and Lifestyle Study (AusDiab) – methods and response rates. *Diabetes Res Clin Pract* 2002; **57**: 119–129.
11. Glümer C, Jørgensen T and Borch-Johnsen K. Prevalence of diabetes and impaired glucose regulation in a Danish population – The Inter99 study. *Diabetes Care* 2003; **26**(8): 2335–2340.
12. Nakagami T, Qiao Q, Carstensen B, Nöhr-Hansen C, Hu G, Tuomilehto J, Balkau B and Borch-Johnsen K. The DECODE–DECODA Study Group. Age, body mass index and Type 2 diabetes – associations modified by ethnicity. *Diabetologia* 2003; **46**(8): 1063–1070.
13. Morrison AS. *Screening in Chronic Disease.* 1985. New York: Oxford University Press.
14. Zweig MH and Campbell G. Receiver-operating characteristic (ROC) plots: a fundamental evaluation tool in clinical medicine. *Clin Chem* 1993; **39**: 561–577.
15. Qiao Q, Keinanen-Kiukaanniemi S, Rajala U, Uusimaki A and Kivela SL. Random capillary whole blood glucose test as a screening test for diabetes mellitus in a middle aged population. *Scand J Clin Lab Invest* 1995; **55**: 3–8.
16. Rolka DB, Narayan KM, Thompson TJ, Goldman D, Lindenmayer J, Alich K, Bacall D, Benjamin EM, Lamb B, Stuart DO and Engelgau MM. Performance of recommended screening tests for undiagnosed diabetes and dysglycaemia. *Diabetes Care* 2001; **24**: 1899–1903.
17. Mortensen HB and Frølund A. Application of a biokinetic model for prediction and assessment of glycated haemoglobins in diabetic patients. *Scand J Clin Lab Invest* 1988; **48**: 595–602.
18. Davidson MB, Schriger DL, Peters AL and Lorber B. Relationship between fasting plasma glucose and glycosylated haemoglobin: potential for false-positive diagnoses of type 2 diabetes using new diagnostic criteria. *JAMA* 1999; **281**: 1203–1210.
19. Jeppsson JO, Kobold U, Barr J, Finke A, Hoelzel W, Hoshino T, Miedema K, Mosca A, Mauri P, Paroni R, Thienpont L, Umemoto M and Weykamp C. Approved IFCC reference method for the measurement of HbA_{1c} in human blood. *Clin Chem Lab Med* 2002; **40**: 78–89.

20. The DECODE-Study Group on behalf of the EDESG. New diagnostic criteria for diabetes mellitus – will they change the phenotype of the diabetic subjects? *BMJ* 1998; **317**: 371–375.
21. The Decoda Study Group on behalf of the International Diabetes Epidemiology Group. Comparison of the fasting and the 2-hour glucose criteria for diabetes in different Asian cohorts. *Diabetologia* 2000; **43**: 1470–1475.
22. Ruige JB, de Neeling JND, Kostence PJ, Bouter LM and Heine RJ. Performance of an NIDDM screening questionnaire based on symptoms and risk factors. *Diabetes Care* 1997; **20**: 491–496.
23. Herman WH, Smith PJ, Thomson TJ, Engelgau MM and Aubert RE. A new and simple questionnaire to identify people at increased risk of undiagnosed diabetes. *Diabetes Care* 1995; **18**: 382–387.
24. Glümer C, Carstensen B, Sandbæk A, Lauritzen T, Jørgensen T and Borch-Johnsen K. A Danish diabetes risk score for targeted screening. *Diabetes Care* 2004; **27**: 727–733.
25. Baan CA, Ruige JB, Stolk RP, Witteman JC, Dekker JM, Heine RJ and Feskens EJ. Performance of a predictive model to identify undiagnosed diabetes in a health care setting. *Diabetes Care* 1999; **22**: 213–219.
26. Griffin SJ, Little PS, Hales CN, Kinmonth AL and Wareham NJ. Diabetes risk score: towards earlier detection of Type 2 diabetes in general practice. *Diabetes Metab Res Rev* 2000; **16**: 164–171.
27. Wilson JMG and Jungner G. *Principles and Practice of Screening for Disease* 1968. Geneva: World Health Organisation.
28. Colagiuri S and Borch-Johnsen K. DETECT-2. Strategies for the early detection of Type 2 diabetes and impaired glucose tolerance. *Diabetes Voice* 2003; **48**: 11–13.
29. Lauritzen T, Griffin S, Borch-Johnsen K, Wareham NJ, Wolffenbuttel BHR and Rutten G for the ADDITION Study Group. The ADDITION study: proposed trial of the cost-effectiveness of an intensive multifactorial intervention on morbidity and mortality among people with Type 2 diabetes detected by screening. *Int J Obesity* 2000; **24**: S6–S11.
30. Sekikawa A, Tominaga M, Takahashi K, Watanabe H, Miyazawa K and Sasaki H. Is examination of fructosamine levels valuable as a diagnostic test for diabetes mellitus. *Diabetes Res Clin Pract* 1990; **8**: 187–192.
31. Rohlfing CL, Little RR, Wiedmeyer H-M, England JD, Madsen R, Harris MI, Flegal KM, Eberhardt MS and Goldstein DS. Use of GHb (HbA_{1c}) in screening for undiagnosed diabetes in the US population. *Diabetes Care* 2000; **23**: 187–191.
32. Hanson RL, Nelson RG, McCance DR, Beart JA, Charles MA, Pettitt DJ and Knowler WC. Comparison of screening-tests for non-insulin-dependent diabetes mellitus. *Arch Intern Med* 1993; **153**: 2133–2140.
33. Little RR, England JD, Wiedmayer HM, McKenzie EM, Pettitt DJ, Knowler WC and Goldstein DE. Relationship of glycosylated haemoglobin to oral glucose tolerance. Implications for diabetes screening. *Diabetes* 1998; **37**: 60–64.
34. Linne Y, Barkeling B and Rossner S. Natural course of gestational diabetes. Long term follow-up of women in the SPAWN study. *BJOG* 2002; **109**: 1227–1231.
35. Simon D, Coignet MC, Thibult N, Senan C and Eschwege E. Comparison of glycosylated haemoglobin and fasting plasma glucose with two-hour post-load plasma glucose in the detection of diabetes mellitus. *Am J Epidemiol* 1985; **122**: 589–593.
36. Ko GT, Chan JC, Yeung VT, Chow CC, Tsang LW, Li JK, So WY, Wai HP and Cockram CS. Combined use of fasting plasma glucose concentrations and HbA_{1c} or fructosamine predicts the likelihood of having diabetes in high risk subjects. *Diabetes Care* 1998; **21**: 1221–1225.
37. Tavintharan S, Chew LS and Heng DM. A rational alternative for the diagnosis of diabetes mellitus in high risk individuals. *Ann Acad Med Singapore* 2000; **29**: 213–218.

38. Peters AL, Davidson MB, Schriger DL and Hasselblad V. A clinical approach for the diagnosis of diabetes mellitus: an analysis using glycosylated haemoglobin levels. Meta-Analysis Research Group on the Diagnosis of Diabetes Using Glycosylates Hemoglobin Levels. *JAMA* 1996; **276**: 1246–1252.
39. Harris MI. Impaired glucose tolerance – prevalence and conversion to NIDDM. *Diabet Med* 1995; S9–S11.
40. Murphy NJ, Boyko EJ, Schraer CD, Bulkow LR and Lainer AP. Use of a reflectance photometer as a diabetes mellitus screening tool under field conditions. *Arctic Med Res* 1993; **52**: 170–174.
41. Ko GT, Chan JC, Lau E, Woo J and Cockram CS. Fasting plasma glucose as a screening test for diabetes and its relationship with cardiovascular risk factors in Hong Kong Chinese. *Diabetes Care* 1997; **20**: 170–172.
42. Lee CH and Fook-Chong S. Evaluation of fasting plasma glucose as screening test for diabetes mellitus in Singaporean adults. *Diabet Med* 1997; **14**: 119–122.
43. Nitiyanant W, Ploybutr S, Sriussadaporn S, Yamwong P and Vannasaeng S. Evaluation of the new fasting plasma glucose cut point of 7.0 mmol/l in detection of diabetes mellitus in the Thai population. *Diabetes Res Clin Pract* 1998; **41**: 171–176.
44. Chang CV, Wu JS, Lu FH, Lee HL, Yang YC and Wen MJ. Fasting plasma glucose in screening for diabetes in the Taiwanese population. *Diabetes Care* 1998; **21**: 1856–1860.
45. Wiener K. Fasting plasma glucose as a screening test for diabetes mellitus. *Diabet Med* 1997; **14**: 711–712.
46. Gatling W and Begley JP. Diagnosing diabetes mellitus in clinical practice: is fasting plasma glucose a good initial test? *Pract Diabetes Int* 2001; **18**: 89–93.
47. Haffner SM, Rosenthal M, Hazuda HP, Stern MP and Franco LJ. Evaluation of three potential screening tests for diabetes mellitus in a biethnic population. *Diabetes Care* 1984; **7**: 347–353.
48. Blunt BA, Barrett-Conor E and Wingard DL. Evaluation of fasting plasma glucose as a screening test for NIDDM in older adults. Rancho Bernardo Study. *Diabetes Care* 1991; **14**: 989–993.
49. Alberti KGMM and Zimmett PZ for a WHO consultation. *Definition, Diagnosis and Classification of Diabetes Mellitus and its Complications; Part 1: Diagnosis and Classification of Diabetes Mellitus*. 1999. Geneva: World Health Organisation.
50. Ko GTC, Chan JCN and Cockram CS. Supplement to the use of a paired value of fasting plasma glucose and glycated haemoglobin in predicting the likelihood of having diabetes. *Diabetes Care* 1998; **21**: 2032–2033.
51. Glümer C, Jørgensen T and Borch-Johnsen K. Targeted screening for undiagnosed diabetes reduces the number of diagnostic tests. Inter99(8). *Diabetic Med* In press, 2004.

7

Screening for Diabetes Mellitus – the World Health Organization Perspective

Gojka Roglic, Rhys Williams and **Stephen Colagiuri**

Introduction

Diabetes and its consequences

The latest World Health Organization (WHO) *Global Burden of Disease* estimates the worldwide burden of diabetes in adults to be around 173 million in the year 2002.[1] Around two-thirds of these live in developing countries. Diabetes is no longer a condition of developed, 'industrialized' or 'Western' countries. Global estimates of the burden of impaired fasting glucose (IFG) are not available, but the number of people with impaired glucose tolerance (IGT) is estimated to be even greater than the number with diabetes.[2,3]

The prevalence of diabetes is rising dramatically in the developing world, with an increasing proportion of affected people in younger age groups. Recent reports describe Type 2 diabetes being diagnosed in children and adolescents.[4–6] This is likely to increase further the burden of chronic diabetic complications worldwide.

Most of the consequences of diabetes result from its macrovascular and microvascular complications. The age-adjusted mortality, mostly due to coronary heart disease (CHD) in many populations, is two to four times higher than in the nondiabetic population,[7] and people with diabetes have a twofold increased risk of stroke.[8] Diabetes is the leading cause of end stage renal failure in many populations in both developed and developing countries.[9] Lower extremity

Prevention of Type 2 Diabetes Edited by Manfred Ganz
 ISBN: 0-470-85733-1

amputations are at least 10 times more common in people with diabetes than in nondiabetic individuals in developed countries,[10] and more than half of all nontraumatic lower limb amputations are due to diabetes. In developed countries, diabetes is one of the leading causes of visual impairment and blindness.[11,12]

People with diabetes require at least two to three times the health care resources of people who do not have diabetes, and diabetes care accounts for up to 15 per cent of national healthcare budgets.[13,14]

Screening for Type 2 diabetes

The main reasons for the current interest in screening for Type 2 diabetes are the following:

- there is a long, latent, asymptomatic period in which the condition can be detected;[15,16]

- a substantial proportion of people with Type 2 diabetes are undiagnosed (Table 7.1);

TABLE 7.1 Recent studies of the prevalence of known and previously undiagnosed diabetes in selected populations

Study	Country	Prevalence of previously undiagnosed diabetes (%)	Prevalence of known diabetes (%)	Ratio of previously undiagnosed to known diabetes
Levitt *et al.*, 1993[42]	South Africa	3.1	3.3	1:1
Mooy *et al.*, 1995[43]	The Netherlands	4.8	3.6	1:1
Park *et al.*, 1995[44]	South Korea	5.1	3.9	4:3
Elbagir *et al.*, 1996[45]	Sudan	2.2	1.3	2:1
Oliveira *et al.*, 1996[46]	Brazil	2.0	5.1	1:2
Mbanya *et al.*, 1997[47]	Cameroon	0.7	0.5	3:2
Ajlouni *et al.*, 1998[48]	Jordan	4.5	8.9	1:2
Harris *et al.*, 1998[49]	USA	2.7	5.1	1:2
Jimenez *et al.*, 1998[50]	Paraguay	3.6	2.9	1:1
Castell *et al.*, 1999[51]	Spain	3.6	6.7	1:2
Shera *et al.*, 1999[52]	Pakistan	7.1	4.0	2:1
Tan *et al.*, 1999[53]	Singapore	4.9	3.5	1:1
Sekikawa *et al.*, 2000[54]	Japan	4.8	5.3	1:1
Ramachandran *et al.*, 2001[55]	India	4.5	10.5	1:2
Amoah *et al.*, 2002[56]	Ghana	4.4	1.9	2:1
Dunstan *et al.*, 2002[57]	Australia	3.7	3.7	1:1
Satman *et al.*, 2002[58]	Turkey	2.3	4.9	1:2
Suvd *et al.*, 2002[59]	Mongolia	1.9	1.2	2:1
Colagiuri *et al.*, 2002[60]	Tonga	13.0	2.1	6:1

- a substantial proportion of newly referred cases of Type 2 diabetes already have evidence of the microvascular complications of diabetes;[17]
- the rising prevalence[18] of Type 2 diabetes world-wide;
- the seriousness of the immediate effects and long-term complications of Type 2 diabetes;
- evidence supporting the efficacy of intensive blood glucose control[19,20] blood pressure control[21] and blood lipid control[22–25] in Type 2 diabetes;
- accumulating evidence that treatment of hypertension and dyslipidaemia (for example lowering LDL cholesterol[22,23]) can prevent cardiovascular disease in people with Type 2 diabetes and
- increasing pressure from professional organizations, lay groups and some diabetes associations to institute screening for Type 2 diabetes.

In light of the above and in response to requests from national and regional health authorities and individual health care professionals for guidance as to what should be their policies for screening for Type 2 diabetes, WHO and the International Diabetes Federation (IDF) brought together, in May 2002, a group of acknowledged experts to make an assessment of the current evidence on this topic and to make recommendations for action. This chapter summarizes the content of the report of this meeting[26] and the contribution of these experts is gratefully acknowledged.

Effects of screening on individuals, health systems and society

Policies and practices for screening for Type 2 diabetes have profound implications for individuals, health systems and society as a whole. Implications for individuals include the following:

- the time and other resources necessary to undergo the screening test (or tests) and any subsequent diagnostic test (or tests);
- the psychological and social effects of the results, whether the screening test proves 'positive' or 'negative' and whether or not the diagnosis of Type 2 diabetes is subsequently made, and
- the adverse effects and costs of earlier treatment of Type 2 diabetes or of any preventive measures instituted as a result of the individual being found to have

diabetes. These may include occupational discrimination and/or increased costs or difficulty in obtaining insurance.

The effects on the health system and society as a whole are the following:

- the costs and other implications (especially in primary care and support services such as clinical biochemistry) of carrying out the screening test (or tests) and the necessary confirmatory test (or tests);
- the additional costs of the earlier treatment of those found to have diabetes or to be at high risk of developing diabetes or cardiovascular disease in the future;
- the implications of false negative and false positive results, which are inevitable given that any initial test will be a screening test and not a full diagnostic test (except in the case of an OGTT with markedly abnormal values) and
- any loss of production as a result of the earlier diagnosis of the condition (from absence from work or reduced job opportunities, for example).

The potential benefits of early detection of Type 2 diabetes are the following:

- enhanced length and/or quality of life, which might result from a reduction in the severity and frequency of the immediate effects of diabetes or the prevention or delay of its long-term complications, and
- any saving or redistribution of health care resources that might be possible as a result of reduced levels of care required for diabetes complications (reduced hospital admissions and lengths of stay etc.).

Screening and prevention – the links

Any programme aimed at the early identification of Type 2 diabetes through screening will also identify individuals with IGT and/or IFG. Thus any policy, whether related to public health or day-to-day clinical practice, must specify what should be done when these conditions are identified.

The prognostic significance of IGT, and to an extent IFG, is being clarified.[27] Also, evidence concerning the effect of interventions in IGT is now available. In particular, interventions aimed at weight reduction and increased physical activity and the use of some pharmacological agents have been shown to be effective in reducing or delaying the transition to diabetes in those with IGT. In general, lifestyle interventions appear to be more effective than medications.[28]

The Diabetes Prevention Program (DPP) Research Group evaluated the cost-effectiveness of the interventions used in their trial.[29] Lifestyle intervention and metformin were both judged to be cost effective within the context of the US. In health-care systems with lower staff and/or medication costs these costs per QALY would be lower and the interventions, all other things being equal, would be more cost effective.

Given this new, encouraging information on the prevention of or delay in the transition from IGT to diabetes, there is at least potential benefit from the detection of this condition through screening. Whether similar benefits will follow from the early detection of diabetes is another issue.

Formulating Policies on Screening for Type 2 Diabetes

Figure 7.1 summarizes the issues that need to be taken into account when formulating a screening policy. Three epidemiological considerations have been included, four of health system capacity and two economic considerations. Each of these should be viewed as a spectrum from, at one end, a clear indication that screening should be instituted to, at the other, clear evidence that it should not. Any population at any one time will be at a given point along each of these spectra. The policy decision as to whether or not to institute screening will be a judgement that cannot, necessarily, be extrapolated to other situations.

In reaching this judgement, public health authorities, clinicians, diabetes associations and others should consider the following.

The aims and objectives of a screening policy

Aims should be clear and relevant to the context of screening individuals at risk of having undiagnosed diabetes or at risk of developing diabetes. These may relate to the immediate effects of diabetes (e.g. infections), to the prevention of microvascular complications, to the prevention of CVD or to a combination of these. Thus, of crucial importance in relation to framing aims and objectives is knowledge about the most important consequences of diabetes in the population being considered.

Epidemiological considerations

The most important epidemiological consideration is the prevalence of undiagnosed Type 2 diabetes: this is known for some countries and regions as a result of field surveys of diabetes using OGTT; where it is unknown, estimates can be made by extrapolation (ratio of previously undiagnosed to known diabetes is likely to be around 1:1 or 2:1 (Table 7.1) but might be as extreme as 1:2 (e.g. Brazil) or 6:1 (Tonga). If unknown, this can be determined by a relatively simple survey. If

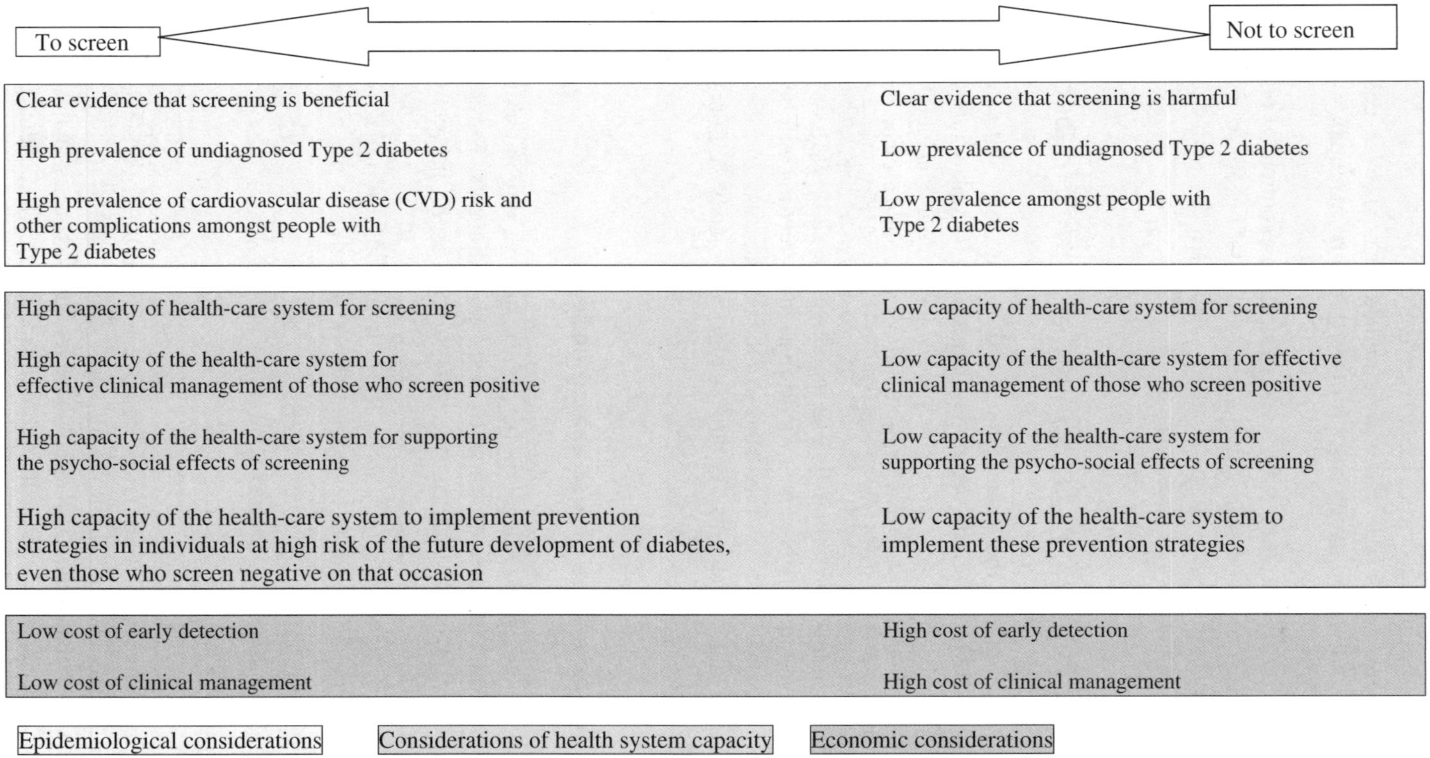

FIGURE 7.1 Considerations relevant to the development of a screening policy

screening of any kind is initiated, data on the numbers of unknown cases identified need to be collected and analysed periodically.

Considerations of health system capacity

The main issues here are the capacity of the system to carry out screening, follow-up and diagnostic testing and its capacity to manage effectively the newly detected cases of diabetes. The system must also be able to support individuals when the results of the screening are known, whether true positives, false positives or false negatives. The identification of people with IGT and IFG is a by-product of screening for type 2 diabetes and any screening policy needs to specify a clear care pathway for such people. Other issues are the capacity of the system to assess individual risks by using routinely available data. The first 'screen' might be made from such data,[30] thus eliminating one attendance by the individual.

Economic considerations

The cost of a screening programme will vary depending on the costs of materials, personnel etc. in any given setting. A large determinant of cost is whether the activity is conducted as a de novo activity or builds on existing health (e.g. primary-care) infrastructure. Clearly, the former is more costly. Also costs in getting the person to the test will vary. Cost of subsequent care will also vary widely (e.g. $10 000/year in the USA versus $100/year in India). It is the second of these (cost of subsequent care) that is the larger component of cost. It may be difficult to build a holistic economic argument since direct costs and indirect costs fall on different public or private sectors and the funding of screening and subsequent treatment may come from different budget lines.

Costs of screening may be reduced if screening uses routinely available information (for example using routine clinical information systems to identify people at high risk of diabetes) or by linking to other screening programmes (for example screening for glucose and lipids on the same fasting blood sample as part of a cardiovascular screening programme). Cost-effectiveness of treating screened individuals may also be increased by screening populations at particularly high risk of preventable adverse outcomes, for example populations with a high risk of cardiovascular disease. However, even the screening of high-risk populations, such as those already known to have hypertension and dyslipidaemia, can be costly.[31]

The choice of a test or tests

This is a judgement dependent upon the characteristics of a test (sensitivity, specificity etc.), the cost of a test in any given context and the capacity of the system to apply the test. Costs are largely driven by the rate of detection of positives (true and false) and the need to follow these up and carry out diagnostic testing.

Competing priorities

There will be competing priorities within diabetes – increased care for people with known diabetes versus identifying new cases; also in the wider health-care context – other health priorities such as communicable diseases; these need to be reassessed on an ongoing basis.

Ethical and political considerations

There is a valid argument for considering it the right of any individual to have diabetes diagnosed. However, this right needs to be weighed against any harm, anxiety etc. that may occur as a result of earlier diagnosis, the harm done to false positive and false negative individuals, and the opportunity cost if screening is carried out because the resources devoted to screening cannot be used for other purposes. No screening programme can be instituted without a political will to do so and this political will to institute screening may run counter to the supporting evidence.

There are also different expectations and ethical imperative depending on how the person comes to the test. In the case of disease the patient comes to seek advice, whereas with screening it is usually the health professional who imposes something on the patient. In addition, there may be medico-legal ramifications of not screening.

Widening the Evidence Base

The need for evidence from randomized controlled trials

The benefits of early detection of Type 2 diabetes through screening are not clearly established. The few available studies suffer from several types of bias that may lead to spurious conclusions regarding the benefits of screening.

The main sources of bias are as follows.

- *Lead time*: the interval between the time of detection by screening and the time that diabetes would have been diagnosed in the absence of screening. Thus lead-time bias prolongs the apparent duration of survival and/or complication-free period simply by advancing the diagnosis.

- *Selection bias*: people who enter screening programmes are volunteers, who are almost always more health conscious than the rest of the population. Thus they are more likely to have a better disease outcome even without screening.

- *Length-time bias*: this relates to the fact that individuals with rapid metabolic deterioration will tend to develop symptoms that prompt them to contact health services. Thus only people with slowly progressing and milder disease remain to be identified by screening. These people are likely to have a better clinical outcome than rapidly progressing cases, regardless of the treatment.

- *Over-diagnosis bias*: occurs when enthusiastic screening results in diagnosing diabetes in people that do not have it. Since nondiabetic individuals have a more favourable life course than persons with diabetes, this difference in the outcome may be erroneously attributed to screening.

Randomized controlled trials (RCTs) are usually regarded as the best means to evaluate the effectiveness of screening and early treatment. They are superior to observational studies because, if randomization is successful, the possible confounding effects of individual attributes and health-related behaviours other than the decision to take up screening can be eliminated.[32]

One of the reasons why data from RCTs that apply available treatment to a screened group, but not a control group, are unavailable is that such studies require long-term follow-up of a large number of participants. The feasibility of RCTs is further decreased by the need to account for people who refuse to participate, as well as for people in the control group who are offered and accept screening outside the programme. Nevertheless, RCTs that can take into account these issues are potentially feasible and should be encouraged.

The need for observational studies

RCTs to evaluate screening for diabetes have not been conducted so far, and even observational studies are scarce, in contrast to screening several other chronic conditions, particularly some of the cancers.

Once a screening method has been shown to be effective in an RCT, cohort studies in the general population could measure how a particular screening programme performs in a specific population. A cohort study could demonstrate the rate of particular outcomes among participants, refusers and noninvited subjects or screened versus nonscreened communities.

In contrast to RCTs and cohort studies, case–control studies estimate the individual's risk reduction if screened, although the protective effect of the screening procedure itself is not quantifiable. Although case–control studies are often regarded with scepticism on account of length-time, lead-time and selection biases, these can largely be accounted for with appropriate design and analysis.[33] Case–control studies cannot replace RCTs for the evaluation of the effect of screening, but they can be used to monitor a programme's effectiveness once screening has been widely introduced.[34]

Recently, the STARD initiative[35,36] has made recommendations for the reporting of studies of diagnostic accuracy. These recommendations include a checklist and flow diagram for the elements (such as the numbers of eligible patients, exclusions, abnormal, normal and inconclusive results etc.) vital to the interpretation of results. By analogy, standardization of the reporting of observational studies of screening would facilitate their interpretation and enable their generalizability to be more easily assessed.

The need for economic evidence

There are only two cost–utility evaluations for Type 2 diabetes, one comparing opportunistic screening and the other comparing mass screening with routine care.[37,38] The US study did not include the benefit of preventing macrovascular complications. The study in Taiwan demonstrated that screening may be cost effective in countries with high diabetes prevalence. There are no studies that have looked at cost–utility of screening for diabetes in populations deemed to be at high risk of Type 2 diabetes.

The use of modelling studies

All issues around the effectiveness of screening for diabetes cannot realistically be resolved by RCTs. The development of less costly and less time-consuming methods is to be advocated. One study used a Markov model to evaluate the efficacy of population screening for diabetes,[39] and another used the Monte Carlo model to estimate the lifetime costs and benefits of opportunistic screening for diabetes.[37] Both indicated there could be economic grounds for screening. Although modelling studies do not provide answers, they direct attention to the right questions, which can then be addressed in empirical studies.

The need for evidence on the psycho-social effects of early detection

Screening may lead to over-diagnosis, inappropriate investigation and treatment, avoidable adverse effects and unnecessary psychosocial and economic costs.[40] Physical harm associated with screening for diabetes may be considered negligible, but psychological and social harm could be more substantial. However, there are limited data specifically examining these issues in diabetes. An explorative study in 40 people participating in the Hoorn study suggests that the psychological impact of screening in newly diagnosed people is limited, with both those who were and those who were not diagnosed with Type 2 diabetes considering the screening procedure positively.[41]

A diagnosis of Type 2 diabetes has potential implications for employment and personal insurance. Treatment with insulin precludes some forms of employment

The Case of Brazil

Brazil recently performed nationwide community screening for diabetes and hypertension as part of its National Re-Organization Plan for the Care of Diabetes and Hypertension. In addition to detection of undiagnosed diabetes, the purpose of the screening programme was twofold:

- to raise public awareness of the importance of diabetes and hypertension, and
- to focus the efforts of primary care and health administrators on the restructuring and capacity building necessary for adequate diagnosis, basic treatment and prevention of complications of diabetes within the primary-care sector as well as for the creation of adequate referral networks.

Following an initial countrywide training of over 13 000 health professionals in the diagnosis and treatment of diabetes, a mass media campaign invited members of the public to participate in capillary glucose testing in March and April of 2001. Over 5300 municipalities participated in the effort.

During the campaign, 21.8 million (73 per cent of those targeted, adults $\geq$40 years of age) were tested with glucose meters. Of these, one per cent (about 0.25 million) had values $\geq$15 mmol/l (270 mg/dl) and were referred directly for medical management. An additional three per cent (about 0.61 million) had glucose screening values above the diabetes cut-off points, and immediately received a referral for confirmatory diagnostic testing.

An additional 12 per cent (3.4 million) were test positive at lower values (fasting $\geq$5.5 mmol/l (100 mg/dl) or nonfasting $\geq$7.8 mmol/l (140 mg/dl)) and were counselled to return within 3 months for further evaluation. Within 6 months of the screening programme, an additional 1.2 million fasting glucose determinations were performed by outpatient laboratories of the National Health System, presumably, in great part, as a result of the diagnostic demand induced by the programme.

Evaluation of the process and costs of this programme are currently contributing to Brazil's effort to shift diabetes prevention and management out of hospitals and into primary care.

The Case of Mexico: 'You Have Diabetes but You Don't Know it'

In Mexico the 2000 National Health Survey demonstrated a prevalence of diabetes of 10.9 per cent among those aged 20 years and over. This meant that in 2000 an estimated 5 million people were suffering diabetes in Mexico.

The Mexican Ministry of Health is conducting continuous diabetes (and hypertension) screening among those aged 20 years and over contacting their medical services for any reason. Volunteers are also evaluated during fairs and diabetes prevention activities such as those commemorating World Diabetes Day in some states. The target population of the government health care plan includes 41 per cent of the Mexican population (about 41 million people in 2001).

The aim of the screening system is to identify those with undiagnosed diabetes to provide early treatment and prevent or delay the onset of long-term complications. It also focuses on the identification of those at high risk of presenting diabetes, aiming to decrease the frequency of known risk factors such as obesity, lack of physical activity and deficient diet. The screening process is divided into two phases. The first one is the identification of individuals at high risk of diabetes through the application of a questionnaire named 'You have diabetes but you don't know it'. This questionnaire has seven questions and includes the calculation of BMI and the measurement of the waist circumference. The questionnaire was validated previously for the Mexican population.

During the second phase, those obtaining scores of 10 or more points in the questionnaire are tested for blood glucose. In cases with capillary fasting blood glucose of 100 mg/dl or capillary non-fasting blood glucose of 140 mg/dl a confirmatory test is required. Confirmation of the diabetes diagnosis includes an oral glucose tolerance test (OGTT) if needed.

Those with newly diagnosed diabetes and also those at risk are referred to different services included in the health system to commence diabetes education and treatment (if indicated). They are also invited to participate in a social group of people called a 'mutual-help group'. Those who obtained scores lower than 10 points in the questionnaire receive counselling about maintaining adequate weight, diet and physical activity. The first evaluation of this plan in 2000 included a pilot of 6186 persons in four states; 43 per cent were considered at high risk of presenting diabetes and 1.6 per cent were diagnosed with diabetes.

The cost of the screening was estimated at US$8.36 per newly diagnosed person with diabetes. In 2001 overall 3 945 885 people were evaluated with the application of the questionnaire, 572 153 people were tested for blood glucose and a total of 273 149 people from 32 states were identified as newly diagnosed with diabetes. Results for 2002 showed that a total of 3 985 860 were evaluated through the application of the questionnaire, 576 825 blood glucose tests were conducted and 313 124 people were diagnosed with diabetes.

and insurance premiums are higher for persons with diabetes. Anxiety caused by false positive results in screening for diabetes is unlikely to be as high as that caused by false positive results in screening for cancer. However, since screening programmes involve a large number of people, even a small adverse effect on quality of life or health-related behaviour could affect public health. Therefore, studies of the psychosocial effects of screening in diabetes are needed to complement studies of effectiveness.

Implementing Policies on Screening for Type 2 Diabetes

Two examples of national policies, from Brazil and Mexico, favouring screening for Type 2 diabetes are given on the following pages. While not necessarily advocating these approaches, the examples are provided here as illustrations of programmes that have been implemented on a large scale.

Conclusions and Recommendations

Conclusions

1. The issue of screening for Type 2 diabetes is important both in terms of individual health, day-to-day clinical practice and public health policy.

2. There is currently no direct evidence* as to whether individuals will or will not benefit from the early detection of Type 2 diabetes through screening.

3. Despite this lack of direct evidence, early detection through screening is already taking place both by inviting individuals from the general population to come forward for screening and, opportunistically, when individuals perceived to be at high risk of developing diabetes attend for health care (usually primary health care) for other reasons.

4. These activities present opportunities for collecting observational data, which, although no substitute for direct RCT evidence, can provide important, circumstantial evidence about efficiency, costs and impact.

5. There is direct evidence that the incidence of diabetes can be reduced in people at high risk of the future development of Type 2 diabetes who may be identified as a result of activities directed towards diabetes detection.

*'Direct evidence' is that from randomized controlled trials (RCTs) specifically designed to answer questions related to early detection through screening.

6. If screening can be shown to be beneficial, the most important *epidemiological considerations* determining whether to screen in any given population will be (1) the prevalence of undiagnosed Type 2 diabetes in that population and (2) the degree to which Type 2 diabetes is associated with risk of cardiovascular disease, diabetes-specific complications and other important health outcomes in that population.

7. The most important *health system considerations* will be its capacity (1) to carry out the screening, (2) to provide effective health care for those who screen positive, (3) to address the psycho-social needs of those who undergo screening and (4) to implement effective prevention in those who, though not confirmed to have diabetes at the time, are at high risk of its future development.

8. The most important *population considerations* will be (1) the acceptability of the screening programme to those invited to attend, (2) the extent to which any lack of acceptability reduces uptake, (3) the psychosocial impact of each screening outcome – positive and negative, 'true' and 'false' – and (4) the ability of those found to be at risk of future development of diabetes to modify this risk.

9. The most important *economic considerations* are (1) the cost of early detection to the health system and to the individual, (2) the extra costs of treatment following early detection and (3) the relative cost effectiveness of early detection compared with that of improving the care of clinically detected (as opposed to screen-detected) cases.

10. The most appropriate protocol for screening for undiagnosed Type 2 diabetes in a particular setting should consider (1) the sensitivity and specificity of the screening methods available, (2) the number of people who will need to be screened, (3) the number of people who will need subsequent diagnostic testing, (4) resource implications and (5) costs.

11. Screening for Type 2 diabetes is a dynamic topic in which new evidence will become available and further considerations will arise over time.

Recommendations

1. Health authorities and professional organizations should formulate policies concerning screening for Type 2 diabetes even if the policy is that screening is not currently to be advocated. In formulating that policy, the benefits and costs to the individual and their well-being are of paramount importance.

2. There is an urgent need for direct RCT evidence on the effects of early detection of Type 2 diabetes through screening. Such evidence should include health outcomes related to diabetes, cardiovascular disease, psychosocial outcomes and economic considerations for individuals, health systems and the wider society. Although RCTs directed to answering these questions may be costly and logistically difficult, there is, in the current state of knowledge, no ethical reason why they should not be undertaken.

3. Since the results of such RCTs will not be available for some time (if ever), there is also an urgent need to develop a framework (or model) that would permit countries to evaluate the cost-effectiveness of earlier detection of diabetes compared with other preventive and therapeutic interventions.

4. Testing apparently unaffected individuals at increased risk of having diabetes when these individuals attend for health care for other reasons (sometimes called 'opportunistic screening') *may* be justified provided (1) the reasons for testing are adequately explained to the individual, (2) the health system has the capacity for the clinical management of those who screen positive, (3) methods with adequate sensitivity and specificity are available, (4) the psycho-social needs of those who screen positive and those who screen negative can be met and (5) the health system can implement effective preventive strategies for those confirmed to be at high risk for the development of diabetes. There is no evidence to justify haphazard screening.

5. If such opportunistic screening is advocated then this should be carried out according to a policy that should (1) be clear and relevant in its aims and objectives, (2) be based as far as possible on sound evidence, (3) take into account the epidemiology of Type 2 diabetes and related cardiovascular disease risk in the population and (4) be sensitive to competing local health priorities.

6. The choice of the method or methods for screening will depend on the resources available, the acceptability of the methods in the population being screened and the levels of sensitivity, specificity etc. that are required. Methods of screening that might be regarded as unacceptable in high-resource settings (e.g. testing for urinary glucose) may be suitable in low-resource settings.

7. Where screening is already taking place, formal evaluation should be integral to these activities. The results of such evaluations could contribute to the general assessment of the value of early detection and should be used in the modification or curtailment of the activities being evaluated.

8. Given the dynamic nature of this topic, policies for screening for Type 2 diabetes must be reviewed from time to time as new evidence accumulates.

References

1. Wild S, Roglic G, Sicree R, Green A and King H. Global burden of diabetes mellitus in the year 2000. *Global Burden of Disease*. 2003. Geneva: WHO.
2. King H and Rewers M. Global estimates for prevalence of diabetes mellitus and impaired glucose tolerance in adults. *Diabetes Care* 1993; **16**: 157–177.
3. *Diabetes Atlas*, 2nd edn. 2003. Brussels: International Diabetes Federation.
4. Rosenbloom AL *et al*. Emerging epidemic of Type 2 diabetes in youth. *Diabetes Care* 1999; **22**: 345–354.
5. Dabelea D *et al*. Increasing prevalence of Type 2 diabetes in American Indian children. *Diabetologia* 1998; **41**: 904–910.
6. Kitagawa T *et al*. Increased incidence of non-insulin dependent diabetes mellitus among Japanese schoolchildren correleates with an increased intake of animal protein and fat. *Clin Paediatr* 1998; **37**: 111–115.
7. Morrish NJ, Wang SL, Stevens LK, Fuller JH and Keen H. WHO Multinational Study Group. Mortality and causes of death in the WHO multinational study of vascular disease in diabetes. *Diabetologia* 2001; **44** (Suppl. 2): S14–S21.
8. Bell DS. Stroke in the diabetic patient. *Diabetes Care* 1994; **17**: 213–219.
9. American Diabetes Association. Diabetic nephropathy. *Diabetes Care* 2002; **25**: S85–S89.
10. Siitonen OI, Niskanen LK, Laakso M, Siitonen JT and Pyörälä K. Lower-extremity amputations in diabetic and nondiabetic patients. *Diabetes Care* 1993; **16**: 16.
11. Anonymous. From the Centres for Disease Control and Prevention. Blindness caused by diabetes. *JAMA* 1996; **276**: 1865–1866.
12. Kuzuya T, Akanuma Y, Akazawa Y and Uehata T. Prevalence of chronic complications in Japanese diabetic patients. *Diabetes Res Clin Practice* 1994; **24** (Suppl.): S159–S164.
13. American Diabetes Association. Economic consequences of diabetes mellitus in the U.S. in 1997. *Diabetes Care* 1998; **21**: 296–309.
14. International Diabetes Federation and World Health Organization. *The Economics of Diabetes and Diabetes Care* 1996. Brussels: International Diabetes Federation.
15. Harris MI, Klein R, Welborn TA and Knuiman MW. Onset of NIDDM occurs at least 4–7 years before clinical diagnosis. *Diabetes Care* 1992; **15**(7): 815–825.
16. Thompson TJ, Engelgau MM, Hegazy M, Ali MA, Sous ES and Badran A *et al*. The onset of NIDDM and its relationship to clinical diagnosis in Egyptian adults. *Diabet Med* 1996; **13**: 337–340.
17. UK Prospective Diabetes Study (UKPDS) Group. The UK Prospective Diabetes Study 30. Diabetic retinopathy at diagnosis of non-insulin-dependent diabetes mellitus and associated risk factors. *Arch Ophthalmol* 1998; **116**: 670–677.
18. King H, Aubert RE and Herman WH. Global burden of diabetes, 1995–2025. *Diabetes Care* 1998; **21**: 1414–1431.
19. Ohkubo Y, Kishikawa H, Araki E, Miyata T, Isami S and Motoyoshi S. Intensive insulin therapy prevents the progession of diabetic microvascular complications in Japanese patients with non-insulin-dependent diabetes mellitus: a randomised prospective 6-year study. *Diabetes Res Clin Practice* 1995; **28**: 103–117.
20. UKPDS Group. Intensive blood glucose control with sulphonylureas or insulin compared with conventional treatment and risk of complications in patients with Type 2 diabetes (UKPDS 33). *Lancet* 1998; **352**: 837–853.
21. UK Prospective Diabetes Study Group. Tight blood pressure control and risk of macrovascular complications in Type 2 diabetes: UKPDS 38. *BMJ* 1998; **317**: 703–713.

22. Pyörälä K, Pedersen TR, Kjekshus J, Faergeman O, Olsson AG and Thorgeirsson G *et al.* Cholesterol lowering with simvastatin improves prognosis of diabetic patients with coronary heart disease. *Diabetes Care* 1997; **20**: 614–620.
23. Goldberg RB, Mellies MJ, Sacks FM, Moye LA, Howard WJ and Davis BR *et al.* Cardiovascular events and their reduction with pravastatin in diabetic and glucose-intolerant myocardial infarction survivors with average cholesterol levels. Subgroup analyses in the cholesterol and recurrent events (CARE) trial. *Circulation* 1998; **98**: 2513–2519.
24. Heart Protection Study Collaborative Group. MRC/BHF Heart Protection Study of cholesterol lowering with simvastatin in 20,536 high-risk individuals: a randomised placebo-controlled trial. *Lancet* 2002; **360**: 7–22.
25. Huang ES, Meigs JB and Singer DE. The effect of interventions to prevent cardiovascular disease in patients with Type 2 diabetes mellitus. *Am J Med* 2001; **111**: 633–642.
26. *Screening for Type 2 Diabetes Mellitus.* Report of a World Health Organization and International Diabetes Federation Meeting. WHO/NMH/MNC/03.1. 2003. Geneva: World Health Organization.
27. International Diabetes Federation. *International Diabetes Federation IGT/IFG Consensus Statement.* Report of an Expert Consensus Workshop. 2001. Brussels: International Diabetes Federation pp. 1–34.
28. Hamman RF. Prevention of Type 2 diabetes. In *The Evidence Base for Diabetes Care,* Williams R, Herman W, Kinmonth AL and Wareham NJ (eds). 2002. Chichester: Wiley, pp. 75–176.
29. *The Cost-Effectiveness of DPP Interventions to Delay or Prevent Type 2 Diabetes.* American Diabetes Association Annual Meeting 2002. San Francisco: American Diabetes Association.
30. Griffin S, Little PS, Hales CN, Kinmonth AL and Wareham NJ. Diabetes risk score: towards earlier detection of Type 2 diabetes in general practice. *Diabetes/Metab Res Rev* 2000; **16**: 164–171.
31. O'Connor PJ, Rush WA, Cherney LM and Pronk NP. Screening for diabetes mellitus in high-risk patients: cost, yield and acceptability. *Effective Clin Pract* 2001; **4**: 271–277.
32. Sasco AJ. Validity of case–control studies and randomized controlled trials of screening. *Int J Epidemiol* 1991; **20**: 1143–1144.
33. Sasco AJ. Lead time and length bias in case–control studies for the evaluation of screening. *J Clin Epidemiol* 1988; **41**: 103–104.
34. Sasco AJ, Day NE and Walter SD. Case–control studies for the evaluation of screening. *J Chron Dis* 1986; **39**: 399–405.
35. Bossuyt PM, Reitsma JB, Burns DE, Gastonis CA, Glasziou PP and Irwig LM *et al.* Towards complete and accurate reporting of studies of diagnostic accuracy: the STARD initiative. *BMJ* 2003; **326**: 41–44.
36. Straus SE. Reporting diagnostic tests. *BMJ* 2003; **326**: 3–4.
37. CDC Diabetes Cost-Effectiveness Study Group. The cost-effectiveness of screening for Type 2 diabetes. *JAMA* 1998; **280**: 1757.
38. Kuo HS, Chang HJ, Chou P, Teng L and Chen THH. A Markov chain model to assess the efficacy of screening for non-insulin dependent diabetes mellitus (NIDDM). *Int J Epidemiol* 1999; **28**: 233–240.
39. Chang H-J, Kuo H-S, Tung T-H, Chou P and Chen TH-H. Evaluation of a population-based screening for Type 2 diabetes: a community-based screening project in Puli, Taiwan. *Prevent Med* 2000; **31**: 396–402.
40. Stewart-Brown S and Farmer A. Screening could seriously damage your health. *BMJ* 1997; **314**: 533–534.

41. Adriaanse MC, Snoek FJ, Dekker JM, van der Ploeg HM and Heine RJ. Screening for Type 2 diabetes: an exploration of subjects' perceptions regarding diagnosis and procedure. *Diabet Med* 2002; **19**: 406–411.
42. Levitt NS, Katzenellenbogen JM, Bradshaw D, Hoffman MN and Bonnici F. The prevalence and identification of risk factors for NIDDM in urban Africans in Cape Town, South Africa. *Diabetes Care* 1993; **16**: 601–607.
43. Mooy JM, Grootenhuis PA, De Vries H, Valkenburg HA, Bouter LM and Kostense PJ *et al.* Prevalence and determinants of glucose intolerance in a Dutch Caucasian population – The Hoorn Study. *Diabetes Care* 1995; **18**: 1270–1273.
44. Park Y, Lee H, Koh, C-S, Min H and Yoo K *et al.* Prevalence of diabetes and IGT in Yonchon County, South Korea. *Diabetes Care* 1995; **18**: 545–548.
45. Elbagir MN, Eltom MA, Elmahadi EMA, Kadam IMS and Berne C. A population-based study of the prevalence of diabetes and impaired glucose tolerance in adults in Northern Sudan. *Diabetes Care* 1996; **19**: 1126–1128.
46. Oliveira JEP, Milech A and Franco LJ. The Cooperative Group for the Study of Diabetes Prevalence in Rio de Janeiro. The prevalence of diabetes in Rio de Janeiro, Brazil. *Diabet Med* 1996; **19**: 663–666.
47. Mbanya JCN, Ngogang J, Salah JN, Minkoulou E and Balkau B. Prevalence of NIDDM and impaired glucose tolerance in a rural and an urban population in Cameroon. *Diabet Med* 1997; **40**: 824–829.
48. Ajlouni K, Jaddou H and Batieha A. Diabetes and impaired glucose tolerance in Jordan: prevalence and associated risk factors. *J Intern Med* 2001; **244**: 317–323.
49. Harris MI, Flegal KM, Cowie CC, Eberhardt MS, Goldstein DE and Little RR *et al.* Prevalence of diabetes, impaired fasting glucose, and impaired glucose tolerance in U.S. adults. The Third National Health and Nutrition Examination Survey, 1988–1994. *Diabetes Care* 1998; **21**: 518–524.
50. Jimenez JTPM, Cañete F, Barriocanal LA, Medina U, Figueredo R and Martinez S *et al.* Prevalence of diabetes mellitus and associated cardiovascular risk factors in an adult urban population in Paraguay. *Diabet Med* 1998; **15**: 334–338.
51. Castell C, Tresserras R, Serra J, Goday A, Lloveras G and Salleras L. Prevalence of diabetes in Catalonia (Spain): an oral glucose tolerance test-based population study. *Diabetes Res Clin Pract* 1999; **43**: 33–40.
52. Shera AS, Rafique G, Ahmend KI, Baqai S, Khan IA and King H. Pakistan National Diabetes Survey. Prevalence of glucose intolerance and associated factors in North West Frontier Province (NWFP) of Pakistan. *J Pakistan Med Assoc* 1999; **49**: 206–211.
53. Tan C-E, Emmanuel SC, Tan B-Y and Jacob E. Prevalence of diabetes and ethnic differences in cardiovascular risk factors. The 1992 Singapore National Health Survey. *Diabetes Care* 1999; **22**: 241–247.
54. Sekikawa A, Eguchi H, Tominaga M, Igarashi K, Abe T and Manaka H *et al.* Prevalence of Type 2 diabetes mellitus and impaired glucose tolerance in a rural area of Japan. The Funagata diabetes study. *J Diabetes Complications* 2000; **14**: 78–83.
55. Ramachandran A, Snehalatha C, Kapur A, Vijay V and Mohan V and Das AK *et al.* High prevalence of diabetes and impaired glucose tolerance in India: National Urban Diabetes Survey. *Diabetologia* 2001; **44**: 1094–1101.
56. Amoah AG, Owusu SK and Adjei S. Diabetes in Ghana: a community based prevalence study in Greater Accra. *Diabetes Res Clin Pract* 2002; **56**: 197–205.
57. Dunstan DW, Zimmet P, Welborn TA, De Courten MP, Cameron AJ and Sicree RA. The rising prevalence of diabetes and impaired glucose tolerance. The Australian Diabetes, Obesity and Lifestyle Study. *Diabetes Care* 2002; **25**: 829–834.

58. Satman I, Aengûl A, Salman S, Tûtûncû Y, Sargin M and Dinccag N *et al.* Population-based study of diabetes and risk characteristics in Turkey: results of the Turkish Diabetes Epidemiology Study. *Diabetes Care* 2002; **25**: 1551–1556.
59. Suvd J, Gerel B, Otgooloi H, Purevsuren D, Zolzaya H and Roglic G *et al.* Glucose intolerance and associated factors in Mongolia: results of a national survey. *Diabet Med* 2002; **19**: 502–508.
60. Colagiuri S, Colagiuri R, Na'ati S, Muimuiheata S, Hussain Z and Palu T. The prevalence of diabetes in the Kingdom of Tonga. *Diabetes Care* 2002; **25**: 1378–1383.

3 Prevention of Type 2 Diabetes

8

Findings from Preventive Type 2 Diabetes Trials

Markolf Hanefeld

There exists now a bulk of evidence that both impaired fasting glucose (IFG) and impaired glucose tolerance (IGT) are not only risk categories for Type 2 diabetes but also risk factors for coronary heart disease.[1–3] Obviously, deterioration of glucose tolerance and intima media thickening (IMT) of the carotid arteries, an established marker of systemic atherosclerosis, develop in parallel.[4,5] The same applies for risk of cardiovascular mortality as consistently shown in numerous prospective studies (Figure 8.1).[6–11] Recently IFG but not IGT has been attributed as a component of the metabolic syndrome by the NCEP criteria.[12] However, as shown in prospective studies comparing the predictive power of IFG and IGT, the latter was by far the better predictor of cardiovascular and all-cause mortality.[13,14]

In the Riskfactors in IGT for Atherosclerosis and Diabetes (RIAD) study the 2 h postchallenge plasma glucose level in multivariate analysis was an independent highly significant predictor of IMT of the common carotid arteries, whereas fasting plasma glucose and HbA_{1c} were not.[15] The difference between IFG and IGT may become even more striking if the new cut-off limit of 5.6 mmol/l (100 mg/dl) for plasma glucose is accepted.[16] As demonstrated in a review by H Gerstein,[17] the risk of cardiovascular disease related to dysglycaemia develops along a continuum starting below the cut-off level of IFG and IGT.

Because of the overwhelming evidence that IGT is a risk factor for both Type 2 diabetes and cardiovascular disease, the pioneering large studies in the primary prevention of diabetes were performed in subjects with elevated postchallenge hyperglycaemia after a 75 g oral glucose tolerance test, diagnostic for IGT according to WHO criteria.[18]

Prevention of Type 2 Diabetes Edited by Manfred Ganz
 ISBN: 0-470-85733-1

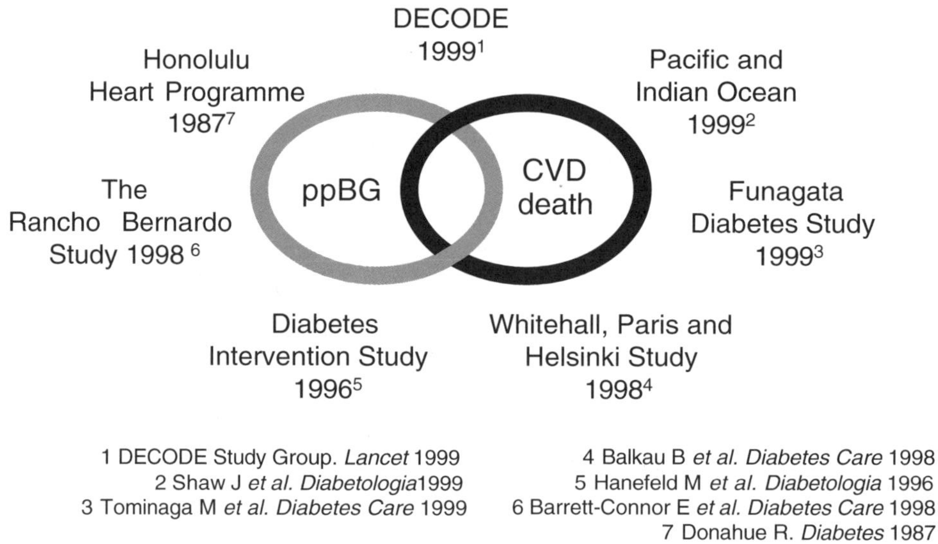

FIGURE 8.1 Prospective studies with postchallenge/postprandial hyperglycaemia as an independent risk factor for cardiovascular disease

The 'Common Soil' Hypothesis – a Rationale for Preventive Measures in Subjects with IGT

In 1984 Jarrett published an article entitled 'Type 2 (non-insulin-dependent) diabetes mellitus and coronary heart disease: chicken, egg or neither'.[19] In the prospective Whitehall Study[20] it was shown for the first time that IGT was associated with a similar prevalence of cardiovascular disease as in patients with known Type 2 diabetes, i.e. macrovascular complications preceded their diabetes.

In 1995 M Stern published a review on diabetes,[21] where he first used the term 'common soil' to explain the phenomenon that macroangiopathy by contrast to diabetes-related microangiopathy can precede diabetes, since both diseases have common genetic and environmental antecedents. As shown in Table 8.1 there is a communality of risk factor for both IGT/Type 2 diabetes and coronary heart disease. Recently, simple scores have been published to identify high-risk people for IFG, IGT and undiagnosed Type 2 diabetes.[22,23] These scores are based on diseases of the metabolic syndrome, family history for diabetes and presence of documented cardiovascular diseases. The data on endothelial dysfunction,[24] intima media thickening[4,5] and increased cardiovascular morbidity and mortality[6–11] in IGT suggest that IGT may be considered as an equivalent of cardiovascular disease as is now accepted for Type 2 diabetes.[25,26] This also explains why the costs of medical treatment for subjects with newly diagnosed diabetes were already twice

TABLE 8.1 Communality of risk factors for Type 2 diabetes and coronary heart disease

CHD	Type 2 diabetes
• Dyslipidaemia	• Dyslipidaemia
• Hypertension	• Hypertension
• IGT/Type 2 diabetes	• CHD
• Abdominal obesity	• Abdominal obesity
• High-fat diet	• High-fat diet
• Low physical activity	• Low physical activity
• IRS*	• IRS*
• Low-grade inflammation	• Low-grade inflammation
• Smoking	

*IRS = insulin resistance.

as high as for those with normal glucose tolerance in the years before diabetes was diagnosed (Figure 8.2).[27] Besides costs for drug treatment of hypertension and dyslipidaemia in subjects with IGT, this is mainly due to costs caused by cardiovascular complications. Thus, the clock starts ticking before diabetes is diagnosed.

This has eminent implications for the search for subjects with IGT as well as the rationale for (primary) prevention. It furthermore raises the question of whether IGT and/or IFG are already diseases in their own right. Challenged by a big bang

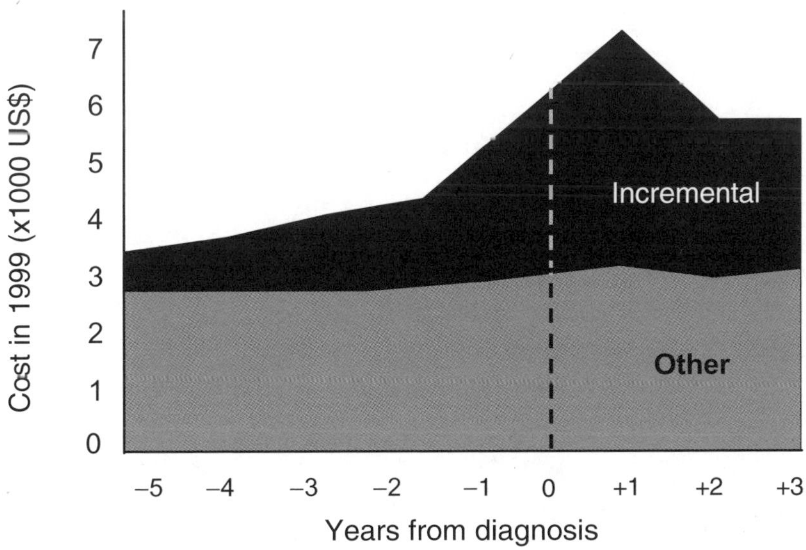

FIGURE 8.2 Costs for treatment of IGT before diabetes is diagnosed[27]

in diabetes prevalence and a high socio-economic burden by its comorbidities and complications in the mid-1990s large-scale prevention studies in subjects with IGT were initiated. At that time primary prevention of Type 2 diabetes was the primary objective; secondary objectives were prevention of diseases of the metabolic syndrome and cardiovascular complications.

Lifestyle Trials with Prevention of Diabetes as the Primary Objective

Overnutrition with a diet high in saturated fat and refined carbohydrate and low physical activity are the major environmental factors that accelerate the conversion of IFG and IGT to Type 2 diabetes. Studies with intensified health education in newly diagnosed Type 2 diabetes sufficiently controlled by diet advice[28] were not successful because the changes in lifestyle achieved were not maintained in the long run. Older studies with lifestyle intervention could not validate the efficacy and safety of lifestyle intervention because of too low numbers of participants and failures in the design, particularly with respect to the control group.

Recently three lifestyle intervention studies have been published, which prove that life behavioural modification is an efficient and safe tool to prevent Type 2 diabetes in subjects with IGT (Table 8.2).

TABLE 8.2 Conversion rate of IGT to Type 2 diabetes in long-term controlled clinical trials

		Conversion to diabetes (%) and relative risk reduction vs. controls						
Study	Years	Controls # (%)	Diet (%)	Exercise (%)	Diet + exercise (%)	Metformin (%)	Acarbose (%)	Orlistat (%)
Da Qing IGT and Diabetes Study[28]	6.0	67.7	43.8 (−31)	41.1 (−46)	46.0 (−42)			
Finnish Diabetes Prevention Study[30]	3.2	23.0			11 (−58)			
US Diabetes Prevention Program[31]	2.8	28.9			14.4 (−58)	21.7 (−31)		
STOP-NIDDM[34]	3.3	42.0					32 (−25 up to −36*)	
XENDOS Study[35]	4.4	9.0						−37.3

#Usual national recommendations for lifestyle modification.
*Two consecutive positive oGTTs.

The Da Qing study[29]

This study, published in 1997, was the first big trial to prove that intervention with diet and exercise significantly reduces the conversion of IGT to Type 2 diabetes. Participants were Chinese in a town near to Beijing. Subjects with IGT ($n = 577$) were randomly allocated either to controls, exercise, diet, or exercise plus diet. The incidence of diabetes versus control group was reduced by 31 per cent with diet, 46 per cent with exercise and 42 per cent by the combination of the two. This study demonstrated that both exercise and diet are effective even among an Asian population with low average body mass index, more traditional eating habits and still rather high physical activity in daily life. This also may explain why the combined effort was not superior to diet and exercise alone. It is also remarkable that the conversion rate to diabetes in the control group was 67.7 per cent.

The Finnish Diabetes Prevention Study (DPS)[30]

This study was the first with an integrated lifestyle approach comprising weight reduction, low-fat diet with a high fibre content, exercise of at least 150 minutes per week and antismoking education. The incidence of newly diagnosed diabetes (two confirmative 75 g OGTTs) was reduced by 58 per cent during the 3.2 years follow-up (Table 8.2). The effect on conversion rate significantly correlated to the positive changes in lifestyle. Diet and exercise changes were closely correlated. Both contributed to the preventive results. Thus, this study provided convincing evidence that lifestyle modification is effective and feasible to prevent diabetes in a European population. Lifestyle modification was associated with beneficial effects on blood lipids and blood pressure. The study was not powered to evaluate the effect of lifestyle improvement on cardiovascular events. This was an open trial without a 'wash-out phase'. Thus it does not answer the question of whether lifestyle modification prevents or delays manifestation of diabetes. With respect to weight-loss maintenance, a continuous increase of weight could be observed in the intervention group after one year follow-up.

The Diabetes Prevention Program (DPP)[31]

This four-arm megatrial was the first published study to compare the efficacy of lifestyle modification, metformin and troglitazone versus a control group (Table 8.2). This study included 3234 probands with all US minorities: Blacks, Hispanics, Asians and native Americans. The intensive lifestyle education was similar to that in the Finnish study. The reduction in the incidence of diabetes in the lifestyle group was exactly the same as in the DPS (Table 8.2). As with the DPS, a reincrease of body weight was observed after one year lifestyle intervention.

What did we learn from these three well controlled trials about efficacy, acceptance and cost-effectiveness of lifestyle intervention? *Efficacy* was high; about every second newly diagnosed Type 2 diabetes could be prevented in comparison with the control group during the trial. The numbers needed to treat to prevent one case with diabetes were 6.9 in the DPP. No data have been published on diabetes incidence and glucose tolerance in the year after trial participation. *Acceptance* and compliance with the lifestyle improvement programme were satisfying: 43 per cent in the DPS and 50 per cent in the DPP reached the targets for weight-loss, 74 per cent and 86 per cent respectively the targets for physical activity. The reincrease in body weight after one year in trial casts some shadow on this positive balance. Thus, it remains open whether a substantial change in eating habits and physical activity during the study can be maintained in this middle-aged and elderly population with IGT and a high prevalence of the metabolic syndrome for a long period of life.

Nothing has been published so far on adherence to lifestyle changes in the time after the trial.

Cost-effectiveness was analysed for the DPP in a recent publication.[32] The authors conclude that the measures to improve lifestyle were as expensive as metformin. However, lifestyle intervention is also beneficial for prevention of comorbidities of the metabolic syndrome and of coronary heart disease.

Thus, by extrapolation lifestyle modification is the first option for prevention of diabetes and presents an integrated approach to correct negative environmental factors as major causes for the big bang in diseases of the metabolic syndrome.

Pharmacological Trials with Prevention of Diabetes as the Primary Objective

Despite the convincing results with lifestyle intervention there remains a need to evaluate drug intervention. Still every second case of diabetes could not be prevented in the lifestyle modification trials. Many people are not able or willing to change their life habits to the extent that was needed in the lifestyle intervention. Long-term results may be poor as shown with the Diabetes Intervention Study (DIS).[33] After 11 years follow-up there was no difference in the control group versus intensified health education.

So far three big studies have been published on medical prevention of Type 2 diabetes.[31,34,35] The TRIPOD study[36] with troglitazone in gestational women and the Chinese Multicenter Clinical Study of Oral Antidiabetic Drugs[37] are further controlled trials that deal with important risk groups with IGT. Older studies with oral antidiabetics will not be considered here because of small numbers of cases and shortcomings in the design.

The Diabetes Prevention Program (DPP)[31]

DPP was the first published megatrial with an oral antidiabetic drug – metformin – showing that diabetes incidence can be reduced significantly (Table 8.2) by medical intervention. The reduction versus control group was 31 per cent after 2.8 years follow-up. Diabetes was diagnosed if 2 h postchallenge plasma glucose was $\geq$200 mg/dl at two consecutive oGTTs or fasting plasma glucose was $\geq$126 mg/dl. The metformin dosage was 2×850 mg/d; 72 per cent in the metformin group and 77 per cent in the placebo group ($p < 0.001$) took at least 80 per cent of the prescribed dosage. Weight loss versus placebo was 2.0 kg. There were only marginal effects on blood lipids and blood pressure. Striking differences were noted with respect to efficacy in subgroups (Table 8.3). Metformin was particularly efficient in obese people, younger ages, male sex and with high fasting plasma glucose. It had no significant effect on postchallenge plasma glucose. Subgroups with low impact were probands >60 years and with BMI <30 kg/m^2. In comparison with lifestyle, metformin was more effective in reducing fasting plasma glucose. No serious side-effects were observed during the study. The number needed to treat was 13.6. No data have been published on effect on cardiovascular complications so far.

By extrapolation metformin was effective, safe and well tolerated. It was not effective in elderly people with BMI below 30 and in subjects with low fasting plasma glucose.

Study to prevent non-insulin dependent diabetes mellitus (STOP-NIDDM)[34,38]

The STOP-NIDDM Trial was an international study undertaken in nine countries, which used acarbose, an α-glucosidase inhibitor, as an oral antidiabetic drug. By contrast to metformin, acarbose specifically reduces postprandial hyperglycaemia by delaying release of glucose from complex carbohydrates in the food. Participants were eligible if they had IGT plus fasting plasma glucose concentration between 5.6 and <7 mmol/l. 1429 subjects were included. The minimal follow-up time was three years. The target dosage was 100 mg acarbose tid. 211 (31 per cent of 682 patients) in the acarbose and 130 (19 per cent) in the placebo group discontinued early. The difference in the discontinuation rate between acarbose and placebo was mainly due to gastrointestinal side-effects associated with acarbose. There was, however, no serious adverse event registered in the acarbose group. The reduction in diabetes incidence was 25 per cent if one diagnostic oGTT was used as reference and 36 per cent if as in the DPS and DPP two consecutive oGTTs diagnostic for diabetes were considered. Further beneficial effects were reduction of blood pressure, a small weight loss and significant effects on blood

TABLE 8.3 Incidence of diabetes in subgroups of subjects with IGT: The Diabetes Prevention Program[31]. Reproduced by permission of the Massachusetts Medical Society

Variable	No. of participants (%)	Incidence			Reduction in incidence (95% CI)		
		Placebo	Metformin	Lifestyle	Lifestyle vs. placebo	Metformin vs. placebo	Lifestyle vs. metformin
		Cases/100 person-years			%		
Overall	3234	11.0	7.8	4.8	58 (48 to 66)	31 (17 to 43)	39 (24 to 51)
Age							
25–44 years	1000	11.6	6.7	6.2	48 (27 to 63)	44 (21 to 60)	8 (−36 to 37)[1]
45–59 years	1586	10.8	7.6	4.7	59 (44 to 70)	31 (10 to 46)	41 (18 to 57)[1]
Sex							
Male	1043	12.5	8.1	4.6	65 (49 to 76)	37 (14 to 54)	46 (20 to 63)
Female	2191	10.3	7.6	5.0	54 (40 to 64)	28 (10 to 43)	36 (16 to 51)
Body mass index[2]							
22 to <30	1045	9.0	8.8	3.3	65 (46 to 77)	3 (−36 to 30)[1]	63 (44 to 76)[1]
30 to <35	995	8.9	7.6	3.7	61 (40 to 75)	16 (−19 to 41)[1]	53 (28 to 70)[1]
Plasma glucose							
In the fasting state							
95–109 mg/dl[3]	2174	6.4	5.5	2.9	55 (38 to 68)	15 (−12 to 36)[1]	48 (27 to 63)
110–125 mg/dl[4]	1060	22.3	12.3	8.8	63 (51 to 72)	48 (33 to 60)[1]	30 (6 to 48)
Two hours after an oral load							
140–153 mg/dl	1049	7.1	4.3	1.8	76 (58 to 86)[1]	41 (11 to 61)	59 (27 to 77)
154–172 mg/dl	1103	10.3	6.6	4.4	60 (41 to 72)[1]	38 (13 to 56)	34 (2 to 56)
173–199 mg/dl	1082	16.1	12.3	8.5	50 (33 to 63)[1]	26 (3 to 43)	33 (9 to 51)

[1] $P < 0.05$ for the test of heterogenicity across strata. Age, body mass index, and plasma glucose were analysed as continuous variables.
[2] The eligibility criterion was a body mass index of at least 22 for Asians and at least 24 for all other persons.
[3] This category includes American Indian participants who had a fasting glucose concentration that was less than 95 mg per decilitre, according to the eligibility criteria.
[4] This category includes 54 participants with a fasting glucose concentration of 126 to 139 mg per deciliter who were enrolled before June 1997, when the eligibility criteria were changed to conform to the diagnostic criteria of the American Diabetes Association, published that year.

lipids. In multivariate analysis acarbose but not reduction of postchallenge hyperglycaemia was a significant determinant of diabetes risk. The authors did not use a mixed meal to directly measure the impact of acarbose on postprandial hyperglycaemia. Interestingly, a subgroup analysis revealed that this drug was particularly effective in elderly women with BMI $< 30\,kg/m^2$. The study did not answer the question of whether it was a delay or prevention of development of diabetes.

In conclusion, acarbose is an effective and safe drug to delay development of Type 2 diabetes in patients with IGT and increased fasting hyperglycaemia diagnostic for IFG if the new ADA cut-off limits for fasting glucose are used. It was particularly effective in elderly moderately overweight subjects.

Prespecified secondary objectives[39] were cardiovascular events and hypertension. For the first time it could be shown that treatment of IGT with acarbose results in a significant reduction of cardiovascular events (Figure 8.3) and of newly diagnosed hypertension (Figure 8.4). The major reduction was in the risk of myocardial infarction (HR 0.09, $p = 0.006$). Acarbose treatment was also associated with a 34 per cent relative risk reduction in the incidence of new cases of hypertension. The number needed to treat to prevent one cardiovascular event would be 40 patients with IGT in 3.3 years. The number needed to treat to prevent one new case of hypertension would be 19. In multivariate analysis acarbose, fasting glucose and systolic blood pressure were the only independent predictors of cardiovascular events. Thus, besides treatment of IGT and correction of postprandial hyperglycaemia, other mechanisms may be involved in the vasoprotective effects of acarbose.

In conclusion, in agreement with the common soil hypothesis treatment of patients with IGT was effective in preventing both Type 2 diabetes and cardiovascular diseases. It remains an open question whether this beneficial effect is only related to strict normalization of postprandial hyperglycaemia or is (also) due to so far unknown specific effects of acarbose.

Xenical in the prevention of diabetes in obese subjects (XENDOS) study[35]

This Swedish study tested the efficacy of orlistat as an adjunct to lifestyle changes in obese subjects with a BMI $> 30\,kg/m^2$. 3305 patients were randomized: 79 per cent with normal glucose tolerance and 21 per cent with IGT. Lifestyle plus placebo was compared with lifestyle plus 120 mg orlistat tid – an intestinal lipase inhibitor. Primary endpoints were time to diabetes and weight loss. 52 per cent with orlistat and 34 per cent with placebo completed the study. Follow-up time was 4 years. The relative risk reduction was 37.3 per cent. The preventive effect was only significant for the subjects with IGT despite the fact that the weight loss was similar (5.8 kg in the subgroup with normal glucose tolerance, 5.7 kg in the

Cardiovascular event	No. of patients Ac ($n = 682$)	Pl ($n = 686$)	Risk red. (%)	p
Coronary heart disease				
myocardial infarction	1	12		0.0226
angina	5	12		0.1344
revascularization	11	20		0.1806
cardiovascular death	1	2		0.6298
Congestive heart failure	0	2		–
Cerebrovascular accident/ stroke	2	4		0.5061
Peripheral vascular disease	1	1		0.9255
Any prespecified cardiovascular event	15	32	49	0.0326

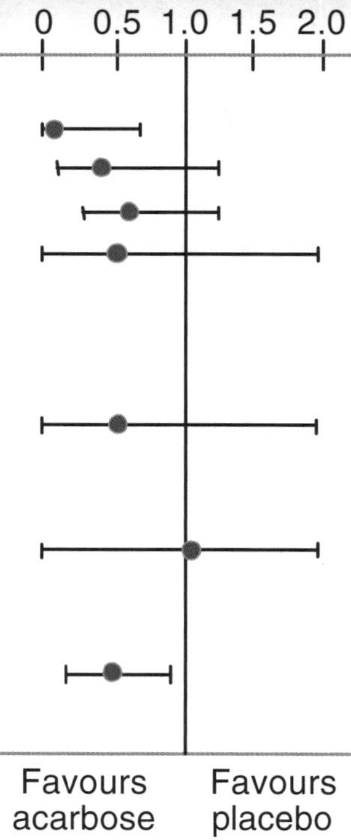

FIGURE 8.3 Effects of treatment of IGT by acarbose on the incidence of major cardiovascular disease[38]. Reproduced from *JAMA*, 2003, **290**, 486–94.

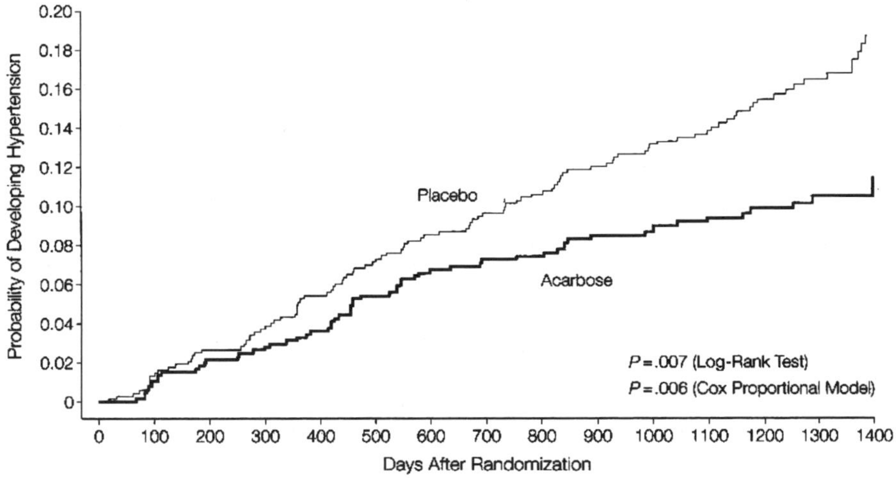

No. at Risk															
Placebo	686	663	646	632	607	593	581	573	562	550	538	458	368	287	196
Acarbose	682	645	617	601	585	570	559	559	552	524	514	435	342	254	178

FIGURE 8.4 Effect of treatment of IGT by acarbose on the incidence of newly diagnosed hypertension[38]. Reproduced from *JAMA*, 2003, **290**, 486–94.

IGT subgroup). Lifestyle intervention was also effective with respect to weight, resulting in a weight loss of 3 kg after 4 years.

Conclusion: orlistat, a weight reducing drug that blocks fat absorption in the small intestine, is a useful adjunct to lifestyle modification for the prevention of Type 2 diabetes. Side-effects were moderate without any serious event. The effects were only seen in patients with IGT.

The TRIPOD (troglitazone in the prevention of diabetes) study[36]

In this study in high-risk Hispanic women the insulin-sensitizing drug troglitazone (400 mg/d) was tested in 266 women with previous gestational diabetes. The follow-up time was 30 months. Troglitazone highly significantly reduced the diabetes rate: annual incidence was 12.1 per cent in the placebo versus 5.4 per cent in the troglitazone group. The preventive effect persisted 8 months after medication was stopped. The investigators also performed intravenous glucose tolerance tests to evaluate effects of troglitazone on both beta cell function and insulin resistance. The protective effect was associated with the preservation of the beta-cell function via improvement of insulin sensitivity.

Conclusions: the TRIPOD study has shown the key role of protection of beta-cell function for the prevention of diabetes by a reduction in the secretory burden by insulin resistance. It was the first study to show the efficacy of prevention after stopping drug treatment. Limitations were the small number of cases and a special group of gestational women.

The multicentre clinical study of oral antidiabetic drugs[37]

This multicentre 3 year prospective trial at Chinese university hospitals included 321 subjects above 25 years with IGT. The participants were divided into control, diet plus exercise, acarbose and metformin groups. By contrast to the DPP, both drugs were more effective in reducing incidence of diabetes as compared with diet plus exercise. The annual incidence rate decreased to two per cent with acarbose, 4.1 per cent with metformin and 8.2 per cent in the diet plus exercise group versus 11.6 per cent in the control group. Only the drug intervention reached significance. Neither the difference between the two drugs nor that between natural incidence in IGT and lifestyle intervention was significant. The participants were lean, with an average BMI between 24.5 and 25.3 kg/m^2. Increased fasting plasma glucose was a non-inclusion criterion. Diet plus exercise modification efforts were moderate and a conventional structured education programme with annual reiteration after initiation was applied.

Conclusion: this Asian population had only a few features of the metabolic syndrome. Life habits were obviously more traditional with respect to nutrition and physical activity. Nevertheless, the natural history revealed a high incidence of diabetes in this IGT population. The benefit for both drugs was more pronounced under these conditions. Both drugs significantly reduced postprandial hyperglycaemia, with a stronger effect of acarbose. Interestingly, the discontinuation rate was similar with acarbose and metformin.

Comparing this study with the DPP, DPS and STOP-NIDDM including people with Western lifestyle, this study demonstrates the importance of environment and genetics for the selection of appropriate intervention measures in subjects with IGT.

Coronary Heart Disease Prevention Trials with Prevention of Diabetes as the Secondary Objective

There are two classes of coronary drugs for which a significant effect on diabetes incidence has been described: statins and ACE/ARB inhibitors.

The west of Scotland coronary prevention study (WOSCOPS)[40,41]

This study in 5974 Scotsmen with hypercholesterolaemia had as primary objective the prevention of coronary heart disease by pravastatin – a statin that was successfully tested in a large secondary prevention study: CARE.[42] 139 of them developed diabetes as diagnosed by fasting plasma glucose $\geq$ 7 mmol/l. Pravastatin resulted in a reduction of newly detected diabetes by 30 per cent ($p = 0.042$). The decrease in myocardial infarction incidences was as expected 34 per cent.[40] Diabetes diagnosis was only based on one fasting plasma glucose measurement.

Conclusion: the authors hypothesized that the surprisingly strong impact on diabetes prevalence at the end of the study might be due to unknown pleiotropic effects of statins, probably anti-inflammatory action.

So far no trials have been published that specifically use statins for prevention of diabetes. It is unknown whether this is a class effect or specific for different statins.

Angiotensin-converting enzyme (ACE) inhibitors, AT_2 receptor blockers (ARBs) and the development of diabetes

The renin–angiotensin system is an important regulator of insulin resistance and seems to be closely related to low-grade chronic inflammation. The first study to show that ACE inhibitors not only prevent coronary heart disease but also reduce the incidence of diabetes was the Heart Outcomes Prevention Evaluation (HOPE) trial.[43] In this randomized controlled trial 5720 patients older than 55 years without known diabetes but with documented vascular disease were included. Follow-up time was 4.2 years. The patients were randomly allocated to 10 mg ramipril/day or placebo. 102 individuals in the ramipril group and 153 with placebo developed diabetes, corresponding to a relative risk reduction of 34 per cent. This outcome result was based on self-reports every 6 months but similar results were noted with initiation of glucose-lowering drugs (RR 0.56 (CI 0.41–0.77)). This reduction in diabetes incidence was in the same range as in primary prevention trials. The data, however, need confirmation by prospective trials with plasma glucose monitoring and application of well defined diagnostic criteria for diabetes.

The beneficial effect of ACE inhibitors on the incidence of newly diagnosed diabetes has been supported by two large trials for the treatment of hypertension comparing ACE inhibitors, beta blockers and diuretics.

The antihypertensive and lipid lowering treatment to prevent heart attack trial (ALLHAT)[44]

This study compared lisinopril, chlorthalidone and amlodipine in a large population of patients with hypertension. Lisinopril intake was associated with a significantly lower incidence of diabetes. The macrovascular outcome was the same as with the other antihypertensive drugs.

The captopril prevention project (CAPPP)[45]

Comparing the ACE inhibitor captopril with conventional antihypertensive treatment (diuretics, beta blockers) in 10 985 Swedish patients with hypertension, a lower incidence of new diabetes with captopril was noted. Captopril and conventional treatment did not differ in preventing cardiovascular morbidity and mortality.

The losartan intervention for endpoint reduction in hypertension study (LIFE)[46]

In this trial the effect of losartan was compared with the beta blocker atenolol in patients with hypertension and left ventricular hypertrophy. The primary objective was cardiovascular morbidity and mortality. The relative cardiovascular risk in the losartan group versus atenolol was 0.87 ($p = 0.021$). New onset of diabetes was 25 per cent less with losartan.

Conclusion: the results with ACE inhibitors and ARBs consistently show a lower incidence of newly diagnosed diabetes. These data are particularly relevant for hypertensive patients at high risk for diabetes. The lower incidence of diabetes with these drugs may improve long-term cardiovascular outcomes.

Summary of trials with diabetes incidence as the secondary objective

The reduction in the incidence of newly diagnosed diabetes in studies for prevention of coronary heart disease observed with statins and ACE inhibitors is similar to those obtained with oral antidiabetics in primary prevention trials for diabetes. It is likely that the preventive action of statins is due to anti-inflammatory properties. Low-grade chronic inflammation seems to contribute to progression of glucose intolerance to overt diabetes. For ACE-inhibiting agents and angiotensin receptor blockers improvement of insulin resistance has been described in some but not all studies. This may well be connected with a down-regulation of proinflammatory adipokines and pro-atherogenic enzymes. Because these results have important clinical and public health implications for large subgroups with the metabolic syndrome and/or cardiovascular diseases, prospective studies have been launched to test the common soil hypothesis for diabetes and atherosclerosis. This could open the gate for an integrated approach of medical prevention of a cluster of diseases.

Studies for Primary Prevention of Diabetes in Progress

The diabetes reduction assessment with Ramipril and Rosaglitazone medication (DREAM) Trial[47]

The primary objective of this multinational study is to determine whether treatment with Ramipril and/or Rosiglitazone will prevent diabetes in subjects with IGT or IFG. Ramipril has shown its potential to reduce the incidence of diabetes in patients with cardiovascular diseases. It has direct effects on the renin–angiotensin system, which in a cascade of events may improve insulin sensitivity and down-regulate subclinical low-grade inflammation. Rosiglitazone is a potent insulin-sensitizing oral antidiabetic drug, which has a possible beta-cell protective effect.[48] Its anti-inflammatory action was described in a recent publication.[49] The primary objective is the conversion to diabetes. Secondary objectives are cardiovascular events. More than 4000 subjects have been randomized. Recruitment was finished in June 2003. The minimal follow-up time will be 3 years after randomization.

The Nateglinide and Valsartan in impaired glucose tolerance outcomes research (NAVIGATOR) trial[50]

NAVIGATOR is a multinational trial with prevention of diabetes and cardiovascular events as primary objectives. The target population are people with IGT and cardiovascular disease or at least one risk factor for cardiovascular disease respectively. As with DREAM a 2×2 factorial design is used to evaluate the efficacy of either Nateglinide or Valsartan or the combination of the two versus placebo. Recruitment for the planned 8000 participants was finished in December 2003. This megatrial is the first with cardiovascular events besides diabetes incidence as the primary objective. The follow-up time will be $\approx$5.5–6 years.

The outcome reduction with an initial glargine intervention (ORIGIN) trial[51]

This multinational trial in patients with IFG, IGT or early diabetes and at least one cardiovascular event uses a 2×2 factorial design with either glargine plus omega 3 fatty acids, insulin glargine plus placebo, standard therapy plus omega 3 fatty acids or standard therapy plus placebo. The primary objective is prevention of cardiovascular complications in subjects with IGT, IFG or early diabetes with a documented cardiovascular disease (myocardial infarction, stroke, vascular surgery etc.) by tight glucose control with early introduction of insulin treatment. The secondary objective in the subgroup with IFG and IGT is prevention of Type 2 diabetes. Specific questions for the omega 3 fatty acids as add-on therapy to insulin and standard therapy are impact on cardiovascular mortality and antiarrhythmic potency. The study will include 10–12 000 patients. A standardized algorithm will be used for titration of insulin to reach the target of 5.3 mmol/l fasting plasma glucose. Recruitment was started in September 2003. The minimal follow-up time in the treatment phase will be 3 years.

ORIGIN is primarily a study to evaluate the efficacy of strict glucose control on incidence of cardiovascular complications. It should answer the question of whether strict glucose control with early introduction of insulin treatment can prevent both cardiovascular complications and diabetes or diabetes progression.

Is Impaired Glucose Tolerance (IGT) a Disease?

The answer to this is a question of high clinical and public health relevance. As shown in the previous chapters, the prevalence of IGT is roughly in the same range as for known diabetes. The risk for diabetes and macroangiopathy increases along a continuum for dysglycaemia.[17] There is no clear difference in diseases related to hyperglycaemia between IGT and newly diagnosed diabetes in many[19,52] but not all studies.[3] IGT and newly diagnosed diabetes share the same underlying pathophysiology: subclinical chronic inflammation (Figure 8.5)[53,54], increased insulin resistance, impaired insulin secretion (Figure 8.6), as described in detail in Chapter 2. From the clinical viewpoint it is important that IGT is associated with a cluster of comorbidities[55] characteristic of the metabolic syndrome. Furthermore, we find in subjects with IGT classical diabetes related diseases that for long have been considered as late complications. Even more important, IGT is associated with an increased risk for cardiovascular morbidity and mortality as previously described in more detail. Pathophysiological studies have shown that postchallenge hyperglycaemia diagnostic for IGT causes endothelial dysfunction that leads to a distinct flow-mediated vasodilation.[56] Furthermore, a rapid increase in all adhesion molecules and NFkB has been noted in CLAMP studies mimicking postprandial hyperglycaemia at a range diagnostic for IGT.[57] The study in critically ill patients by van den Berghe and co-workers[58] has proven that a perfect normalization of glucose concentration to a level of 5–6 mmol/l improves short- and long-term survival significantly. These impressive results have been attributed to improved endothelial function. Direct evidence of clinical benefit of treatment of IGT was provided by the STOP-NIDDM trial, which has shown an impressive reduction in cardiovascular events and newly diagnosed hypertension.[37]

In summary, epidemiological, pathophysiological and clinical findings suggest that IGT is a risk category that shares in many aspects the characteristics of newly diagnosed diabetes. Thus, the answer 'to the question to be or not to be a disease' is not simple. At present, an expert panel of the IDF defines IGT: 'Neither IFG nor IGT are considered clinical entities in their own right, but as risk categories for the future development of diabetes and CVD. They represent metabolic state intermediate between normal glucose homeostasis and diabetic hyperglycaemia'. However, extrapolating the present evidence, IGT may well be considered as a disease or condition that should be treated. As we have learned from the history of

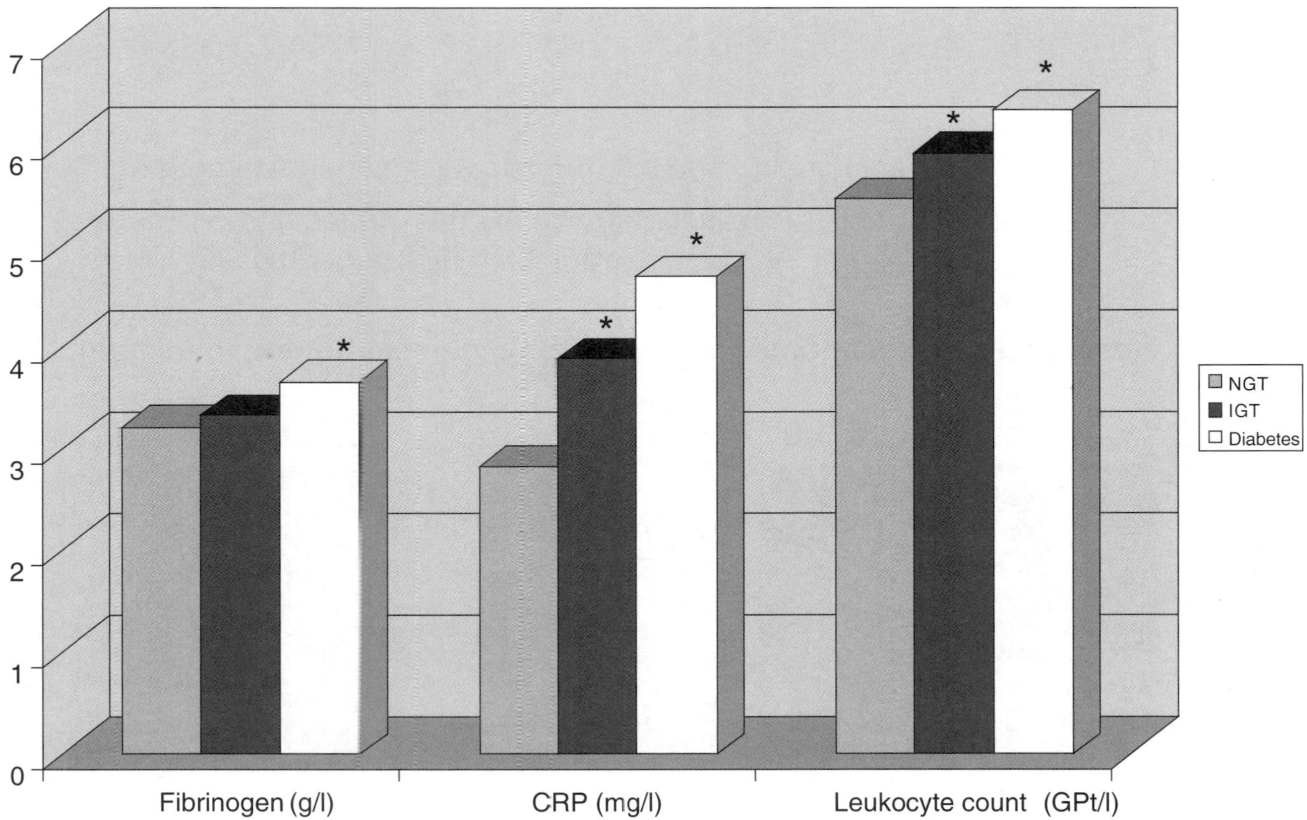

FIGURE 8.5 Low-grade inflammation by categories of glucose tolerance in a high-risk population for diabetes: the RIAD Study[54]

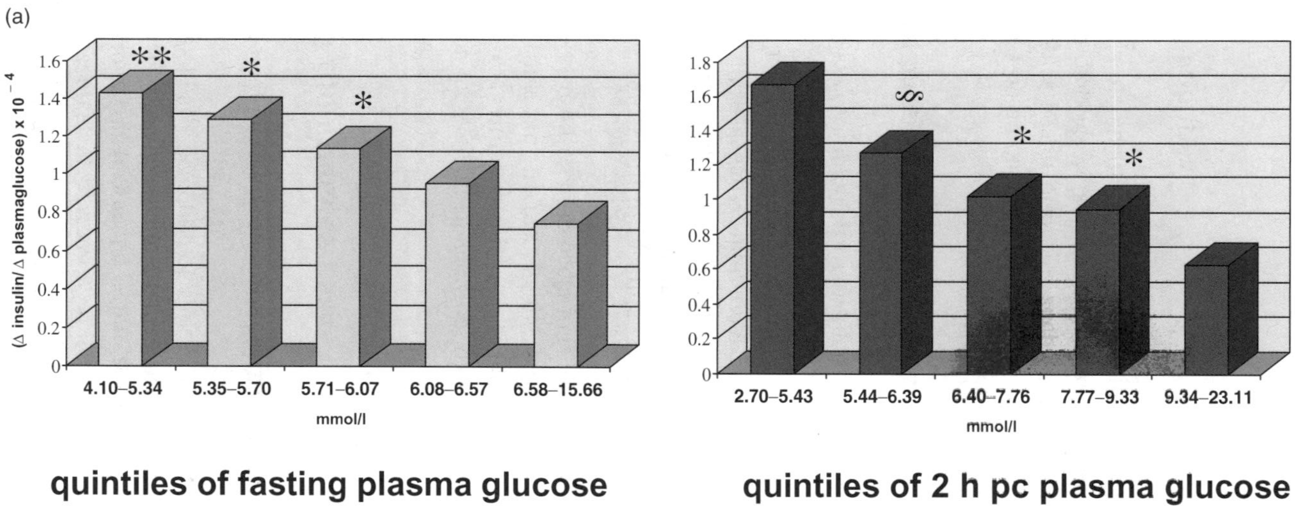

* $p < 0.05$ comparing with 5thquintile

** $p < 0.05$ comparing with 4th and 5thquintiles

§§ $p < 0.05$ comparing with 2nd, 3rd, 4th and 5thquintiles

FIGURE 8.6 (a) Insulin secretion

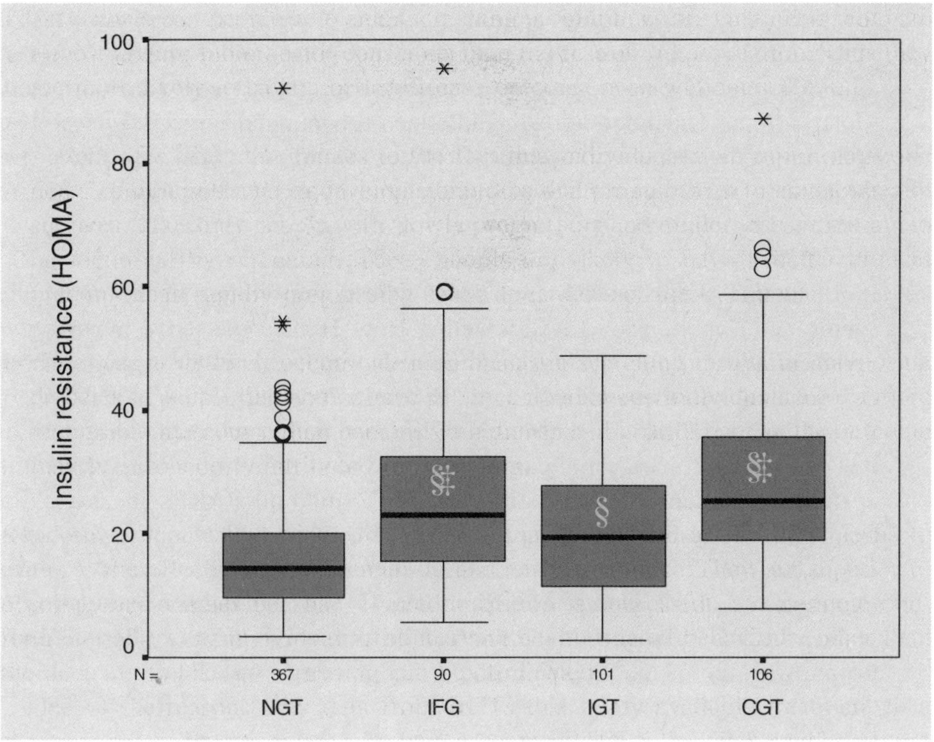

§ ANOVA lg $p < 0.001$ vs. NGT; ‡ANOVA lg $p < 0.05$ vs. IGT

FIGURE 8.6 (b) insulin resistance (HOMA-IR) in a high-risk population for Type 2 diabetes:The RIAD Study[55]

the lipid hypothesis with mild hypercholesterolaemia, the decision should be based on the global risk.

Who Should be Treated (and How)?

If we consider treatment of IGT with our present knowledge the decision can only be based on the global risk. Not least, it should be remembered that any IGT needs a second confirmative oGTT. There are three constellations that could speak in favour of medical intervention in the case of confirmed IGT if lifestyle intervention is not possible or fails: (1) association with cardiovascular disease, (2) comorbidities of the metabolic syndrome and (3) combined hyperglycaemia.

(1) There is consistent evidence from study in critically ill patients,[58] the DIGAMI study[59] and STOP-NIDDM that a strict normalization of fasting and postprandial hyperglycaemia has beneficial effects on endothelial

function, progression of intima media thickness[60] and incidence of myocardial infarction.[38,59] Therefore, it is reasonable that postprandial glucose levels of >8, <11 mmol/l plasma glucose diagnostic for IGT need to be corrected. Most national and international guidelines recommend target levels of two hour postprandial hyperglycaemia <8 mmol/l. Studies are under way to prove the benefit of perfect control of postprandial hyperglycaemia in IGT and in patients with diabetes.

(2) IFG and IGT are frequently associated with comorbidities of the metabolic syndrome. Hypertension, dyslipidaemia (low HDL-cholesterol, hypertriglyceridaemia), android obesity and albuminuria escalate the risk for both development of atherosclerosis and diabetes. Considering the global risk in subjects with IGT plus two diseases of the metabolic syndrome, correction of IGT seems to be an essential part of coronary heart prevention. Vice versa, it is a strong argument to use statins and ACE inhibitors/ARBs as drugs for treatment of dyslipidaemia and hypertension respectively since they also lower the risk for diabetes. Metformin should be particularly useful in the treatment of obese young people with IGT and the metabolic syndrome, whereas acarbose seems to be more efficient in moderately obese elderly people with the metabolic syndrome.

(3) People with IFG plus IGT have an annual conversion rate of ≈10 per cent to diabetes. They share the same cardiovascular risk and prevalence of diabetes-related diseases as newly diagnosed asymptomatic Type 2 diabetes. Therefore, prevention with oral antidiabetics (acarbose, metformin) with evidence of preventive power should be considered if lifestyle fails to normalize glucose tolerance.

It should be re-emphasized that lifestyle modification in any case is the first option. Drug intervention should only be considered if lifestyle modification is not possible or accepted or if lifestyle is not effective despite best efforts after 6 months follow-up.

Thus, at present treatment of IGT is a rational approach for special high-risk groups for diabetes and cardiovascular disease. This recommendation requires confirmation by controlled prospective trials. The studies under way will (hopefully) answer most of the open questions up to the end of this decade.

Do we Treat Type 2 Diabetes too Late?

If we accept that IGT at least in patients with cardiovascular disease and/or the metabolic syndrome has to be treated then the answer should be 'yes'. However, the IDF still considers IFG and IGT as risk categories for diabetes and cardiovascular disease.[18] Already epidemiological data from the Whitehall Study,[19] the Diabetes Intervention Study[28,33] and the UK-PDS[61] have convincingly shown that newly diagnosed diabetes is associated with an excessive prevalence of cardiovascular disease and also with a remarkably high prevalence of diabetes-related diseases such as nephropathy and retinopathy. These studies used $\geq$7.8 mmol/l fasting plasma glucose as the cut-off limit. This was the major reason to bring down the cut-off limit to 7 mmol/l (126 mg/dl). Recently published data[62] with this cut-off limit on in-hospital mortality in patients with undiagnosed diabetes show that hyperglycaemia was present in 38 per cent of patients admitted to a community teaching hospital in Atlanta, USA. 26 per cent had a history of diabetes; 12 per cent were undiagnosed. Newly discovered diabetes was associated with a 16 per cent mortality rate versus three per cent with prior history of diabetes and 1.7 per cent in subjects with normal glucose tolerance ($p < 0.01$ for both). The multimorbidity in patients with newly diagnosed diabetes as shown in a meta-analysis with 90 000 patients with 12.4 year follow-up requires early and strict control of hyperglycaemia and of associated risk factors such as hyperlipidaemia, hypertension and microalbuminuria.[63] The high cardiovascular complication rate and omnipresence of the metabolic syndrome in newly diagnosed diabetes – at the same level as for known diabetes – was also shown in a practice network study in the Basque Country, Spain.[64] On the other hand, we cannot ignore the fact that no intervention studies have been performed comparing the outcomes in patients detected by screening versus cohorts with known diabetes. This seems to be critical in patients aged 70 and over, where the long-term risk by hyperglycaemia is not strikingly different from those with normal glucose levels.

Thus, intervention trials with early diabetes are needed, particularly for the elderly. In any case, the existing evidence already calls for intensified case finding and opportunistic screening including pp glucose measurements in high-risk groups.[65] The newly diagnosed Type 2 diabetes patients need an optimal control of hyperglycaemia as well as of coexisting cardiovascular risk factors. The encouraging results with primary prevention in IGT subjects are strong arguments for early therapy.

References

1. European Arterial Risk Policy Group on behalf of the International Diabetes Federation European Region. A strategy for arterial risk assessment and management in Type 2 (non-insulin-dependent) diabetes mellitus. *Diabet Med* 1997; **14** (7): 611–621.
2. The DECODE Study Group. Glucose tolerance and mortality: comparison of WHO and American Diabetes Association diagnostic criteria. European Diabetes Epidemiology Group. Diabetes epidemiology: collaborative analysis of diagnostic criteria in Europe. *Lancet* 1999; **21**: 617–621.
3. Saydah SH, Miret and M Sung J *et al.* Postchallenge hyperglycemia and mortality in a national sample of U.S. adults. *Diabetes Care* 2001; **24** (8): 1397–1402.

4. Hanefeld M, Koehler C, Schaper F, Fücker K, Henkel E and Temelkova-Kurktschiev Th. Meal time plasma glucose is an independent risk factor for increased intima-media thickness in non-diabetic individuals. *Atherosclerosis* 1999; **144**: 229–235.
5. Temelkova-Kurktschiev T, Henkel E, Koehler C, Karrei K and Hanefeld M. Subclinical inflammation in newly detected Type II diabetes and impaired glucose tolerance. *Diabetologia* 2002; **45**: 151.
6. Barrett-Connor E and Ferrara A. Isolated postchallenge hyperglycemia and the risk of fatal cardiovascular disease in older women and men. The Rancho Bernardo Study. *Diabetes Care* 1998; **21** (8): 1236–1239.
7. Rodriguez BL, Lau N, Burchfiel CM, Abbott RD, Sharp DS, Yano K and Curb JD. Glucose intolerance and 23-year risk of coronary heart disease and total mortality: the Honolulu Heart Program. *Diabetes Care* 1999; **22** (8): 1262–1265.
8. Qureshi AI, Giles WH and Croft JB. Impaired glucose tolerance and the likelihood of nonfatal stroke and myocardial infarction: the Third National Health and Nutrition Examination Survey. *Stroke* 1998; **29** (7): 1329–1332.
9. Malmberg K, Norhammar A, Wedel H and Ryden L. Glycometabolic state at admission: important risk marker of mortality in conventionally treated patients with diabetes mellitus and acute myocardial infarction: long-term results from the Diabetes and Insulin-Glucose Infusion in Acute Myocardial Infarction (DIGAMI) study. *Circulation* 1999; **99** (20): 2626–2632.
10. Shichiri M, Kishikawa H, Ohkubo Y and Wake N. Long-term results of the Kumamoto Study on optimal diabetes control in Type 2 diabetic patients. *Diabetes Care* 2000; **23** (Suppl. 2): B21–B29.
11. Hanefeld M. Postprandial hyperglycaemia: noxious effects on the vessel wall. *Int J Clin Pract Suppl* 2002; **129**: 45–50.
12. Cleeman JI. Executive Summary of the Third Report of the National Cholesterol Education Program (NCEP) Expert Panel on Detection, Evaluation, and Treatment of High Blood Cholesterol in Adults (Adult Treatment Panel III). *JAMA* 2001; **285** (19): 2486–2497.
13. DECODE Study Group and European Diabetes Epidemiology Group. Is the current definition for diabetes relevant to mortality risk from all causes and cardiovascular and noncardiovascular diseases? *Diabetes Care* 2003; **26** (3): 688–696.
14. De Vegt F, Dekker JM and Stehouwer CD *et al.* The 1997 American Diabetes Association criteria versus the 1985 World Health Organization criteria for the diagnosis of abnormal glucose tolerance: poor agreement in the Hoorn Study. *Diabetes Care* 1998; **21**: 1686–1690.
15. Temelkova-Kurktschiev TS, Koehler C, Henkel E, Leonhardt W, Fuecker K and Hanefeld M. Postchallenge plasma glucose and glycemic spikes are more strongly associated with atherosclerosis than fasting glucose or HbA_{1c} level. *Diabetes Care* 2000; **23** (12): 1830–1834.
16. Anand SS, Razak F and Vuksan V *et al.* Diagnostic strategies to detect glucose intolerance in a multiethnic population. *Diabetes Care* 2003; **26** (2): 290–296.
17. Gerstein HC and Yusuf S. Dysglycaemia and risk of cardiovascular disease. *Lancet* 1996; **347** (9006): 949–950.
18. Unwin N, Shaw J, Zimmet P and Alberti KG. Impaired glucose tolerance and impaired fasting glycaemia: the current status on definition and intervention [review]. *Diabet Med* 2002; **19** (9): 708–723.
19. Jarrett RJ, Keen H and McCartney P. The Whitehall Study: ten year follow-up report on men with impaired glucose tolerance with reference to worsening to diabetes and predictors of death. *Diabet Med* 1984; **1** (4): 279–283.
20. Jarrett RJ and Shipley MJ. Type 2 (non-insulin-dependent) diabetes mellitus and cardiovascular disease – putative association via common antecedents; further evidence from the Whitehall Study. *Diabetologia* 1988; **31** (10): 737–740.

21. Stern MP. Diabetes and cardiovascular disease. The 'common soil' hypothesis [review]. *Diabetes* 1995; **44** (4): 369–374.
22. Lindstrom J and Tuomilehto J. The diabetes risk score: a practical tool to predict Type 2 diabetes risk. *Diabetes Care* 2003; **26** (3): 725–731.
23. Stern MP, Williams K and Haffner SM. Identification of persons at high risk for Type 2 diabetes mellitus: do we need the oral glucose tolerance test? *Ann Intern Med* 2002 **136** (8): 575–581.
24. Ceriello A, Taboga C, Tonutti L, Quagliaro L, Piconi L, Bais B, Da Ros R and Motz E. Evidence for an independent and cumulative effect of postprandial hypertriglyceridemia and hyperglycemia on endothelial dysfunction and oxidative stress generation: effects of short- and long-term simvastatin treatment. *Circulation* 2002; **106** (10): 1211–1218.
25. Haffner SM. Coronary heart disease in patients with diabetes. *N Engl J Med* 2000; **342** (14): 1040–1042.
26. Grundy SM and Benjamin IF and Burke GL *et al.* Diabetes and cardiovascular disease: a statement for healthcare professionals from the American Heart Association. *Circulation* 1999; **100** (10): 1134–1146.
27. Nichols GA, Glauber HS and Brown JB. Type 2 diabetes: incremental medical care costs during the 8 years preceding diagnosis. *Diabetes Care* 2000; **23** (11): 1654–1659.
28. Hanefeld M, Fischer S, Schmechel H, Rothe G, Schulze J, Dude H, Schwanebeck U and Julius U. Diabetes Intervention Study. Multi-intervention trial in newly diagnosed NIDDM. *Diabetes Care* 1991; **14** (4): 308–317.
29. Pan XR, Li GW, Hu YH, Wang JX, Yang WY, An ZX, Hu ZX, Lin J, Xiao JZ, Cao HB, Liu PA, Jiang XG, Jiang YY, Wang JP, Zheng H, Zhang H, Bennett PH and Howard BV. Effects of diet and exercise in preventing NIDDM in people with impaired glucose tolerance. The Da Qing IGT and Diabetes Study. *Diabetes Care* 1997; **20** (4): 537–544.
30. Tuomilehto J, Lindstrom J, Eriksson JG, Valle TT, Hamalainen H, Ilanne-Parikka P, Keinanen-Kiukaanniemi S, Laakso M, Louheranta A, Rastas M, Salminen V and Uusitupa M. Finnish Diabetes Prevention Study Group. Prevention of Type 2 diabetes mellitus by changes in lifestyle among subjects with impaired glucose tolerance. *N Engl J Med* 2001; **344** (18): 1343–1350.
31. Knowler WC, Barrett-Connor E, Fowler SE, Hamman RF, Lachin JM, Walker EA and Nathan DM. Diabetes Prevention Program Research Group. Reduction in the incidence of Type 2 diabetes with lifestyle intervention or metformin. *N Engl J Med* 2002 **346** (6): 393–403.
32. Diabetes Prevention Program Research Group. Within-trial cost-effectiveness of lifestyle intervention or metformin for the primary prevention of Type 2 diabetes. *Diabetes Care* 2003; **26** (9): 2518–2523.
33. Hanefeld M, Fischer S, Julius U, Schulze J, Schwanebeck U, Schmechel H, Ziegelasch HJ and Lindner J. The DIS-Group: Risk factors for myocardial infarction and death in newly detected NIDDM: the Diabetes Intervention Study, 11-year follow-up. *Diabetologia* 1996; **39**: 1577–1583.
34. Chiasson JL, Josse RG, Gomis R, Hanefeld M, Karasik A and Laakso M. Acarbose for prevention of Type 2 diabetes mellitus: the STOP-NIDDM randomised trial. *Lancet* 2002; **359**: 2072–2077.
35. Torgerson JS, Hauptman J, Boldrin MN and Sjostrom L. Xenical in the prevention of diabetes in obese subjects (XENDOS) study: a randomized study of orlistat as an adjunct to lifestyle changes for the prevention of Type 2 diabetes in obese patients. *Diabetes Care* 2004; **27** (1): 155–161.
36. Azen SP, Peters RK, Berkowitz K, Kjos S, Xiang A and Buchanan TA. TRIPOD (troglitazone in the prevention of diabetes): a randomized, placebo-controlled trial of troglitazone in women with prior gestational diabetes mellitus. *Control Clin Trials* 1998; **19** (2): 217–231.

37. Wenying Y *et al.* The preventive effect of acarbose and metformin on the progression to diabetes mellitus in the IGT population: 3-year multicenter prospective study. *Chin J Endocrin Metab* 2001; **17**: 131–136.
38. Chiasson JL, Josse RG, Gomis R, Hanefeld M, Karasik A, Laakso M and STOP-NIDDM Trial Research Group. Acarbose treatment and the risk of cardiovascular disease and hypertension in patients with impaired glucose tolerance: the STOP-NIDDM trial. *JAMA* 2003; **290** (4): 486–494.
39. Chiasson JL, Gomis R, Hanefeld M, Josse RG, Karasik A and Laakso M. The STOP-NIDDM Trial: an international study on the efficacy of an alpha-glucosidase inhibitor to prevent Type 2 diabetes in a population with impaired glucose tolerance: rationale, design, and preliminary screening data. Study to Prevent Non-Insulin-Dependent Diabetes Mellitus. *Diabetes Care* 1998; **21** (10): 1720–1725.
40. Shepherd J, Cobbe SM, Ford I *et al.* Prevention of coronary heart disease with pravastatin in men with hypercholesterolemia: West of Scotland Coronary Prevention Study Group. *N Engl J Med* 1995; **333**: 1301–1307.
41. Freeman DJ, Norrie J and Sattar N *et al.* Pravastatin and the development of diabetes mellitus: evidence for a protective treatment effect in the West of Scotland Coronary Prevention Study. *Circulation* 2001; **103** (3): 357–362.
42. Sacks FM, Pfeffer MA and Moyé La *et al.* The effects of pravastatin on coronary events after myocardial infarction in patients with average cholesterol levels: the Cholesterol and recurrent events investigators. *N Engl J Med* 1996; **335**: 1001–1009.
43. Yusuf S, Gerstein H and Hoogwerf B *et al.* Ramipril and the development of diabetes. *JAMA* 2001; **286**: 1882–1885.
44. The ALLHAT Collaborative Research Group. Major outcomes in high-risk hypertensive patients randomized to angiotensin-converting enzyme inhibitor of calcium channel blocker vs. diuretic. *JAMA* 2002; **288**: 2981–2997.
45. Hansson L, Lindholm LH and Niskanen L *et al.* Effect of angiotensin-converting-enzyme inhibition compared with conventional therapy on cardiovascular morbidity and mortality in hypertension: the Captopril Prevention Project (CAPPP) randomized trial. *Lancet* 1999; **353**: 611–616.
46. Dahlof B, Devereux RB and Kjeidsen SE *et al.* Cardiovascular morbidity and mortality in the losartan intervention for endpoint reduction in hypertension study (LIFE): a randomized trial against atenolol. *Lancet* 2002; **359**: 995–1003.
47. NDEP and United States Department of Health and Human Service. Websites http://www.dream-ctn.org.
48. Diamant M and Heine RJ. Thiazolidinediones in Type 2 diabetes mellitus: current clinical evidence. *Drugs* 2003; **63** (13): 1373–1405.
49. Haffner SM, Greenberg AS and Weston WM *et al.* Effect of rosiglitazone treatment on nontraditional markers of cardiovascular disease in patients with Type 2 diabetes mellitus. *Circulation* 2002; **107** (16): 679–684.
50. The NAVIGATOR Trial Steering Committee. Nateglinide and valsartan in impaired glucose tolerance outcomes research: rationale and design of the NAVIGATOR trial [Abstract]. *Diabetes* 2002; **51**: A116.
51. Hanefeld M and Niemoeller E. Outcome reduction with an initial glargine intervention: Die Origin-Studie: Eine multinationale, multizentrische Studie zur Untersuchung der kardiovaskulären Risikoreduktion mit Insulin Glargin bei Hochrisikopatienten mit Type-2-Diabetes [poster]. *Diabetes Stoffwechsel* 2003; **12** (Suppl. 1): 113 (P-114).
52. Koehler C, Temelkova-Kurktschiev T, Henkel E, Schaper F, Fuecker K and Hanefeld M. Is the newly suggested fasting plasma glucose cut-off point for the diagnosis of diabetes the right one? *Diabetologia* 1999; **42** (5): 635–636.

53. Hanefeld M. Postprandial hyperglycaemia: noxious effects on the vessel wall. *Int J Clin Pract Suppl* 2002; **129**: 45–50.
54. Temelkova-Kurktschiev T, Henkel E and Koehler C *et al.* Subclinical inflammation in newly detected Type II diabetes and impaired glucose tolerance. *Diabetologia* 2002; **45** (1): 151.
55. Hanefeld M, Schaper F and Koehler C *et al.* Insulin secretion and insulin sensitivity pattern is different in isolated impaired glucose tolerance and impaired fasting glucose – The Risk Factor in Impaired Glucose Tolerance for Atherosclerosis and Diabetes Study. *Diabetes Care* 2003; **26**: 868–874.
56. Kawano H, Motoyama T and Hirashima O *et al.* Hyperglycemia rapidly suppresses flow-mediated endothelium-dependent vasodilation of brachial artery. *J Am Coll Cardiol Cardiol* 1999; **34** (1): 146–154.
57. Schiekofer S, Andrassy M and Chen J *et al.* Acute hyperglycemia causes intracellular formation of CML and activation of ras, p42/44 MAPK, and nuclear factor kappaB in PBMCs. *Diabetes* 2003; **52** (3): 621–633.
58. van den Berghe G, Wouters P and Weekers F *et al.* Intensive insulin therapy in the critically ill patients. *N Engl J Med* 2001; **345** (19): 1359–1367.
59. Malmberg K, Ryden L and Hamsten A *et al.* Effects of insulin treatment on cause-specific one-year mortality and morbidity in diabetic patients with acute myocardial infarction. DIGAMI Study Group. Diabetes Insulin–Glucose in Acute Myocardial Infarction. *Eur Heart J.* 1996; **17** (9): 1337–1344.
60. Hanefeld M, Chaisson JL and Koehler C *et al.* Acarbose slows progression of intima-media thickness of the carotid arteries in subjects with impaired glucose tolerance. *Stroke* 2004; **35** (5): 1073–1078.
61. Turner RC, Millns H and Neil HAW *et al.* for the United Kingdom Prospective Diabetes Study Group. Risk factors for coronary artery disease in non-insulin dependent diabetes mellitus: United Kingdom prospective diabetes study (UKPDS: 23). *BMJ* 1998; **316**: 823–828.
62. Umpierrez GE, Isaacs SD and Bazargan N *et al.* Hyperglycemia: an independent marker of in-hospital mortality in patients with undiagnosed diabetes. *J Clin Endocrinol Metab* 2002; **87** (3): 978–982.
63. Viberti G. The need for tighter control of cardiovascular risk factors in diabetic patients. *J Hypertens Suppl* 2003; **21** (Suppl. 1): S3–S6.
64. Arteagoitia JM, Larranaga MI and Rodrigues JL *et al.* Incidence, prevalence and coronary heart disease risk level in known Type 2 diabetes: a sentinel practice network study in the Basque country, Spain. *Diabetologia* 2003; **46** (7): 899–909.
65. Borch-Johnsen K, Lauritzen T, Glumer C and Sandbaek A. Screening for Type 2 diabetes – should it be now? *Diabet Med* 2003; **20** (3): 175–181.

9

A Paradigm Shift is Needed in the Primary Prevention of Type 2 Diabetes

Jaakko Tuomilehto

Primary Prevention of Type 2 Diabetes – the Current Paradigm

The primary prevention of Type 2 diabetes is based on the facts that (a) currently available treatments for diabetes are only partially successful in preventing complications, (b) the disease itself is degenerative and progressive, (c) secondary prevention is very costly, and (d) risk factors and natural history of Type 2 diabetes are known. Nevertheless, the primary prevention of Type 2 diabetes has not been considered to be a part of the everyday medical practice. The paradigm regarding the primary prevention of Type 2 diabetes has until now been centred around the questions 'Can Type 2 diabetes really be prevented?', 'Do both lifestyle modification and pharmacotherapy lead to reduced rates of Type 2 diabetes in high-risk subjects?' and 'Does Type 2 diabetes prevention work in different ethnic groups?'.

Today, evidence that we can prevent or delay the development of Type 2 diabetes is strong. In 2001, the results of the Diabetes Prevention Study (DPS) conducted in Finland were published.[1] A total of 522 persons with IGT were individually randomized to either an intensive lifestyle or a control intervention. During an average of 3.2 years of follow-up, diabetes incidence was reduced by 58 per cent in the intensive lifestyle group compared with the control group and the trial had to be closed prematurely. As a result, the Diabetes Prevention Program (DPP) in the US carried out an interim analysis and reported in 2002 results from their lifestyle intervention similar to that used in the Finnish study.[2] A total of 3234 persons from 27 centres were followed for 2.8 years, on average. The study arm

Prevention of Type 2 Diabetes Edited by Manfred Ganz
 ISBN: 0-470-85733-1

comparing standard lifestyle with intensive lifestyle intervention found a 58 per cent reduction in diabetes incidence. Additional data from the non-randomized Malmö feasibility study[3] and the Chinese Da Qing study,[4] both these studies also comprising subjects with IGT, also indicated that lifestyle intervention leads to a reduced risk of Type 2 diabetes.

Pharmacological interventions have also provided compelling evidence. One study arm of the DPP found that those who received metformin (and standard lifestyle), compared with standard lifestyle only, had a 31 per cent reduction in diabetes.[2] The STOPP-NIDDM trial conducted in Canada, Israel and Europe randomized 1429 persons (mean age 54.5 years, all with IGT) to either acarbose or placebo and followed them up for 3.3 years on average, and reported a 25 per cent reduction in incidence of diabetes.[5] In the TRIPOD trial Hispanic GDM women were randomized to placebo or the insulin-sensitizing drug troglitazone using a double-blind design.[6] During a median follow-up of 30 months on trial medication, the average annual incidence of Type 2 diabetes was 12.1 per cent in women randomized to troglitazone and 5.4 per cent in the placebo group ($p < 0.01$). Another Chinese study on IGT used both acarbose and metformin, showing that both these treatments lowered the risk of diabetes in relatively lean Chinese subjects with IGT.[7] The XENDOS (*Xenical in the Prevention of Diabetes in Obese Subjects*) trial used a weight loss agent, orlistat, compared with weight reduction with lifestyle alone for the prevention of Type 2 diabetes over a period of four years.[8] Overweight (BMI $\geq$ 30 kg/m^2) subjects aged 30–60 years of whom 21 per cent had IGT at baseline received lifestyle counselling every 2 weeks for the first 6 months of the study and thereafter monthly. At four years mean weight reduction was 3.0 kg in the placebo group and 5.8 kg in the orlistat group. Cumulative incidence of Type 2 diabetes was 9.0 per cent in the placebo group and 6.2 per cent in the orlistat group, with a 37 per cent risk reduction in the orlistat group compared with the placebo group.

These studies have formed the basis for the current paradigm in prevention of Type 2 diabetes.

1. People with IGT will benefit from preventive interventions.

2. Lifestyle intervention will result in greater benefits than interventions with antidiabetic drugs, but the combination of lifestyle intervention and antiobesity drug therapy may be the most efficacious.

3. To apply this knowledge from the RCTs in the population at large it would be necessary to screen for 2 hour post-challenge glucose to identify subjects with IGT.

4. The intervention in people with IGT will not necessarily prevent Type 2 diabetes, but may postpone its onset age.

Re-Defining the Paradigm of Primary Prevention of Type 2 Diabetes

Earlier, it was obvious that we did not know enough about the efficacy and the feasibility of the primary prevention of Type 2 diabetes and, without a sufficient data basis supporting the prevention, the discussion was accompanied with subtitles such as 'dream or reality', etc.[9] In the present, we know that prevention of Type 2 diabetes works; the need to prove it no longer exists. Whether Type 2 diabetes will eventually be prevented and the disease will become uncommon is far from obvious. All earlier studies that now provide the evidence basis for the primary prevention of Type 2 diabetes were carried out in subjects with IGT. IGT is an intermediate state from normoglycaemia to Type 2 diabetes and it is associated with an increased risk of cardiovascular disease and death.[10,11] Therefore, IGT may be considered not as a risk factor for Type 2 diabetes but rather a state preceding it.[12] There are other factors that may be considered as aetiological risk factors. To what extent the efforts to influence modifiable risk factors of Type 2 diabetes when blood glucose levels are still normal will influence the risk of Type 2 diabetes is not known. Due to these unresolved issues, it is now the time to redefine the paradigm of Type 2 diabetes prevention.

The new paradigm of prevention may include the following issues.

1. Population approach for the primary prevention of Type 2 diabetes in the community.

2. Definition of people at high risk of Type 2 diabetes.

3. Prevention of Type 2 diabetes in high-risk subjects before they have IGT.

4. The essential role of primary prevention actions for the prevention or postponement of complications of Type 2 diabetes.

5. Controlling costs of diabetes care.

I will summarize the main points of these issues in the following sections.

New Paradigm – A Population Approach for Prevention of Type 2 Diabetes

The basic principle of the population approach for the disease prevention is that preventive actions (a) are implemented in the entire community, (b) do not rely on identification of high-risk subjects and (c) will aim at reducing the risk of Type 2 diabetes at any level of risk, resulting in a shift of the entire distribution of modifiable risk factors towards lower levels.

In the population approach health information plays a central role. Information about the disease and its risk factors is essential, particularly how to control the risk factors in practice. Information must be systematic and repetitive.

Another cornerstone of the population approach is the modification of the environment. The introduction of policies, facilities and support services to promote the way of life that helps in making choices that are desirable will have the greatest impact on the entire population's lifestyles. This can often also include pricing policies, either tax on unhealthy choices or price reduction on choices wanted. If only unhealthy choices are available, it is not possible to achieve lifestyle changes that are required for the prevention of Type 2 diabetes. For, instance if schools only have vending machines with soft drinks and snacks and do not serve normal healthy food choices, it is not possible to get children to eat healthy food. Similarly, if no light traffic lanes or pavements for pedestrians exist but only streets for motor vehicles, it is not possible to get people to achieve commuting physical activity that is one of the most cost- and time-efficient ways to practice regular physical activity. Environmental changes are mostly carried out by other sectors of the society than the health sector, but it is the role and the responsibility of people in the health sector to act as experts and opinion leaders to make others aware of the problems and their potential solutions.

New Paradigm – Who is at High Risk?

By definition, persons at high risk for developing Type 2 diabetes are non-diabetic, but have a probability of getting Type 2 diabetes higher than the average in the population. Some people may think they have a high risk, typically if there is a positive family history of Type 2 diabetes or if a person is very obese, but usually people are not aware of their high-risk status or cannot quantify the level of risk. Much debate has been around early detection of undiagnosed Type 2 diabetes and we still lack RCT data on this question, and thus the evidence for screening for asymptomatic Type 2 diabetes is missing.[13] Recently, much attention has been around intermediate states such as IGT, since people with IGT will often become diabetic[12] and have an increased risk of death and cardiovascular disease (CVD).[10,11]

There are three general approaches for detecting people at high risk for Type 2 diabetes. The first is based on measuring blood glucose levels to detect non-diabetic people whose fasting or post-challenge blood glucose is located in the upper part of the glucose distribution. Since hyperglycaemia is a progressive condition, such people obviously have a higher probability to progress to Type 2 diabetes than those whose glucose levels are at the lower end of the distribution. We have to remember that Type 2 diabetes simply means that blood glucose concentration is above a certain threshold (more or less arbitrarily defined), and thus people whose glucose is near the threshold will be the most likely to progress to Type 2 diabetes. This means that the risk of Type 2 diabetes can be somewhat quantified: the higher the glucose the higher the risk. However, the rate of progression is not constant. Thus, if we measure blood glucose today and follow the cohort of people for several years, the largest number of new cases of Type 2 diabetes comes from the group of people whose glucose levels were considered normal at baseline. Therefore, having normal blood glucose does not mean that a person will not be at risk for Type 2 diabetes. Obviously this strategy would detect cases of undiagnosed diabetes, too, and could be also called screening for undetected diabetes.

The second approach is to rely on demographic (age, sex, socio-economic status, ethnic group etc.) and clinical characteristics and previous laboratory tests (avoiding the need for new laboratory or glycaemia testing) to estimate the probability of future Type 2 diabetes. Obviously the data available will be crude, not uniform from person to person and subject to biases and random errors. Risk quantification can be attempted but due to the data quality it will be very difficult and therefore the interpretation of the information available will be very subjective and the likelihood of both false positive and false negative conclusions is high. Also, there may be practical and logistic problems; for instance, laboratory data may not be available at the location where the subject is visiting the clinic, etc. This approach will not provide information about current glycaemic status and will not pick up undetected Type 2 diabetes.

The third approach uses questionnaire-type information on factors that can be considered to provide information of the presence and the degree of a number of a etiological factors for Type 2 diabetes, modifiable or non-modifiable. The parameters included in the questionnaire will be summed up either by computer or on paper and the summary score will give the risk probability. In principle, this approach can include any number of variables, but in practice it is necessary to restrict the items to the most important ones. Actually, the relative gain in introducing more factors into the final prediction model is marginal after the main factors are included. Also, if this kind of questionnaire is to be used by lay people, it is necessary to concentrate on the basic issues and avoid applications that require computer-based calculations. As shown by the Finnish Diabetes Risk Score, the accuracy of 10 year prediction of Type 2 diabetes was as high as 85 per cent.[14] This approach offers a practical screening method to identify people who are at risk of developing Type 2 diabetes. In order to develop such a risk estimation formula or score it is necessary to estimate the relative weights for different parameters included in the formula. This requires prospective data with multivariate analysis. The Finnish diabetes risk score was developed in such a way. Although this risk score may be to some extent population specific, it includes variables that are common risk factors for Type 2 diabetes in any population and therefore it may suit other populations as well, although cut points for body mass index and waist circumference may need to be adjusted. This is inexpensive, easy to apply and suitable for population-wide applications. Since no laboratory measurements are made in this approach, it leaves current glycaemic status ambiguous. However, this approach will serve as primary and cost-efficient screening tools, identifying a subgroup of the population in whom glycaemic testing may be targeted. A high risk score value indicates not only a high risk for developing Type 2 diabetes but also a high probability of having asymptomatic Type 2 diabetes. In addition to the Finnish diabetes risk score, other attempts to develop such methods with variable approaches have been reported.[15–21]

In summary, today we have a good possibility not only to detect asymptomatic Type 2 diabetes but also to determine the probability of quantifying the risk of Type 2 diabetes with inexpensive and non-invasive methods.

New Paradigm – True Primary Prevention: Targeting People Before Their Blood Glucose Values are Abnormal

The convincing results from the RCTs demonstrating the great potential for the prevention or postponement of Type 2 diabetes have been based on subjects who had IGT.[1–5,7] Thus, they already had abnormal glucose tolerance and one can argue whether these have been true primary prevention studies or whether these actually dealt with secondary prevention of hyperglycaemia. The primary prevention of Type 2 diabetes at best would mean to keep genetically or otherwise susceptible individuals normoglycaemic, not only preventing Type 2 diabetes from developing. Also, it has been shown that the risk of cardiovascular disease is already increased in people with IGT,[10,11] indicating that a lesser degree of hyperglycaemia is already deleterious to health. This suggests that the prevention of hyperglycaemia in general, not only at the level that is currently considered as Type 2 diabetes, is important. Thus far there are no data to show that it is possible to prevent the progression to Type 2 diabetes among high-risk subjects whose glucose levels are normal. What we know is that we can identify such high-risk subjects using easy tests such as history of Type 2 diabetes or Diabetes Risk Score.[14–21] Then, the additional questions remain: can we keep glucose levels normal in such people and, if so, how and for how long may they be able to avoid Type 2 diabetes? At the population level we know from recent history that in families who now have Type 2 diabetes earlier generations did not always have the disease, although by definition some of the family members carried Type 2 diabetes susceptibility genes. Everyday life in the past required considerable physical activity and obesity was still uncommon, thus keeping the genetically susceptible individual free of Type 2 diabetes. This has been probably best illustrated among the Pima Indians, among whom clinical diabetes was proven uncommon early in the 20th century.[22]

It would be important to demonstrate that this approach works in practice. While clinical trials on this question may not be carried out in the near future, data from community-based Type 2 diabetes prevention programmes such as the one recently started in Finland[23] will provide necessary data that can be useful for this assessment.

New Paradigm – Prevention of Complications of Type 2 Diabetes by Preventing Type 2 Diabetes Itself

Type 2 diabetes is a serious disease; not necessarily only due to high blood glucose but also due to multiple complications that are common in diabetic patients, they suffer a lot during their years with Type 2 diabetes. Most of the human tissues will be damaged from hyperglycaemia, either directly or mostly through other processes initiated or stimulated by hyperglycaemia. It is still unclear how acute and late complications of diabetes could be most effectively prevented. While the prevention of acute complications must always include the prevention of hypo- and hyperglycaemia, there has been a debate on the extent to which the control of blood glucose levels helps in preventing cardiovascular disease in Type 2 diabetes.[24] It is commonly known that a considerable proportion of Type 2 diabetes patients have cardiovascular disease already at the time of diagnosis[25,26] and that the risk of coronary or stroke death in Type 2 diabetes patients is equally high as in patients with previous myocardial infarction or stroke.[27] In many countries Type 2 diabetes is becoming the most common cause of end-stage renal disease and renal replacement therapy.[28] In principle, hyperglycaemia results in pathological processes in all tissues of the human body and, therefore, multiple complications occur. It has been also shown that excessive prandial glucose excursions that usually mark the early stages of the development of Type 2 diabetes acutely trigger a large number of reactions that increase cardiovascular risk. Acute glucose excursions are accompanied by a series of alterations in the coagulation system that is likely to increase the risk of thrombosis in diabetic patients.[29–35] The mechanisms by which acute hyperglycaemia may affect atherogenic process probably involve both nonenzymatic labile glycation[36] and the production of free radicals.[37] In labile glycation, glucose binds through a nonenzymatic bond with amino groups of circulating or vessel wall proteins, which subsequently rearrange to form the more stable Amadori-type early glycosylation products. These products continue to rearrange and will form advanced glycosylation end products (AGEs).[38] Once formed, AGE protein adducts are virtually irreversible. AGEs promote atherosclerotic effects through various non-receptor-mediated mechanisms (e.g. through extracellular matrix, functional alterations of regulatory proteins, lipoprotein modifications) and receptor-mediated mechanisms (e.g. inflammation promotion, induction of cellular proliferation, endothelial dysfunction).

The most convincing evidence of increased CHD risk related to abnormal glucose tolerance was provided by the DECODE study. In this project, individual data from many prospective cohort studies have been analysed jointly.[10,39–41] Death rates from all causes, CVD and CHD, were higher in diabetic subjects diagnosed by 2hPG criteria than in those not meeting these criteria. Significantly increased mortality was also observed in subjects with IGT, whereas there was no difference in mortality between subjects with IFG and those with normal fasting glucose. Multivariate Cox proportional hazard analyses showed that elevated 2hPG was an independent predictor of mortality from all causes, CVD and CHD, but elevated FPG alone was not. A high 2hPG was found to be associated with an increased risk of death, independent of the level of FPG, whereas increased mortality in people with elevated FPG was largely due to the simultaneous elevation of 2hPG. On the other hand, FPG did not add any predictive information once 2hPG was in the model. The largest absolute number of excess CVD deaths was observed in subjects with IGT, especially those with IGT but normal fasting glucose. The association between glucose and the incidence of CHD was assessed in five Finnish cohorts belonging to the DECODE study.[42] Multivariate Cox regression analyses showed that the hazard ratio for one standard deviation increase in 2hPG and FPG after logarithmic transformation was 1.17 (95 per cent CI 1.05–1.30) and 1.05 (0.94–1.17) for CHD incidence, respectively.

It is clear from sub-group analyses of controlled trials that antihypertensive drug treatment in hypertensive patients with diabetes[43–46] and statin therapy in those who have high serum cholesterol[47,48] are efficient ways to prevent CHD in diabetic patients. In addition, it is currently recommended that patients with Type 2 diabetes should receive acetosalicylic acid treatment if not contraindicated.[49] The multifactorial, aggressive approach to influence the multiple risk factors for CHD in diabetic patients has recently been well demonstrated by the Steno-2 study.[50] Diabetes is one of the strongest factors in vascular pathology through multiple pathways, not exclusively by hyperglycaemia, and hyperglycaemia may activate other pathophysiological pathways.[51] Thus, it is important that several if not all of these metabolic abnormalities are corrected, or preferably prevented, in diabetic patients. Otherwise, it seems inevitable that they will continue to suffer from disproportionate rates of cardiovascular disease, in particular in women.[52]

The most logical way to prevent the negative health consequences of Type 2 diabetes seems to be the prevention of Type 2 diabetes itself. Since hyperglycaemia is the necessary although not sufficient condition for microvascular complications of Type 2 diabetes, they can be fully prevented by preventing diabetes. However, to what extent it is possible to prevent the development of CVD in people with asymptomatic hyperglycaemia is not known, since we lack trial data on this question. What is known, however, is that the worsening of hyperglycaemia can be effectively halted by lifestyle intervention[1,2] and certain antidiabetic drugs.[2,5] Whether this will then also result in a delay in the development of cardiovascular disease is still unclear. The recent analyses of the STOP-NIDDM trial data have revealed statistically significant reductions in cardiovascular event rates in patients receiving acarbose compared with placebo.[53] Since acarbose specifically reduces postprandial glucose excursions, this is the first demonstration that lowering postprandial glucose may lead to a reduction in cardiovascular events. Such controlled clinical outcome trials among subjects with asymptomatic hyperglycaemia are now underway, but the results from these will only be available after several years. Meanwhile, the only way to make clinical treatment decisions in such subjects is to make inferences from the observational epidemiological data and pathophysiological studies.

New Paradigm – How Could Money for Diabetes Care be Allocated in A More Efficient Way?

Diabetes is a very costly disease. In Western countries 10–15 per cent of the total health budget goes to treatment of diabetes and its complications.[54,55] Most of it, 60–70 per cent, is used to treat cardiovascular and renal complications of Type 2 diabetes,[56] i.e. the tertiary prevention of Type 2 diabetes. Money spent for the secondary prevention of Type 2 diabetes, i.e. for case-finding, diagnosis and clinical management of patients with Type 2 diabetes, is much less than needed for treatment of complications. According to the clinical trial data on the prevention of Type 2 diabetes in subjects with IGT, 10–20 IGT subjects need to be managed with reinforced lifestyle intervention for a year in order to prevent one case of Type 2 diabetes.[57] Thus, such intervention is extremely efficient and also cost effective. How much money is currently used from national health budgets of developed countries for the primary prevention of Type 2 diabetes? Almost nothing. Even in Finland, where the first national Type 2 diabetes prevention programme has been launched,[23] only about 1 million Euros per year have been allocated for it, in comparison to about 550 million Euros used for diabetes care in Finland,[58] i.e. 0.18 per cent of all costs of diabetes care. At the same time, in Western countries health administrators and decision makers are distressed because there is not enough money for health care. Consequently, the strategy in many countries at the national and local level has been to cut preventive health care in order to assure tertiary care. Such a formula will never be able to solve the problem of imbalance between the health care resources available and the demand. It is obvious that the allocation of funds for the prevention and care of Type 2 diabetes is completely distorted.

Without effective implementation of the primary prevention of Type 2 diabetes health care budgets cannot be properly managed in the future. The situation is worst in developing countries, where Type 2 diabetes today is already almost as big a health problem as in developed countries, and in some of them even bigger. Since their resources for secondary and tertiary prevention of Type 2 diabetes are very limited, patients are suffering from severe complications without care, relying on their relatives. This in turn will impact the development of the country and leads to inefficient use of workforce. It has been estimated that during the next 15 years there will be a 30–50 per cent increase in the number of patients with Type 2 diabetes,[59] and at the same time the number of Type 2 diabetes patients with duration sufficient to produce late complications will increase drastically. This will mean that the costs of the secondary and tertiary prevention of Type 2 diabetes will probably double, reaching then 20–30 per cent of the total health care costs. Governments seem not be too worried about this, although some high officers sometimes express their concern of a potential Type 2 diabetes epidemic in their speeches.

An effective lifestyle intervention programme such as used in the DPS will definitely postpone the development of Type 2 diabetes and, most likely, to the corresponding degree also its late complications. Thus, the need for the secondary and tertiary prevention of Type 2 diabetes would decrease. My simple and non-scientific calculations based on the Finnish DPS results on the potential for prevention of Type 2 diabetes in high-risk subjects[1] and the costs of Type 2 diabetes care in Finland[58] indicate that every Euro used for such a primary prevention programme will in 10–20 years' time save about 100 Euros. Thus, if we would use only 20 million Euros for Type 2 diabetes prevention now (about 3.5 per cent of all annual costs of diabetes care), we would save as much as 2 billion Euros in the future. This should be a rather attractive investment, but obviously it would take some time before the savings would materialize. Actually, since I am talking about primary prevention, the savings would never be seen on the accounts of health administration.

Comment

At present, we know that Type 2 diabetes can be very effectively prevented in high-risk subjects in all ethnic groups and in different cultural settings. In addition, we know how to identify high-risk subjects for Type 2 diabetes. So, it should be easy and simple to prevent Type 2 diabetes worldwide. However, things are not so simple. First, we must acknowledge that knowing is not enough; it is necessary to apply the knowledge. What has happened since the data from the above-mentioned RCTs on Type 2 diabetes prevention in people with IGT have been considered by the medical community and by diabetes experts? In the United States, the Expert Committee on Diagnostic Criteria for diabetes reduced the lower cut-point of impaired fasting glucose from 6.1 mmol/l to 5.6 mmol/l and still consider an oral glucose tolerance test virtually not necessary.[60] In China, IGT is considered as a condition where certain antidiabetic drugs may be used. In Finland, a national Type 2 diabetes programme based on lifestyle intervention in people at high risk has been launched.[23] In Sweden, no formal recommendations have been proposed.

It is interesting to note that China, still considered as a developing country (but developing very fast), which has been renowned for its healthy diet and high level of physical activity, both of which are deteriorating with the fast development, chose a pharmacologic model. Similarly interesting is that Finland, which has a high level of medical technology, is basing Type 2 diabetes prevention on lifestyle issues. It is not easy to understand why the US strategy is to screen for fasting plasma glucose and label subjects on that basis 'prediabetic' when all the intervention studies with excellent results have been based on IGT, i.e. elevated 2 hour glucose. This strategy certainly does not apply the knowledge from the successful intervention trials that even showed in the US that the risk reduction by lifestyle intervention worked equally well in ethnic minority groups (Native American Indians, African Americans and Asian/Pacific origin people) and in Caucasians,[2] even though this was questioned during the trial.[61]

The new paradigm for the prevention of Type 2 diabetes should be based on the population strategy. A mass epidemic requires a mass prevention strategy. It should include all sectors of the society. Type 2 diabetes, a disease that results from genetic susceptibility and unhealthy lifestyle, cannot be prevented population-wide without such broad efforts. The population strategy can however be effective only when supported simultaneously by adequate services for people at high risk. During the past few decades it has been demonstrated that the CVD risk in the middle-aged population can be effectively prevented. While the management of high-risk subjects for CVD has dramatically improved, the changes in risk factor levels in the community have not been restricted to the high end of the risk factor distributions but the entire distributions of serum cholesterol and blood pressure have moved downwards.[62] The majority of the CVD cases always arise from the middle of the risk factor distribution where people have intermediate risk – be it blood pressure, cholesterol or 2 hour glucose – because there are so many people in the middle of the distribution (39). Since there will never be sufficient resources to lower the risk in this bulk of individuals with intermediate risk with medical services, the only way is to apply the population strategy.

Type 2 diabetes has its origin in genetic susceptibility[63] and in early development[64] and childhood. If we agree that genetic susceptibility is the necessary condition for Type 2 diabetes to develop, we can estimate its magnitude best by observing the lifetime risk of Type 2 diabetes in various populations. The cumulative incidence or its crude indicator, the prevalence, shows the proportion of people genetically susceptible. Since Type 2 diabetes develops slowly with a long asymptomatic period, the true prevalence can only be estimated by using the OGTT. The data for some specific populations such as the American Indians, Pacific Islanders and Asian Indians clearly show that in age groups over 50 or 60 years the prevalence of Type 2 diabetes is over 50 per cent.[65] The recent data from the DECODE study also shows that the prevalence in Europeans aged 70 years or above is over 50 per cent.[66] When over 20 per cent of the elderly populations have IGT, it means that the vast majority of humans may have an abnormal glucose tolerance during their lifetime, indicating that the majority of people probably carry genes permitting Type 2 diabetes to develop. This will further stress the importance of the population strategy in the primary prevention of Type 2 diabetes.

There are now simple and inexpensive questionnaire-based screening tools to detect people at high risk for Type 2 diabetes.[14–21] Most of them are non-invasive, and can be easily applied population-wide to make people themselves aware of their level of risk, or be used by the health-care sector systematically. It is not yet clear how these ‘diabetes risk scores’ are best applied as a part of Type 2 diabetes prevention at the population level. Screening for diabetes and glucose tolerance by testing the level of glycaemia biochemically has been debated and found to be neither reliable nor cost-effective.[67,68] Also, no screening efforts with subsequent intervention studies have been performed for asymptomatic diabetes in order to evaluate possible advantages and disadvantages of screening. Therefore, intensified case-finding among health-care users and opportunistic screening in high-risk groups can be encouraged.[69]

Now the simple and reliable risk scores are available, the screening issue can be reconsidered. People who have a high-risk score value at screening may not have diabetes or even impaired glucose regulation, but they still have elevated risk of developing Type 2 diabetes in the future and their risk of premature mortality is also increased.[70] This group is the target group for true primary prevention of hyperglycaemia and Type 2 diabetes.

It is obvious that the preventive measures against Type 2 diabetes should start during the intrauterine period and continue throughout life from early childhood on. People born small and thin and becoming heaviest within their birth cohort during childhood have the highest lifetime risk of Type 2 diabetes.[64] When the relative weight and obesity in childhood have increased continuously, this has a major effect on the overall risk of Type 2 diabetes and, in particular, to the age of onset of its severe complications. Therefore, efforts to reverse this increasing obesity trend in young people, which is further associated with decreasing levels of physical activity, are urgently needed. Without reversing these unfavourable trends, it is not possible to prevent Type 2 diabetes effectively in the future. Although it may be argued that is difficult or not possible to reverse these trends in obesity and physical inactivity in childhood, without trying the pessimism and nihilism is not justified. Fortunately, we have some data on this issue. In 1992, the education ministry in Singapore commenced a ‘trim and fit’ programme for school children to reduce obesity and improve physical fitness.[71] Overweight students, parents and teachers were targeted. Nutrition education was integrated into the curriculum, special exercise programmes were established (for the overweight) and food and beverages available in the school environment were controlled. By 2000 the prevalence of obesity declined from 17 to 15 per cent in 11–12 year olds and 16 to 13 per cent in 15–16 year olds. Similar programmes are urgently needed elsewhere, too.

References

1. Tuomilehto J, Lindström J and Eriksson J *et al.* Prevention of Type 2 diabetes mellitus by changes in lifestyle among subjects with impaired glucose tolerance. *N Engl J Med* 2001; **344**: 1343–1350.
2. Knowler WC, Barrett-Connor E and Fowler SE *et al.* Reduction in the incidence of Type 2 diabetes with lifestyle intervention or metformin. *N Engl J Med* 2002; **346**: 393–403.
3. Eriksson KF and Lindgärde F. Prevention of Type 2 (non-insulin-dependent) diabetes mellitus by diet and physical exercise. The 6-year Malmo feasibility study. *Diabetologia* 1991; **34**: 891–898.
4. Pan XR, Li GW and Hu YH *et al.* Effects of diet and exercise in preventing NIDDM in people with impaired glucose tolerance: the Da Qing IGT and Diabetes Study. *Diabetes Care* 1997; **20**: 537–544.
5. Chiasson JL, Josse RG, Gomis R, Hanefeld M, Karasik A and Laakso M, for The STOP-NIDDM Trial Research Group. Acarbose for prevention of Type 2 diabetes mellitus; the STOP-NIDDM randomised trial. *Lancet* 2002; **359**: 2072–2077.
6. Buchanan TA, Xiang AH and Peters RK *et al.* Preservation of pancreatic B-cell function and prevention of Type 2 diabetes by pharmacological treatment of insulin resistance in high-risk Hispanic women. *Diabetes* 2002; **51**: 2796–2803.
7. Wenying Y, Lixiang L and Jinwu Q *et al.* The preventative effect of acarbose and metformin on the progression to diabetes mellitus in the IGT population: a 3-year multicentre prospective study. *Chin J Endocrinol Metab* 2001; **17**: 131–135.
8. Torgerson JS, Hauptman J, Boldrin MN and Sjostrom L. Xenical in the Prevention of Diabetes in Obese Subjects (XENDOS) Study: a randomized study of orlistat as an adjunct to lifestyle changes for the prevention of Type 2 diabetes in obese patients. *Diabetes Care* 2004; **27**: 155–161.
9. Tuomilehto J, Alberti KGMM and Mazze R (eds). Primary prevention of non-insulin-dependent diabetes mellitus: a dream or reality? In *Frontiers of Diabetes Research: Current Trends in Non Insulin Dependent Diabetes Mellitus*. Amsterdam: Elsevier, 1989, pp. 101–115.
10. DECODE Study Group. Glucose tolerance and cardiovascular mortality: comparison of fasting and 2-hour diagnostic criteria. *Arch Intern Med* 2001; **161**: 397–405.
11. Qiao Q, Lindström J, Valle TT and Tuomilehto J. Progression to clinically diagnosed and treated diabetes from impaired glucose tolerance and impaired fasting glycaemia. *Diabet Med* 2003; **20**: 1027–1033.
12. Unwin N, Shaw J, Zimmet P and Alberti KG. Impaired glucose tolerance and impaired fasting glycaemia: the current status on definition and intervention. *Diabet Med* 2002; **19**: 708–723.
13. Engelgau MM, Narayan KMV and Herman WH. Screening for Type 2 diabetes. *Diabetes Care* 2000; **23**: 1563–1580.
14. Lindstrom J and Tuomilehto J. The diabetes risk score: a practical tool to predict Type 2 diabetes risk. *Diabetes Care* 2003; **26**: 725–31.
15. Herman WH, Smith PJ, Thompson TJ, Engelgau MM and Aubert R. A new and simple questionnaire to identify persons at increased risk for undiagnosed diabetes mellitus. *Diabetes Care* 1995; **18**: 382–387.
16. Ruige JB, de Neeling JN, Kostense PJ, Bouter LM and Heine RJ. Performance of an NIDDM screening questionnaire based on symptoms and risk factors. *Diabetes Care* 1997; **20**: 491–496.
17. Baan CA, Ruige JB, Stolk RP, Witteman JC, Dekker JM and Heine RJ *et al.* Performance of a predictive model to identify undiagnosed diabetes in a health care setting. *Diabetes Care* 1999; **22**: 213–219.

18. Griffin S, Little P, Hales C, Kinmonth A and Wareham N. Diabetes risk score: towards earlier detection of Type 2 diabetes in general practice. *Diabetes Metab Res Rev* 2000; **16**: 164–171.
19. Lawrence J, Bennett P, Young A and Robinson A. Screening for diabetes in general practice: cross sectional population study. *BMJ* 2001; **323**: 548–551.
20. Rolandsson O, Hägg E, Nilson M, Hallmans G, Mincheva-Nilsson L and Lernmark Å. Prediction of diabetes with body mass index, oral glucose tolerance test and islet cell autoantibodies in a regional population. *J Intern Med* 2001; **249**: 279–288.
21. Stern MP, Williams K and Haffner SM. Identification of persons at high risk for Type 2 diabetes mellitus: do we need the oral glucose tolerance test? *Ann Intern Med* 2002; **136** (8): 575–581.
22. Bennett PH, Burch TA and Miller M. Diabetes mellitus in American (Pima) Indians. *Lancet* 1971; **ii**: 125–128.
23. Finnish Diabetes Association. Programme for the prevention of Type 2 diabetes in Finland http://www.diabetes.fi/english/prevention/programme/index.html. 2003. Tampere.
24. Heine RJ and Dekker JM. Beyond postprandial hyperglycaemia: metabolic factors associated with cardiovascular disease. *Diabetologia* 2002; **45**: 461–475.
25. Haffner SM, Stern MP, Hazuda HP, Mitchell BD and Patterson JK. Cardiovascular risk factors in confirmed prediabetic individuals. Does the clock for coronary heart disease start ticking before the onset of clinical diabetes. *JAMA* 1990; **263**: 2893–2898.
26. McPhillips JB, Barrett-Connor E and Wingard DI. Cardiovascular disease risk factors prior to the diagnosis of impaired glucose tolerance and non-insulin dependant diabetes in a community of older adults. *Am J Epidemiol* 1990; **131**: 443–453.
27. Haffner SM, Lehto S, Ronnemaa T, Pyorala K and Laakso M. Mortality from coronary heart disease in subjects with Type 2 diabetes and in nondiabetic subjects with and without prior myocardial infarction. *New Engl J Med* 1998; **339**: 229–234.
28. *United States Renal Data System: 1999 Annual Data Report*. MD: Bethesda. National Institute of Diabetes and Digestive and Kidney Diseases.
29. Jones RL and Peterson CM. Reduced fibrinogen survival in diabetes mellitus. A reversible phenomenon. *J Clin Invest* 1979; **63**: 485–493.
30. Jones RL. Fibrinopeptide-A in diabetes mellitus. Relation to levels of blood glucose, fibrinogen disappearance, and hemodynamic changes. *Diabetes* 1985; **34**: 836–843.
31. Ceriello A, Giugliano D, Quatraro A, Dello Russo P, Marchi E and Torella R. Hyperglycemia may determine fibrinopeptide a plasma level increase in humans. *Metabolism* 1989; **38**: 1162–1163.
32. Ceriello A, Giugliano D, Quatraro A, Dello Russo P and Torella R. Blood glucose may condition factor VII levels in diabetic and normal subjects. *Diabetologia* 1998; **31**: 889–891.
33. Ceriello A, Giacomello R, Stel G, Motz E, Taboga C, Tonutti L, Pirisi M, Falleti E and Bartoli E. Hyperglycemia-induced thrombin formation in diabetes. The possible role of oxidative stress. *Diabetes* 1995; **44**: 924–928.
34. Ceriello A, Taboga C, Tonutti L, Giacomello R, Stel L, Motz E and Pirisi M. Post-meal coagulation activation in diabetes mellitus: the effect of acarbose. *Diabetologia* 1996; **39**: 469–473.
35. Sakamoto T, Ogawa H, Kawano H, Hirai N, Miyamoto S, Takazoe K, Soejima H, Kugiyama K, Yoshimura M and Yasue H. Rapid change of platelet aggregability in acute hyperglycemia. Detection by a novel laser-light scattering method. *Thromb Haemost* 2000; **83**: 475–479.
36. Ceriello A, Quatraro A and Giugliano D. New insights on non-enzymatic glycosylation may lead to therapeutic approaches for the prevention of diabetic complications. *Diabet Med* 1992; **9**: 297–299.

37. Ceriello A, Bortolotti N, Falleti E, Taboga C, Tonutti L, Crescentini A, Motz E, Lizzio S, Russo A and Bartoli E. Total radical-trapping antioxidant parameter in NIDDM patients. *Diabetes Care* 1997; **20**: 194–197.
38. Mullarkey CJ, Edelstein D and Brownlee M. Free radical generation by early glycation products: a mechanism for accelerated atherogenesis in diabetes. *Biochem Biophys Res Commun* 1990; **173**: 932–939.
39. DECODE Study Group. Will new diagnostic criteria for diabetes mellitus change phenotype of patients with diabetes? Reanalysis of European epidemiological data. DECODE Study Group on behalf of the European Diabetes Epidemiology Study Group. *BMJ* 1998; **317**: 371–375.
40. DECODE Study Group. Glucose tolerance and mortality: comparison of WHO and American Diabetes Association diagnostic criteria. The DECODE Study Group. European Diabetes Epidemiology Group. Diabetes Epidemiology: collaborative analysis of diagnostic criteria in Europe. *Lancet* 1999; **354**: 617–621.
41. DECODE Study Group. Is the current definition for diabetes relevant to mortality risk from all-cause and cardiovascular and non-cardiovascular disease? *Diabetes Care* 2003; **26** 688–696.
42. Qiao Q, Pyorala K, Pyorala M, Nissinen A, Lindstrom J, Tilvis R and Tuomilehto J. Two-hour glucose is a better risk predictor for incident coronary heart disease and cardiovascular mortality than fasting glucose. *Eur Heart J* 2002; **23**: 1267–1275.
43. Curb JD, Pressel SL, Cutler JA, Savage PJ, Applegate WB, Black H, Camel G, Davis BR, Frost PH, Gonzalez N, Guthrie G, Oberman A, Rutan GH and Stamler J. Effect of diuretic-based antihypertensive treatment on cardiovascular disease risk in older diabetic patients with isolated systolic hypertension. Systolic Hypertension in the Elderly Program Cooperative Research Group. *JAMA* 1996; **276**: 1886–1892.
44. UK Prospective Diabetes Study Group. Tight blood pressure control and risk of macrovascular and microvascular complications in Type 2 diabetes: UKPDS 38. UK Prospective Diabetes Study Group. *BMJ* 1998; **317**: 703–713.
45. Tuomilehto J, Rastenyte D, Birkenhager WH, Thijs L, Antikainen R, Bulpitt CJ, Fletcher AE, Forette F, Goldhaber A, Palatini P, Sarti C and Fagard R. Effects of calcium-channel blockade in older patients with diabetes and systolic hypertension. Systolic Hypertension in Europe Trial Investigators. *New Engl J Med* 1999; **340**: 677–684.
46. The ALLHAT Officers and Coordinators for the Collaborative Research Group. Major outcomes in high-risk hypertensive patients randomized to angiotensin-converting enzyme inhibitor or calcium channel blocker vs diuretic: The Antihypertensive and Lipid-Lowering Treatment to Prevent Heart Attack Trial (ALLHAT). *JAMA* 2002; **288**: 2981–2997.
47. Pyorala K, Pedersen TR, Kjekshus J, Faergeman O, Olsson AG and Thorgeirsson G. Cholesterol lowering with simvastatin improves prognosis of diabetic patients with coronary heart disease. A subgroup analysis of the Scandinavian Simvastatin Survival Study (4S). *Diabetes Care* 1997; **20**: 614–620.
48. Heart Protection Study Collaborative Group. MRC/BHF Heart Protection Study of cholesterol lowering with simvastatin in 5963 people with diabetes: a randomised placebo-controlled trial. *Lancet* 2003; **361**: 2005–2016.
49. American Diabetes Association. Aspirin therapy in diabetes. *Diabetes Care* 2002; **25**: S78–S79.
50. Gaede P, Vedel P, Larsen N, Jensen GV, Parving HH and Pedersen O. Multifactorial intervention and cardiovascular disease in patients with Type 2 diabetes. *New Engl J Med* 2003; **348**: 383–393.
51. Heine RJ and Dekker JM. Beyond postprandial hyperglycaemia: metabolic factors associated with cardiovascular disease. *Diabetologia* 2002; **45**: 461–475.

52. Orchard TJ. The impact of gender and general risk factors on the occurrence of atherosclerotic vascular disease in non-insulin-dependent diabetes mellitus. *Ann Med* 1996; **28**: 323–333.
53. Chiasson JL, Josse RG, Gomis R, Hanefeld M, Karasik A and Laakso M. Acarbose treatment and the risk of cardiovascular disease and hypertension in patients with impaired glucose tolerance: the STOP-NIDDM trial. *JAMA* 2003; **290**: 486–494.
54. American Diabetes Association. Economic costs of diabetes in the U.S. in 2002. *Diabetes Care* 2003; **26**: 917–932.
55. Jönsson B. Diabetes—the cost of illness and the cost of control. *Acta Med Scand* 1983; **671** (Suppl. I): 19–27.
56. Williams D, Tuomilehto J and Björk S. *The Economics of Diabetes Care. An International Perspective.* 2000. London: Blackwell.
57. Tuomilehto J and Lindström J. The major diabetes prevention trials. *Curr Diabetes Rep* 2003; **3**: 115–122.
58. Kangas T. The consumption and direct costs of health care services among persons with diabetes in Helsinki. A case-controlled cross-sectional study of the fiscal year 1997. *KELA Sosiaali- ja terveysturvan tutkimuksia* 67. 2002. Helsinki.
59. King H, Aubert RE and Herman WH. Global burden of diabetes, 1995–2025: prevalence, numerical estimates, and projections. *Diabetes Care* 1998; **21**: 1414–1431.
60. American Diabetes Association. The Expert Committee on the Diagnosis and Classification of Diabetes Mellitus. Follow-up report on the diagnosis of diabetes mellitus. *Diabetes Care* 2003; **26**: 3160–3167.
61. Tataranni PA and Bogardus C. Changing habits to delay diabetes. *N Engl J Med* 2001; **344**: 1390–1392.
62. Kuulasmaa K, Tunstall-Pedoe H, Dobson A, Fortmann S, Sans S, Tolonen H, Evans A, Ferrario M and Tuomilehto J, for the WHO MONICA Project. Estimation of contribution of changes in classic risk factors to trends in coronary-event rates across the WHO MONICA Project populations. *Lancet* 2000; **355**: 675–687.
63. McCarthy M. Progress in defining the molecular basis of Type 2 diabetes mellitus through susceptibility-gene identification. *Human Mol Genet* 2004; **13**: R33–R41.
64. Forsén T, Eriksson J, Tuomilehto J, Reunanen A, Osmond C and Barker D. The fetal and childhood growth of persons who develop Type 2 diabetes. *Ann Intern Med* 2000; **133**: 176–182.
65. De Courten M, Bennett PH, Tuomilehto J and Zimmet P. Epidemiology of NIDDM in non-Europids. In *International Textbook of Diabetes Mellitus*, 2nd edn, Alberti KGMM, Zimmet P, DeFronzo RA and Keen H (eds). 1997. London: Wiley, pp. 143–170.
66. The DECODE Study Group. Age- and sex-specific prevalences of diabetes and impaired glucose regulation in 13 European cohorts. *Diabetes Care* 2003; **26**: 61–69.
67. Enelgau M, Narayan V and Herman WH. Screening for Type 2 diabetes. *Diabetes Care* 2000; **23**: 1563–1580.
68. American Diabetes Association. Diabetes care. Screening for Type 2 diabetes. *Diabetes Care* 2003; **26**: 521–524.
69. Borch-Johnsen K, Lauritzen T, Glumer C and Sandbaek A. Screening for Type 2 diabetes – should it be now? *Diabet Med* 2003; **20**: 175–181.
70. Spijkerman A, Griffin S, Dekker J, Nijpels G and Wareham NJ. What is the risk of mortality for people who are screen positive in a diabetes screening programme but who do not have diabetes on biochemical testing? Diabetes screening programmes from a public health perspective. *J Med Screen* 2002; **9**: 187–190.
71. Toh CM, Cutter J and Chew SK. School based intervention has reduced obesity in Singapore. *BMJ* 2002; **324**: 427.

10

The Behaviour Change Process

Frank J. Snoek and **Richard R. Rubin**

Introduction

Type 2 diabetes has been long linked with behavioural factors, in particular sedentary behaviour and unhealthy dietary habits. Based on the results from three randomized controlled prevention trials, we now can conclude that effective lifestyle intervention can prevent or delay the progression to Type 2 diabetes in groups at high risk, such as overweight people with impaired glucose tolerance.[1–3] Moreover, the Diabetes Prevention Program (DPP) convincingly demonstrated that lifestyle intervention is more effective in reducing the incidence of Type 2 diabetes than blood glucose lowering medication in people at risk, and that this effect is robust across gender and ethnicity. Based on these results, the American Diabetes Association (ADA) recommends to offer counselling on weight loss as well as instruction on increasing physical activity to all those identified as having 'pre-diabetes'.[4] Besides face-to-face programmes for individuals identified as being at risk for Type 2 diabetes, community-oriented interventions are needed to promote healthy lifestyles and reduce the risk of Type 2 diabetes in the general population. The dramatically increasing prevalence of overweight in Western societies, and particularly among children and adolescents in minority groups, is a public health issue that warrants an 'ecological' approach, targeting lifestyle changes at the individual, organizational and community levels.[5] In this chapter we will focus on behaviour change strategies on the individual level, building on evidence from health psychology literature and the large diabetes prevention trials. While behaviour change is in essence an individual process, we should acknowledge the importance of cultural and social norms that impact on individuals' attitudes,

Prevention of Type 2 Diabetes Edited by Manfred Ganz
 ISBN: 0-470-85733-1

health beliefs and self-care behaviours.[6,7] Certainly, contextual factors play an important role, affecting the entire population exposed to them. By affecting policies of companies, schools, government agencies and other organizations whose decisions influence many people, it may be possible to change the unhealthy environment and thereby change lifestyle behaviours at a population level.[8] For example, the pricing of health foods in supermarkets and the food contents of vending machines at schools and work sites influence eating behaviours. Making sports facilities available for individuals of lower economic status can increase physical activity and thereby reduce obesity rates.[9,10]

The large diabetes prevention trials have proven that the onset of diabetes can be delayed by means of lifestyle changes. The question we now face is how this encouraging finding can be translated and disseminated in the real world, i.e. outside research settings. How can lifestyle modification be effectively achieved and maintained in people identified as having pre-diabetes, either by routine examination or screening? What are the key elements of successful lifestyle counselling? Clearly, simply telling people they need to eat less and exercise more is not enough. In order to be effective lifestyle counsellors, we need to appreciate the complexity of the behaviour change process and understand the factors that mediate changes in lifestyle.

Readiness to Change

Lifestyle interventions can only be effective in so far as participants sign up and actively engage in the programme. For the purpose of the three major diabetes prevention trials, potential participants were actively recruited, screened and stimulated to join the programme. In daily practice obviously the situation is different. Still, once a person at risk has been identified as having pre-diabetes, either by screening or clinical examination, he or she can be stimulated to engage in a lifestyle programme by informational mailings, referrals and personal communication. Informing people of the positive results from the Finnish Diabetes Study (FDS) and Diabetes Prevention Program (DPP) can help to raise their awareness and willingness to consider lifestyle changes, and can reinforce their current efforts towards a healthier lifestyle. One cannot, however, force people to be motivated. The intention to make behavioural changes in order to gain the demonstrated health benefits needs to be intrinsic, i.e. must come from the person him- or herself, based on informed choice.[11]

We cannot assume, however, that all people at risk for Type 2 diabetes are intrinsically motivated and ready to make the necessary changes in their lifestyle. Social cognition theories, such as the health belief model,[12] theory of planned behaviour[13] and self-regulation theory,[14] predict that in order for people to be motivated to make changes in their lifestyle they need to perceive themselves as at risk and see more benefits from making the required changes than 'costs'. This points to the importance of risk perception and perceived seriousness regarding diabetes and related complications. Studies that have explored risk perception in diabetes suggest overall relatively low levels of awareness in people with an increased risk for developing Type 2 diabetes.[15–17] Importantly, people with impaired glucose tolerance generally do not experience clear signs and symptoms from their condition that prompt them to seek medical advice.[18] Even if people with pre-diabetes do appreciate the risks and potential health benefits from lifestyle changes, they may not come into action, due to lack of self-confidence or self-efficacy.[19] Particularly in the area of weight loss, failing to lose or maintain weight over time is a common experience, negatively impacting people's self-confidence to achieve the necessary changes in dietary behaviour, which ultimately may result in a psychological state of 'learned helplessness'.[20]

In tailoring intervention strategies to the needs of people at risk for developing diabetes, it is important to distinguish between those not aware or appreciative of the health risks involved and with no intention to make changes in their lifestyle ('precontemplators') and persons who are aware and 'ready to change', but unsure about their capability to meet the behavioural demands.[21] In the latter case, enhancing the person's sense of self-efficacy in the area of lifestyle change, rather than communicating risk information, should be the first step of the intervention (see Figure 10.1).

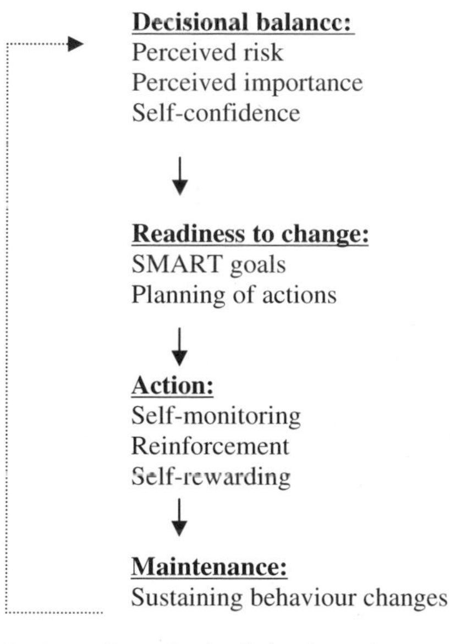

FIGURE 10.1 Steps in the behaviour change process

Goal Setting

Goal setting has been recognized as an important element in the process of behaviour modification. The likelihood of behaviour changes to occur is greatest when based on goals that are 'SMART', i.e. specific, measurable, agreed, realistic and time limited.[22] Successful change counselling involves helping participants use pro-active coping skills, such as setting realistic, individual goals and planning concrete actions.[23]

It is important to note that the Da Qing, Finnish Diabetes Study and Diabetes Prevention Program set multiple but fairly modest, and specific, goals with regard to weight loss, dietary changes and physical activity, which were tailored to the individual. With regard to weight loss, participants in the Da Qing study with a BMI > 25 were encouraged to lose weight (until they reached a BMI of 23) at a rate of 0.5 to 1.0 kg/month. This would represent a weight loss of about eight per cent. In the FDS the weight loss goal for all participants was five per cent of baseline body weight and seven per cent in the DPP. Participants in the DPP were encouraged to lose weight at the rate of 1–2 pounds each week during the first 20–24 weeks of the intervention.

As to calorie consumption, in the Da Qing and FDS the goals for total fat and saturated fat were <30 per cent and <10 per cent respectively. In the DPP the goal was <25 per cent of calories as fat. The DPP set total daily calorie goals as well. All interventions encouraged use of low-fat milk and meat products, soft margarines and vegetable oils high in mono-unsaturated fatty acids, to decrease the percentage of total fat and saturated fat in participants' diets. They were also encouraged to increase the amount of fibre, by eating more whole-grain cereals, fruits and vegetables.

All studies set clearly defined goals for physical activity. Participants in the Da Qing exercise and combined diet and exercise group were asked to increase their daily activity by the equivalent of at least 20 minutes of brisk walking a day if they were over 50 years old and had cardiovascular disease or arthritis, or at least twice that amount if they were younger and had no risk factors. The goal for physical activity in the FDS was lower; participants were encouraged to exercise at a moderate level for 30 minutes a day (equivalent to brisk walking). The goal for DPP participants was lower still; they were encouraged to exercise at a moderate level for about 20 minutes a day, adding up to 150 minutes per week.

Supporting Behaviour Change

Literature pertaining to weight loss and physical activity in adults suggests that theory-based, multi-component behaviour change programmes are most promising.[8,24] Typical elements of such programmes are patient goal setting, written diet and exercise prescriptions, use of self-monitoring techniques (food and activity records), individual and/or group counselling, frequent contact with staff and follow-ups.

All three diabetes prevention programmes asked participants to keep records of what they ate for purposes of self-monitoring. These records were also used to make periodic adjustments in individual meal plans to better meet individual needs. All interventions provided substantial support to help participants reach their activity goals, including individual guidance in choosing activities, and supervised, individually tailored, exercise sessions. Frequent staff contact was an important element of all three interventions.

In the DA Qing study, diet arm participants received individual counselling from physicians concerning daily food intake (frequency unspecified). In addition, counselling sessions in small groups at diet arm clinics were offered weekly for 1 month, monthly for 3 months, and every 3 months for the rest of the study (6 years).

In the FDS, participants had a total of about 20 sessions with a nutritionist (seven during the first year of the study), as well as an unspecified number of individual and group exercise sessions. The dietary advice was tailored to each subject on the basis of 3 day food records completed four times a year. FDS participants also received individual guidance on increasing their levels of physical activity. Endurance exercise (e.g. walking, jogging and swimming) was recommended as a way to increase aerobic capacity and improve cardio-respiratory fitness. Supervised, progressive, individually tailored circuit type training sessions were also offered with the aim of improving the functional capacity and strength of the large muscle groups.

The DPP was the most intensive in terms of contact with clinic staff, where participants had 16 individual sessions with their case manager during the first 24 weeks of the study, twice monthly contact during the duration of the study, optional supervised exercise sessions twice each week and 'healthy living' classes offered for 4–6 weeks four times each year.

The 16 individual sessions were based on a core curriculum covering diet, exercise and behaviour modification, designed to help participants achieve their goals. Subsequent individual sessions and group sessions with the case manager were designed to reinforce the behavioural changes.

Changes and Maintenance

A closer look at the behavioural outcomes of the diabetes prevention trials can help us identify the behavioural changes that mediated the physiological benefits observed in the participants of the lifestyle interventions. In the FDS, participants in the intervention group changed their eating (consumption of fat, improved quality of fat, increased consumption of fibre) and increased their activity more than those in the control arm. Among those who met four of the five goals set for the intervention, none developed diabetes. Participants who reached this goal included 49 in the intervention and 15 in the control group.

In the DPP daily energy intake decreased significantly more in the lifestyle intervention group than in the placebo group (−450 kcal versus −249 kcal) and average percentage of daily calories as fat did as well (−6.6% versus −0.8%). Changes in self-reported physical activity followed the same pattern, with an increase of MET hr/week of +7.8 versus 1.8.

In the Da Qing study the only significant behavioural change observed was an increase in daily exercise in the combined diet and exercise arm. In the FDS and DPP, mean BMI decreased significantly more from baseline to follow-up in the intervention arms compared with the control arms (−4.2 kg versus −0.8 kg and −5.6 kg versus −0.1 kg respectively). During the course of the study of the FDS, mean OGTT fasting and 2 hour glucose levels fell significantly. In the DPP intervention group, mean OGTT fasting glucose levels at the end of the study were essentially identical to those at baseline, while these levels increased significantly in the control arm.

It is uncertain at this point to what extent adherence to the lifestyle recommendations that have shown to be protective of developing Type 2 diabetes will be maintained by the participants over time. The efficacy data from the DPP show that 50 per cent of the participants in the lifestyle intervention group had achieved the goal of weight loss of at least seven per cent at 6 months, and 38 per cent at the most recent visit. The proportion of participants who met the goal of at least 150 minutes of physical activity per week declined from 74 per cent at 6 months to 58 per cent at the most recent visit. Literature on long-term effects of weight loss programmes suggest that we may expect participants to face increasing difficulty maintaining the weight loss achieved in the course of the prevention trial more so, perhaps, if we take into account the progressive nature of the metabolic syndrome. Generally speaking, a patient entering a face-to-face programme combining weight loss, exercise and behaviour modification will lose on average 10 per cent of his or her weight over the course of 20–26 weeks. After 1 year follow-up, however, a participant has typically regained 30 per cent of the initial weight loss, and at 3–5 year follow-up most of the participants are back to baseline. These findings should warn us against unrealistic expectations, and underscore the importance of continuing contacts with staff, by telephone, e-mail and/or face to face, combined with participation in community-based healthy eating programmes.

Research into the long-term effects of physical exercise programmes provides a more positive picture, possibly due to the flexibility of activity goals that make it easier to fit into people's daily routine in a way that accommodates their lifestyle and life demands.[25] This also offers good opportunities for long-term maintenance of weight loss, if subjects can gradually increase moderate physical activity up to 5 hours per week.[26]

Implications

The diabetes prevention trials have conclusively demonstrated that primary prevention of Type 2 diabetes is possible by means of a non-pharmacological intervention in persons with IGT. Implementing effective lifestyle interventions in primary care could therefore significantly help reduce the incidence of Type 2 diabetes, and all the associated human and social costs. From an economic point of view, primary prevention of diabetes by lifestyle strategies targeted to those identified as being at risk is likely to be cost effective. From the DPP it was calculated that lifestyle interventions would cost approximately $750 per participant per year, although the incremental costs are greater from a societal perspective. The costs of the lifestyle intervention could be reduced by improving the efficiency of utilization of staff time by using group visits.[27]

Implementing lifestyle counselling in primary care clearly requires an active role for the primary care physician, although more research is needed to confirm the efficacy of counselling by clinicians in primary care to improve physical activity.[28] An important issue in this context is whether busy clinicians can afford to spend time on behaviour change counselling as part of their clinical routine. Obviously, time restraints are to be considered. However, one could argue that in elderly patients at risk, who have much to gain and often visit their primary care physician for prevention-oriented reasons, there are ample 'teachable moments' at which lifestyle advice can be introduced without burdening the consultation.[29] Also, as pointed out by Estabrooks *et al.*,[30] lifestyle interventions need not be delivered entirely by physicians. Delegation of responsibility and time spent on intervention activities can be accomplished by enlisting trained practice assistants, nursing staff and volunteers to participate in the delivery.

Perhaps the major barrier in translating the message from the diabetes prevention trials is insufficient knowledge among the general public and primary care physicians alike of the clinical significance of impaired glucose tolerance as a risk factor for developing Type 2 diabetes. Many primary care physicians at this point seem reluctant to screen for pre-diabetes.[31] As pointed out earlier in this chapter, awareness campaigns and tailored public health education programmes are warranted to reach those at risk and inform them of the possibility of preventing diabetes or at least delaying the onset of the disease by years. Although the long-term benefits of lifestyle counselling in people with pre-diabetes are still to be established, we can expect substantial positive health effects, in particular on cardiovascular risks. A recent prospective study in adults with established diabetes demonstrated that walking for at least 2 hours a week resulted in a striking 39 per cent reduction of all-cause mortality and a 34 per cent reduction of CVD mortality across persons of varying age, race and body mass index.[42] In other words, once people have developed diabetes, they will continue to benefit from adhering to a relatively straightforward lifestyle recommendation. Still, initiation and maintenance rates of physical activity in the general population are disappointing, in both the US and many European countries.[33,34] This is particularly disturbing given the increasing prevalence of obesity among children and adolescents. With McGinnis[35] we can conclude that 'The potential for gain against the toll from diabetes is great, but only if we pair aggressive clinical interventions with equally aggressive community action fundamental to broad lifestyle changes'.

References

1. Pan XR, Li GW, Hu YH, Wang JX, Yang WY, An ZX, Hu ZX, Lin J, Xiao JZ, Cao HB, Liu PA, Jiang XG, Jiang YY, Wang JP, Zheng H, Zhang H, Bennett PH and Howard BV. Effects of diet and exercise in preventing NIDDM in people with impaired glucose tolerance. The Da Qing IGT and Diabetes Study. *Diabetes Care* **1997**; **20**: 537–544.
2. Tuomiletho J, Lindstorm J, Riksson JG, Valle TT, Hamalainein H, Ilanne-Parikka P, Keinanen-Kiukaaniemi S, Laakso M, Louheranta A, Rastas M, Salminen V and Uusitupa M. Prevention of Type 2 diabetes mellitus by changes in lifestyle among subjects with impaired glucose tolerance. *New Engl J Med* 2001; **344**: 1343–1350.
3. Knowler WC, Barrett-Connor E, Fowler SE, Hamman RH, Lachin JM, Walker EA and Nathan D for the Diabetes Prevention Program Research Group. Reduction in the incidence of Type 2 diabetes with lifestyle intervention or metformin. *New Engl J Med* 2002; **346**: 393–403.
4. American Diabetes Association and National Institute of Diabetes, Digestive and Kidney Diseases. The prevention or delay of Type 2 diabetes. Position statement. *Diabetes Care* 2002; **25**: 742–749.
5. Fisher EB, Walker EA, Bostrom A, Fischhoff B, Haire-Joshu D and Bennett-Johnson S. Behavioral science research in the prevention of diabetes. *Diabetes Care* 2002; **25**: 599–606.
6. Kumanyika SK. Special issues regarding obesity in minority populations. *Ann Intern Med* 1993; **119**: 650–654.
7. Kafatos A, Manios Y, Markatji I, Giachetti I, Vaz de Almeida MD and Engstrom LM. Regional, demographic and national influences on attitudes and beliefs with regard to physical activity, body weight and health in a nationally representative sample in the European Union. Special Issue Pan European survey of consumer attitudes to physical activity, body weight and health. *Public Health Nutr* 1999; **2** (1A): 87–95.
8. Wing RR, Goldstein MG, Acton KJ, Birch LL, Jakicic JM, Sallis JF, Smith-West D, Jefert RW and Surwit RS. Behavioral science research in diabetes. Lifestyle changes related to obesity, eating behavior, and physical activity. *Diabetes Care* 2001; **24**: 117–123.
9. Hill J and Peters J. Environmental contributions to the obesity epidemic. *Science* 1998; **280**: 1371–1374.
10. Humpel N, Owen N and Leslie E. Environmental factors associated with adults' participation in physical activity. A review. *Am J Preventive Med* 2002; **22**: 188–199.
11. Williams GC, Grow VM, Freedman ZR, Ryan RM and Deci EL. Motivational predictors of weight loss and weight loss maintenance. *J Personality Social Psychol* 1996; **70**: 115–126.
12. Janz N and Becker MH. The health belief model: a decade later. *Health Ed Q* 1984; **11**: 1–47.
13. Azjen I. The theory of planned behavior. *Organizational Behavior Human Decision Processes* 1991; **50**: 179–211.
14. Leventhal H, Nerenz DR, Steele DJ, Taylor SE and Singer JE. Illness representations and coping with health threats. In *Handbook of Psychology and Health*, Baum A (ed.). 1984. Killsdale, NJ: Erlbaum, pp. 219–252.
15. Farmer AJ, Levy TC and Turner RC. Knowledge of risk of developing diabetes among siblings of Type 2 patients. *Diabet Med* 1999; **16**: 233–237.

16. Harwell TS, Dettori N, Flook BN, Priest L, Williamson, DF, Helgerson SD and Gohdes D. Preventing Type 2 diabetes: perceptions of risk and prevention in a population-based sample of adults > or = 45 years of age. *Diabetes Care* 2001; **24**: 2007–2008.
17. Adriaanse MC, Snoek FJ, Dekker JM, Spijkerman AMW, Nijpels G, van der Ploeg HM and Heine RJ. Perceived risk for Type 2 diabetes in participants in a stepwise population-screening programme. *Diabet Med* 2003; **20**: 210–215.
18. Murphy E and Kinmonth AL. No symptoms, no problem? Patients' understandings of non-insulin dependent diabetes. *Family Practice* 1995; **12**: 184–192.
19. Schwarzer R and Fuchs R. Self-efficacy and health behaviours. In *Predicting Health Behaviour*, Connor M and Norman P (eds). 1996. Buckingham: Open University Press, pp. 163–196.
20. Seligman MEP. *Helplessness*. 1975. San Francisco: Freeman.
21. Prochaska JO, Norcross JC and DiClemente CC. *Changing for Good* 1994. New York.: Morrow.
22. Doherty Y, James P and Roberts S. Stage of change counselling. In *Psychology in Diabetes Care*, Snoek FJ, Skinner TC (eds). 2000. Chichester: Wiley, pp. 99–139.
23. Aspinwall LG. A stitch in time: self-regulation and proactive coping. *Psychol Bull* 1997; **121**: 417–436.
24. Kahn EB, Ramsey LT, Brownson RC, Heath GW, Howze EH, Powell KE, Stone EJ, Rjab MW and Corso P. The Task Force on Community Preventive Sciences. The effectiveness of interventions to increase physical activity. A systematic review. *Am J Preventive Med* 2002; **22** (4S): 73–102.
25. Kriska A. Striving for a more active community. Lessons learned from Diabetes Prevention Program and beyond. *Am J Preventive Med* 2002; **22** (4S): 6–7.
26. American College of Sports Medicine. Appropriate intervention strategies for weight and the prevention of weight regain for adults. *Med Sci Sports Exercise* 2001; **33**: 2145–2156.
27. Herman WH, Brandle M, Zhang P, Wiiliamson DF, Matulik MJ, Ratner RE, Lachin JM and Engelgau MM; Diabetes Prevention Research Group. Costs associated with the primary prevention of Type 2 diabetes mellitus in the diabetes prevention program. *Diabetes Care* 2003; **26**: 36–47.
28. Eden KB, Orleans CT, Mulrow CD, Pender NJ and Teutsch SM. Does counseling by clinicians improve physical activity? A summary of the evidence for the US Preventive Services Task Force. *Ann Intern Med* 2002; **137**: 208–215.
29. Petrella RJ, Koval JJ, Cunningham DA and Paterson DH. Can primary care doctors prescribe exercise to improve fitness? The StepTest Exercise Prescription (STEP) Project. *Am J Preventive Med* 2003; **24**: 316–322.
30. Estabrooks PA, Glasgow RE and Dzewatowski DA. Physical activity promotion through primary care. *JAMA* 2003; **22**: 2913–2916.
31. Wylie G, Hungin AP and Neely J. Impaired glucose tolerance: qualitative and quantitative study of general practitioners' knowledge and perceptions. *BMJ* 2002; **324**: 1190–1196.
32. Gregg EW, Gerzoff RB, Caspersen CJ, Williamson DF and Narayan KMV. Relationship of walking to mortality among US adults with diabetes. *Arch Intern Med* 2003; **163**: 1440–1447.
33. Centers for Disease Control and Prevention. Physical activity trends – United States, 1990–1998. *MMWR Morbidity Mortality Weekly Rep* 2001; **150**: 166–169.
34. Vaz de Almeida MD, Graca P, Alfonso C, D'Amicis A, Lappalainen R and Damkjaer S. Physical activity levels and body weight in nationally representative sample in the European Union. Special Issue Pan European survey of consumer attitudes to physical activity, body weight and health, *Public Health Nutr* 2 (1A): 105–114.
35. McGinnis J. Diabetes and physical activity. Translating evidence into action. *Am J Preventive Med* 2002; **22** (4S): 1–2.

4 Prevention of Complications of Type 2 Diabetes

11

Preventive Disease Management – Risk Stratification as a New Tool in the Hands of General Practitioners

Thomas Konrad

Chronic Diseases, Health-Care Systems, Internet and Economic Burden: From Intervention to Prevention

Chronic diseases, such as cardiovascular disease (CVDs) and diabetes mellitus Type 2 (Type 2 diabetes) are increasing world wide, especially in the Western world and developing countries with growing economic prosperity. The causes for this epidemiological and economic disaster are simple to define: over-nutrition and physical inactivity. In British youth aged 11–16 years, waist circumference, representing central fatness, has increased much faster than body mass index over 10–20 years. In other words, the commonly used body mass index has therefore systematically underestimated the prevalence of obesity in young people.[66] The higher the fat the higher the risk for getting Type 2 diabetes.[85] Thus, the Western societies will have a never-ending stream of new young patients with incurable, cost-intensive diseases. According to research in the USA, Americans tend to put on weight gradually: about 2 pounds (0.9 kg) a year from age 20 to 40 years. Communities and health experts are cooperating against obesity by moving people into safe and activity-friendly environments.[59] The increased personal and medical burden but above all the economic disaster caused

Prevention of Type 2 Diabetes Edited by Manfred Ganz
 ISBN: 0-470-85733-1

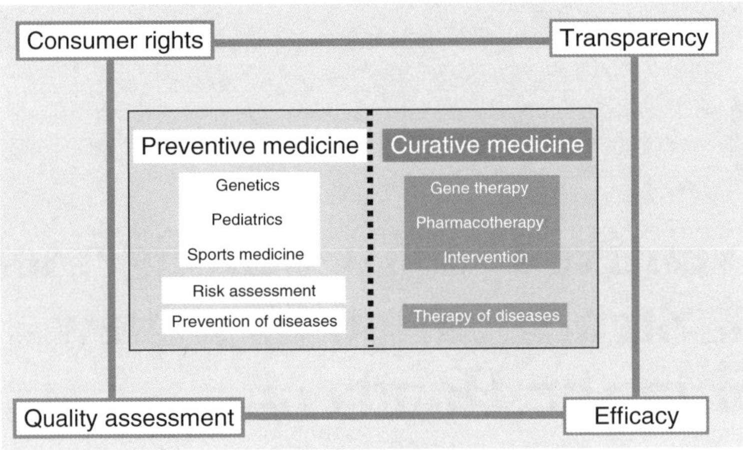

FIGURE 11.1 The framework of preventive and curative medicine

by Type 2 diabetes will force all societies to reorganize public health in the coming years. The concept of effectiveness in the diagnosis and therapy of chronic diseases has come to dominate the health-care debate. Recommendations and guidelines of medical societies should provide effective but cost-sparing therapies for chronically ill subjects.[1,11,44,72] Access to the internet, direct information for the consumer from pharmaceutical industries and other health-care providers will empower consumers and influence their demand for qualified health-care services. The empowered, well informed consumer and consumer rights will occupy the key role in health-care systems and should be considered as landmarks for every decision in preventive medicine (Figure 11.1).

In the next few years, societies have to decide how much health-care is the right amount, but it must be mentioned that every penny spent on health-care means one less spent on some other consumable item. Therefore, while health expenditures increase with growth, reducing these expenditures may be a key to economic growth and a source of economic advantage.[78] These economic relations may profoundly influence ethic and medical decisions today and in the future.

Gene testing and advances in biotechnology will become driving forces in medical practice. The likely increases in availability of DNA-based tests and demand by consumers or patients for genetic information and advice mean that practitioners in primary care will need to become genetically literate. Genetic testing, the economic burden of chronic diseases, enhanced consumerism and the internet will shift health-care systems from cure to prevention.

The general notion has evolved that the intensity of preventive efforts should be adjusted to the subject's risk for developing CVD, i.e. the higher the risk, the more aggressive the intervention should be. Such a procedure seeks to achieve a

TABLE 11.1 The characteristics of curative and preventive medicine

	Curative medicine	Preventive medicine
Driving forces	Symptoms/clinical signs	Knowledge/family care
Primary incentive	Less pain	Quality of life
Status	Illness	Risk
Protagonist	Active physician	Active consumer/patient
Costs	Short time: very high costs	Long time: low costs
Therapy	Costs orientated	Effectiveness
Resonance	Spectacular	Modest

reasonable balance among three factors: efficacy, safety and costs of intervention.[35] The initiation of specific risk-reduction therapies means that clinicians move secondary prevention strategies across the boundary into high-risk primary prevention.[40,82] Extending therapy to a nondiseased population may also have important ethical and economic implications: a widespread unselected treatment with statins for example may lead to perceptions of illness and only a few would receive a benefit. The West of Scotland Coronary Prevention study (WOSCOP) showed that of 10 000 patients treated with a statin for five years, 9755 would receive no benefit.[26,62] To reduce the costs for therapeutic intervention in chronic illness, the early detection of high-risk subjects will be the most suitable and convincible tool to reduce costs and to prevent the disease (Table 11.1). A clearly defined strategy to detect high-risk persons and to motivate them to change their life habits must be the first step in preventive care in order to avoid a growing medicalization.[27]

Basics of Preventive Medicine: Risk Stratification, Genetic Testing and Information

The causes for the increasing rate of patients with CVD or Type 2 diabetes are clearly detected: physical inactivity and over-nutrition. In this context, what will be the role of genetics? Can consumers await more than the information about an individual statistic risk, meaning more motivation for changes in lifestyle and behaviour, more responsibility for individual health? Just telling people that they are at risk of developing a disease is rarely sufficient to change behaviour. Providing people with personalized information on risk is not new. The question is whether responses will be any different if the information is based on DNA. Such responses depend on pre-existing perceptions and on the way the information is presented.

Genetic risk information could both increase and decrease motivation by strengthening the belief that current behaviour, combined with a genetic predisposition, is putting a person at increased risk of disease. On the other hand, given a common perception that genetic risk is immutable, a sense of fatalism might decrease the motivation for changing lifestyle. This reaction might well be caused by the general belief that genetically conferred risk is serious and immutable.[65] People who have or perceive a family history of CVD or Type 2 diabetes are not more or less likely than other people to engage in behaviours that reduce the risk of heart disease, such as not smoking or being physically active. Perceiving a family history of heart disease was associated with a sense of fatalism in fewer than 15 per cent of participants in a population based survey of over 2000 adults.[5,50,61]

In complex disease a person's susceptibility genotype and environmental history combine to establish present health status, and the genotype's norm of reaction determines future health trajectory.[86] How a genetic component may influence the individual risk can be estimated by family studies in which the disease risk in relatives of a patient is compared with the general risk of disease in the population. Stratification of risk by degree of relatedness and comparisons with unrelated individuals living in the same household can help to distinguish between genetic and nongenetic familial effects. Recently, especially spouses have been found to be higher risk for CVD and Type 2 diabetes when living in households with patients affected by such diseases.[57,60]

Large-population based studies of the predisposition for hypertension, Type 2 diabetes and other chronic diseases have however shown that large geographical and temporal variations in the occurrence of many diseases indicate a major role of the environment. The environment is understood to encompass everything nongenetic, from the intrauterine environment to physical and chemical effects and to behavioural and social aspects (Figure 11.2).[56] Many genes act through several

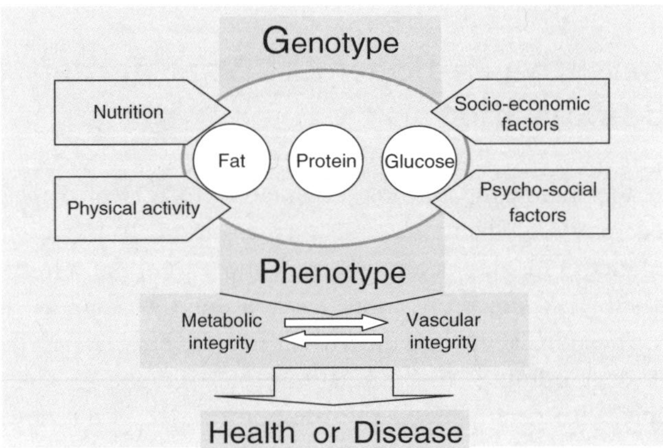

FIGURE 11.2 The factors influencing the balance between health and disease. The environmental factors and the genotype's norm of reaction determine future health or disease

intermediate phenotypes in CVD, blood lipids, haemostatic factors and blood pressure to increase disease risk. In other words, genotype poorly predicts phenotype.

In summary, as with all information on risk, behaviour is more likely to be changed if the information is presented as a part of an intervention that is known to be effective in changing behaviour. Today, the first issue for primary care practitioners is the risk assessment of modifiable parameters, i.e. describing the phenotype of an individual.

Principles of Assessment of Risk Factors in Clinical Practice for Cardiovascular Diseases and Diabetes Mellitus Type 2: Consequences for the Individual Life

Global risk assessment has become an accepted component of clinical guidelines and recommendations in medicine. The American Heart Association (AHA) and the American College of Cardiology (ACC) have published joint recommendations for medical intervention in patients with cardiovascular diseases (CVD)[37,41,75] and more recently for the prevention of other forms of atherosclerotic diseases, such as diabetes mellitus Type 2.[75] The guidelines are provided by the National Cholesterol Education Program (NCEP[15]) and the American Diabetes Association.[41] The risk status of persons without CVD or without diabetes (prediabetes[3]) varies greatly, and this variability mandates a range in the intensity of interventions. Effective primary prevention in these persons thus requires an assessment of risk to categorize patients for selection of appropriate interventions. Given these facts, prevention programs have been started in most Western countries to create tools for reducing the incidence of chronic diseases.[36,64,97]

The basic concept of prevention is risk assessment. The pathway from assessment of risk to reduction of risk basically involves three steps.

(a) Measurement of risk factors and collection of clinical data relevant to patient risk.

(b) Interpretation of risk-related data with estimation of risk in absolute terms (risk of an event per year) as well as relative terms (low, intermediate, or high compared with others of the same age and sex).

(c) On the basis of the estimated risk, intervention occurs to minimize risk or to prevent risk factor development in the future.[32]

The Framingham Heart Study as well as the Prospective Cardiovascular Münster (PROCAM) study[4,97] has taken the lead in developing the concept of risk factors for the prevention of cardiovascular diseases and has been widely used by practitioners. Both population-based studies have clearly shown that risk factors for the development of premature vascular disease often coexist and act synergistically in terms of coronary risk. The term risk factor describes those characteristics found in healthy individuals that are independently related to the subsequent occurrence of CVD. It includes modifiable lifestyles and biochemical and physiological characteristics as well as nonmodifiable personal characteristics, such as age, gender and family history of early-onset CVD.[21]

The first step in preventive medicine is to estimate the individual risk considering three categories: absolute, relative and attributable risk. *Absolute risk* defines the probability of developing CHD over a finite time. A high *short-term* risk might be defined as a probability of a fatal or nonfatal myocardial infarction of at least 20 per cent in the next 10 years, whereas high *long-term* risk considers a longer period over more than 10 years. The relative risk is the ratio of absolute risk for CVD in an individual with risk factors compared with a person at a standard level of risk.[35] The estimation of the *relative risk* may result from the application of 'risk calculators' for the Framingham or PROCAM study in a single person at the same age without major risk factors or by considering the population-based average risk.[37] Attributable risk is the difference in absolute risk between an individual under consideration and that of a control group. Attributable risk typically is low in young adulthood and rises with age.[35]

Risk status in persons without clinically manifest CVD or other clinical forms of atherosclerotic disease is determined by a *two-step procedure* as supposed by NCEP.[15]

- *First*, the number of risk factors is counted. Risk factors can be divided into causal, conditional and predisposing risk factors (Table 11.2[41]). About 85 per cent of excess risk for an CVD in the whole US population can be explained by the sum of major risk factors.[2]

- *Second*, for persons with multiple risk factors (more than two), 10 year risk assessment is carried out with Framingham scoring to identify individuals whose short-term (10 year) risk warrants consideration of intensive treatment. Estimation of the 10 year CVD risk adds a step to risk assessment beyond risk factor counting, but this step is warranted because it allows better targeting of intensive treatment to people who will benefit from it.[35,37,41]

Problems and limitations of risk assessment and stratification in clinical practice

All the well known population-based studies have restrictions and limitations. One simple explanation is the fact that a longer time period passes before the data and results are commonly used in clinical practice and, therefore, the risk

TABLE 11.2 Major independent, predisposing and conditional risk factors[35,41]

Causal risk factors
Cigarette smoking
Elevated blood pressure
Elevated serum (and LDL) cholesterol
Low serum HDL cholesterol
Diabetes mellitus
Advanced age
Predisposing risk factors
Obesity[1]
Abdominal obesity[2]
Physical inactivity
Family history of premature coronary heat disease
Insulin resistance
Male
Ethnic characteristics
Psychosocial/socioeconomic factors
Conditional risk factors
Elevated serum triglycerides
Small LDL particles
Elevated serum lipoprotein (a)
Plasminogen activator inhibitor I (PAI1)
Fibrinogen
Homocysteine

[1]Body mass index >30 kg/m^2.
[2]Waist circumference: men, >102 cm/40 in; women, >88 cm/35 in.

profile in such a population could be completely changed. Some risk assessment tools, including the Framingham Risk Score, find no increase in CVD in post-menopausal women, in contrast to other epidemiological data sets.[32,72] The PROCAM risk function cannot be used to predict coronary risk in women and its generalization to other populations is unknown.[72]

All available procedures for the assessment of individual risk for CVD cannot delineate the influence of risk factors in the different stage of atherogenesis; instead, they provide a summation of effects. Framingham investigators[97] assign no quantitative scores to either predisposing risk factors or conditional risk factors. If these additional factors are independently causative, Framingham scoring will underestimate the true absolute risk. Furthermore, age has an overwhelming impact as a risk factor in older persons.[35] The major Framingham risk factors include some components of the metabolic syndrome or pre-diabetes but not all. Thus, the aggregate risk carried by patients with insulin resistance may be underestimated by the Framingham score. The Framingham score system, due to the heterogeneity of the explored population (six US cohorts of white and black people, but not those of Japanese, Hispanic or Native American origins), cannot be easily transferred to other countries.[36] As shown for British men, currently recommended risk scoring methods from Framingham prediction equations overestimate the risk of coronary mortality by 47 per cent and of fatal plus nonfatal coronary mortality by 47 per cent.[10]

Insulin resistance, a key risk factor in the development of Type 2 diabetes and for CVD,[47,49,52] is completely lacking in all available risk scores.[38] New risk factors, such as impaired glucose tolerance, homocysteine, plasminogen activator inhibitor 1, high-sensitivity C-reactive protein and fibrinogen are not included in the available risk equations. It is uncertain whether such newer markers would improve risk assessment and treatment selections.

A number of noninvasive imaging modalities have expanded the understanding of the atherosclerotic process and facilitated noninvasive assessment of the coronary and peripheral vasculature. Such techniques may allow us to measure and to monitor atherosclerosis in asymptomatic individuals and to identify appropriate candidates for aggressive preventive therapies. Age alone is not a particularly good indicator of the severity of coronary atherosclerosis for individuals. Quantitative risk assessment for individuals should thus be improved if coronary plaque burden can be assessed more directly.[22,33,74]

Acceptance of risk profiles: physicians' ignorance and patients' noncompliance

Unfortunately, studies show that physicians frequently fail to collect these simple and well accepted data elements in the course of medical care. Routine calculations of the risk of coronary heart disease in primary care are hampered by poor availability of data on risk factors.[67] Interpretation of risk factor data assessed by Framingham scoring also poses problems: physicians cannot readily interpret the results.[32] Survey data show that physicians frequently fail to achieve target levels for optimal risk reduction in high-risk subjects with diabetes as well as in those with arterial hypertension and hypercholesterolaemia.[34,93] Similar results have been shown for general practitioners' knowledge and perceptions of impaired glucose tolerance (IGT). Although IGT carries a 50 per cent risk of progression to Type 2 diabetes within 10 years of diagnosis and a doubling of risk of developing CVD, the awareness of the clinical significance among general practitioners is low. If they have detected IGT in subjects they are uncertain how best to manage and follow up those patients.[99]

Practitioners must realize that people at high risk for Type 2 diabetes as well as those already suffering from Type 2 diabetes are not aware of having a very serious chronic illness with irreversible vascular damage. Therefore, a further problem consists in the patient compliance or lack of appropriate follow-up, which can lead to inadequate risk factor control:[32] risk is not painful.

Medicine has developed a body of knowledge on health risks and the ways in which they can be effectively managed. The question is, therefore, how to communicate risk to subjects not aware of a sneaking disease such as Type 2 diabetes or CVD? Web-based risk calculators are among the newest information resources available to people who want to understand the health risk they face. Thus, the new communication technology gives a greater access to health information than ever before, and doctors need to be aware that they are just one source of information. Individuals evaluate the trustworthiness of sources and the relevance of information for their everyday lives.[81,83]

Requirements on a strategy of preventive care in clinical practice: quality assessment, transparency, effectiveness and consumer rights

The several steps in preventive care strategies have been clearly developed for cardio-vascular diseases only. Similar to the tendencies and requirements in curative medicine, guidelines and clearly defined procedures in the assessment and the reduction of risk as well as the proof of cost effectiveness in preventive care are obligatory. Such guidelines should assist primary care providers in their assessment, education, management and follow-up of patients who are at risk for but who have not yet manifested CVD or Type 2 diabetes. Different aspects and a clearly defined procedure however should be considered if preventive care should fulfil the conditions as described.

The informative content should also include backgrounds published by the popular press and other mass media, such as television: the mass of partially confounding and inconsistent information influences the understanding of medical processes. In the face of the empowered, well informed consumer, practitioners must become qualified guides in the confounding market of health care products in the future. Therefore, practitioners occupy a key position in every health-care system.

Preventive Disease Management for Diabetes Mellitus Type 2 and Cardiovascular Diseases: Phenotyping – the Early Detection of Insulin Resistance and Endothelial Dysfunction

Practice is a melting pot of individuals coming from different populations, having heterogeneous psychosocial and socio-economic environments. Only practitioners have a close relationship to them and are partially integrated in their family life. The early detection of first-degree relatives of patients with CVD and Type 2 diabetes is the *first step* in risk assessment. A family-centred approach to primary prevention is emphasized, in as much as it recognises both the genetic and behavioural causes of the well established familial aggregation of heart disease, stroke and diabetes.[75] Familial history for diabetes and heart diseases implicate the genetic background of an individual for the manifestation of these diseases. Whether the individual is susceptible to these diseases depends on the presence of early metabolic and vascular changes for Type 2 diabetes and CVD. A large body of epidemiological and pathological data documents that Type 2 diabetes is an independent risk factor for CVD in both men and women[38] and has to be considered as an atherosclerotic risk equivalent.[47] Type 2 diabetes and atherosclerotic cardiovascular disease share common metabolic antecedents, including impaired glucose tolerance, hypertension, dyslipidemia, hypercoagulopathy and abdominal obesity. These physiologic risk factors tend to cluster with one another, in large part because they are thought to be manifestations of an underlying insulin resistance syndrome (IRS) or prediabetes.[29] Diabetes mellitus Type 2 should be recognized as cardiovascular disease because atheroscleropathy and hyperglycaemia could be early and late manifestations, respectively, in the natural progressive history of Type 2 diabetes.[12,45] The genetic background (i.e. family history) and the causative relationship of the pathogenesis of cardiovascular diseases and diabetes must be incorporated in risk assessment strategies. The subsequent simple but clear information of these subjects about the risk for these diseases represents the *second step* in preventive care.

Insulin resistance and endothelial dysfunction are closely related: defining *pre*-diabetes and *pre*-atherosclerosis

Both insulin sensitivity and insulin secretion define the risk for Type 2 diabetes of an individual. Individuals who have low insulin secretion but normal insulin sensitivity have a threefold, those with good insulin secretion but low insulin sensitivity have a fivefold and finally those with low insulin secretion and insulin sensitivity have a 20-fold risk for developing Type 2 diabetes.[42] The causes of increased atherogenicity of the prediabetic state appear however to be related more to insulin resistance itself than to decreased insulin secretion.[43] Cross-sectionally, insulin resistance has been associated with a variety of risk factors for CVD, including elevated triglycerides, dense low-density lipoprotein cholesterol levels, decreased high-density lipoprotein (HDL) cholesterol levels,[84,88] and haemostatic markers such as fibrinogen concentrations. Several studies have suggested that subclinical inflammatory processes may also be associated with insulin resistance (IRAS).[24]

Insulin resistance can be evaluated in daily practice by intravenous glucose tolerance tests,[58] oral glucose tolerance tests,[91] homeostasis model assessment[9] or different scoring systems.[63,90] It has been demonstrated in some investigations that a combination of family history, fasting glucose, and total proinsulin identifies individuals with high risk of disease progression; a more specific and predictive value of intact proinsulin or the split products has been described by other scientific publications. Also, recent presentations indicate a potential value for fasting intact proinsulin to become a marker of insulin resistance, e.g. to identify patients eligible for an insulin sensitizer therapy, or to monitor treatment success during sensitizer treatment. Summarizing all scientific literature, intact and/or total proinsulin may become an important diagnostic tool in Type 2 diabetes, e.g. for the identification of high-risk patients, disease progression, treatment success and identification of insulin resistance (see the literature in reference 77). Insulin resistance apparently predates the commonly assessed risk factors. Therefore, the detection of insulin resistance relatively early in life offers the opportunity to identify at an early stage those subjects at higher risk for the development of dyslipidaemia, arterial hypertension and, ultimately, diabetes mellitus Type 2.[28,46,98]

Insulin resistance is associated with impaired vascular reactivity or elasticity, defined as endothelial dysfunction (ED, Figure 11.3[48]). The assessment of both insulin sensitivity and endothelial function represents the *third and most important step* in the prevention of vascular diseases. Because ED occurs even in the absence of angiographically defined disease, endothelial damage has been implicated as preceding and probably contributing to the development of atherosclerosis. In general, ED predicts cardiovascular events.[48] Aging and nutrition are examples of some influencing factors.[23] ED is characterized by a reduction of the bioavailability of vasodilatators, in particular nitric oxide, whereas endothelium-derived contracting factors are increased. This imbalance leads to an impairment of endothelium-dependent vasodilatation, which represents the functional characteristics of ED. The functional impairment of the endothelium is followed by a specific state of 'endothelial activation': a proinflammatory, proliferative and procoagulatory milieu favours all stages of atherogenesis.[18,20,94]

Changes in body composition influence endothelial-dependent vasoreactivity in children and adults.[12,76,87,89] Therefore, the endothelial function reflects metabolic states as well. There is also evidence that there may be a discrete genetic

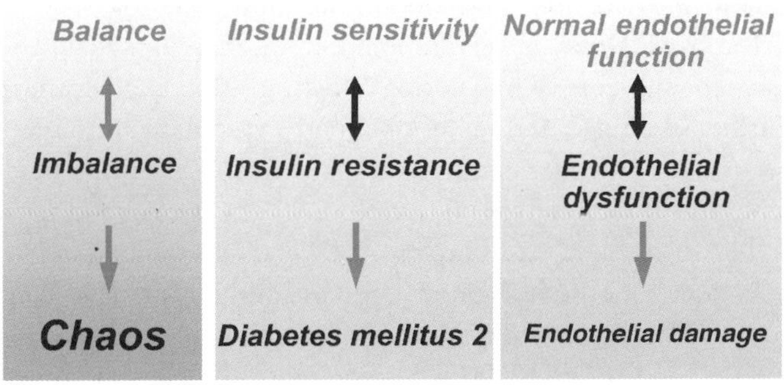

FIGURE 11.3 The balance and imbalance of metabolism and vascular reactivity: the close relation of insulin sensitivity and endothelial function

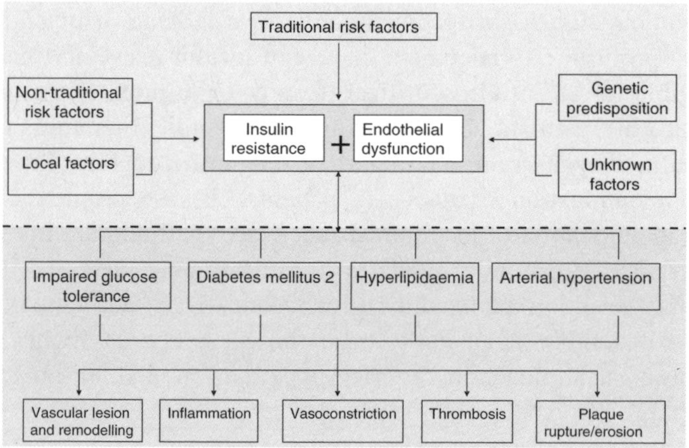

FIGURE 11.4 The key role of both insulin resistance and endothelial dysfunction in the context of risk stratification (modified from reference 8)

determinant of this endothelial dysfunction as judged from studies of first-degree relatives of patients with Type 2 diabetes or those with coronary artery disease.[13,14] Endothelial dysfunction may be regarded as a marker of inherent atherosclerotic risk in an individual and describes the transition from subclinical cardiovascular disease to overt clinical disease.[73] Endothelial integrity depends on the balance of all cardiovascular risk factors and vasculoprotective elements in a given individual, including yet-unknown variables and genetic predisposition: endothelial dysfunction is the risk of risk factors.[8] Coronary endothelial vasomotor dysfunction has been shown to correlate closely with endothelial dysfunction measured in large peripheral arteries.[17] If ED persists over longer time, reactive thickening of smooth muscle cells of the arterial wall follows. As reported recently after analysing the impact of single IRS components on carotid intima media thickness (IMT), a synergy between cardiovascular risk factors and atherosclerosis exists. This evaluation of IMT in a subgroup of the ARIC study provides a basis for using clinical parameters to identify individuals at high risk for IRS-related atherosclerosis.[31] Moreover, there is an association of insulin resistance and carotid arteriosclerosis in subjects with normal fasting glucose and normal glucose tolerance[53] further evidence that metabolism and vascular morphology are closely related.

Both morphological parameters of pathological changes of the vascular wall can be analysed by ultrasound techniques.[16,71] The flow-mediated vasodilatation (FMD) reflects the endothelium-dependent vasodilatation and can be assessed by high-frequency ultrasound imaging of the brachial artery.[16] The two parameters are closely related.[80] FMD and IMT as well represent an integrated view of all known and unknown risk factors. They inform about early functional impairment and subsequently reactive morphologic alterations of the vascular wall. Standard risk factor detection will identify only 59 per cent of men at risk of myocardial infarction over a five year period.[17] However, educational aspects must also be considered: the screened subject directly realizes the influence of metabolic disorder on the 'living' vascular bed and, therefore, these procedures may improve the understanding of his own individual biology and enhance the motivation for changing lifestyle.[80] Medical education of physicians applying these techniques is obligatory to guarantee a high quality of the ultrasound measurements and valid results.[16,54]

Integrative *Preventive* Care: Community-Based Strategy to Avoid Chronic Diseases

Public health perspectives will be influenced by higher migration rates of different populations from different countries with different risk profiles for chronic diseases, increases of obesity in children and young people, sedentary lifestyle and social–political factors such as unemployment and low levels of education. Taking these facts together, lifetime risk for diabetes in the United States will increase in the next 40 years to about one in three for males and two in five for females, even higher among minority populations.[70] A community-based network is required to develop strategies for avoiding the financial collapse caused by enormous expenses for health-care. Most communities have transport systems built around the car, but more physical activities must be incorporated in daily life: safe routes to school, bicycle trails, more parks for running and playing children etc.[59]

Initiatives of the European Society for Preventive Medicine: the school project, the practice project, the city project

The understanding of enhancing preventive efforts in all industrialized countries has induced a large variety of initiatives widely spread in cities and communities. Nevertheless, a sustained effort and a long duration of these strategies are required to be efficient. A clearly defined procedure with exactly defined information about the goals of all efforts undertaken in future for preventing diseases is the first key step for successful preventive care with a high degree of acceptance by a population. The new European Society for Preventive Medicine (ESPM, www.e-s-p-m.org) is the result of an initiative of practitioners, nutrition consultants and people from sporting institutions to develop an evaluated procedure for health-care consumers to practice preventive care in their daily life. A general recommendation for preventing diseases must be applicable in real life by consumers not by specialists in medical care only. The public becomes numbed from countless heath warnings; public health suffers from too much advocacy.[7] ESPM has focused their activities on three main issues: back pain, diabetes mellitus Type 2 and cardiovascular diseases. Therefore, the first project is on the way to determine early markers for these chronic diseases in young people in a German cohort: muscle composition of the back and abdomen, insulin sensitivity and endothelial function. A second project initiated by the ESPM is a quality-based risk stratification and information programme for practices: the 'Prevent! Disease Management Program© (PDMP)' allows a clearly defined risk stratification on the basis of the combined consideration of insulin sensitivity, endothelial function and family history as described in this chapter. The third project consists in a city project: a community-based integrative health-care programme. Health-care should overcome social and economic impediments in a community.

The school project: impact of body weight, physical activity, smoking and nutrition on insulin sensitivity and endothelial function

Obesity in children and young adults leads to early major psychosocial, pulmonary, gastrointestinal, renal, musculoskeletal and endocrine effects and will affect their quality of life as severely as cancer.[19] The first metabolic imbalance of obesity is insulin resistance. The pattern of changes in insulin resistance during puberty and the factors influencing these changes have not been completely defined. All children become more insulin resistant at the time of puberty. While prepubertal children and postpubertal young adults are equally sensitive to insulin, adolescents are insulin resistant compared with either these groups. Thus, insulin resistance appears to be a transient physiological stage of normal development. Body mass index and anthropometric measures of fatness are the main influencing factors of insulin resistance during Tanner stages of puberty.[68] Low-grade systemic inflammation, i.e. higher white blood cells and C-reactive protein concentrations, reflects subclinical atherosclerosis in overweight children.[95] The atherosclerotic process begins in childhood and develops inconspicuously for many decades before cardiovascular complications, such as myocardial infarction or stroke, occur in middle and late age.

The Frankfurt preatheroclerosis–prediabetes screening in adolescents and young adults – 'test to be fit study'

Childhood obesity has reached epidemic levels in the European countries, and the increased levels of obesity have been implicated as contributing to the alarming increase in diabetes mellitus Type 2 emerging during adolescence. 71 per cent of German adults will become obese in the next 3 years, in Spain about 69 per cent and in Italy about 59 per cent.[96] These observations suggest that the trend of decreasing cardiovascular disease in adults observed over the past 50 years may be reversed as the current population of overweight children and adolescents become adults.[88] Obese, hypertensive and diabetic children often originate from families with cardiovascular disease. These children have higher body mass index and higher lipoprotein (a) and apolipoprotein B concentrations.[30] Physical fitness, nutrition and smoking affect a variety of metabolic and vascular components, finally leading to impairment of different metabolic and vascular pathways.[25,51,69,92]

Current data, however, presenting the impact of smoking, nutrition and physical fitness on insulin sensitivity and endothelial function in adolescents and young adults in Germany are completely lacking. Therefore, it is of economic and social interest for European societies to evaluate the early changes in metabolic and cardiovascular systems in the transition phase from adolescence to adult life to initiate population-based preventive care strategies to avoid the economic disaster of these chronic diseases. The assessment of environment (i.e. family history of diabetes mellitus Type 2 or myocardial infarction) and of lifestyle factors such as physical activity, nutrition and professional activities may help to identify characteristic risk factors in early adult life and will allow us to initiate clearly defined preventive strategies. The European Society for Preventive Medicine (ESPM) initiated a study with different professional schools in order to determine first, the influence of familial and professional environment, lifestyle and physical activity on insulin sensitivity and endothelial function in adolescents and young adults and second, the impact of daily physical activity on muscular strength of the spine and abdomen in adolescents and young adults in comparison with earlier data held from the Sport University of Cologne (Dr. Achim Denner, FPZ-Concept©, Cologne). Endothelial dysfunction occurs in wide variety of pathophysiological settings such as diabetes, hypercholesterolaemia and arterial hypertension; it is associated with and precedes atherosclerosis. Endothelium-dependent dilatation is impaired in young healthy subjects with a family history of premature coronary disease[14] and is closely related to folate status,[87] obesity and hyperleptinaemia[87] in children. As in adults, thickening of the intima media of the carotis describes a higher cardiovascular risk profile in children and young adults as well.[55,79] The detailed evaluation of the results of this study will provide further information and recommendations for preventive strategies in young people.

The city project: a community-based integrative health-care programme

The diabetes prevention programmes established in Finland have demonstrated how preventive care should be established: planning and implementing of comprehensive clinical and community-based programmes to change lifestyle.[39] However, these programmes cannot be directly transferred from population to population because the environmental factors, nutrition and traditional lifestyle vary greatly.

The public health approach most often used focuses on maximizing participations in screening rather than on informed participation. Screening programmes may benefit populations, but only a few individuals will benefit. The net effect of any population-based preventive strategy depends on

(a) the number of people participating

(b) their baseline level of risk

(c) changes of risk achieved by interventions after testing

(d) a policy of informed choice to realize a partnership of practitioners with patients seeking help to change their behaviour[64]

(e) a proper scientific evaluation

(f) a dialogue between physician and patient to enable an informed decision about possible interventions[11]

(g) health-care organizations and insurers will consider the incentive systems to motivate their clients.

The term integrative medicine is often used to refer to a blend of the best conventional and complementary and alternative medicine. Health however is an emergent property of an individual as a complex system.[6] Any preventive care strategy in a community should be incorporated/integrated in the different institutions accompanying an individual during her or his life (Figure 11.5). People

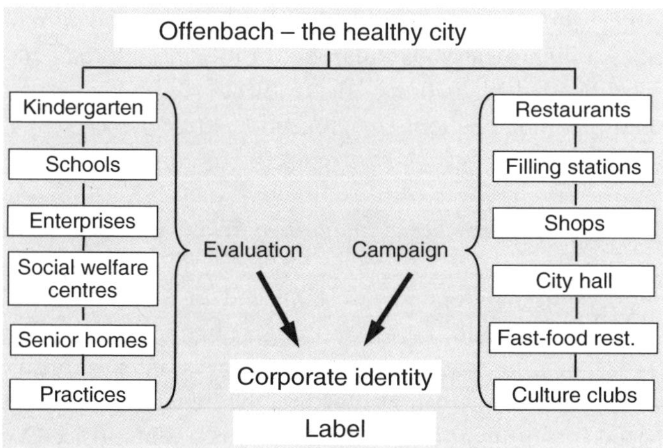

FIGURE 11.5 'The Offenbach project': evaluation in different institutions of individuals' lives and a campaign to promote health-care information in the community

working in these institutions are the protagonists of prevention in a community and guarantee a sustained effectiveness of a longer period. Thus, a circulating information system will be installed to repeat the *effective* recommendations derived from data of the evaluated community.

Summary

- The future challenges on practitioners provoked by advances in biotechnology, enhanced consumerism, the economic burden of chronic diseases and cost effectiveness of preventive strategies require an integrated development of a tool that incorporates all or most measures of risk that are already available.

- Risk factor scoring is widely used in clinical decisions. Limitations of such scores must however be considered and regular updating of the prediction algorithms is needed to avoid over-estimation of the individual risk. New markers and new noninvasive techniques must continuously be evaluated for their consistency and included in the risk assessment.

- Preventive care strategies must be more readily incorporated into clinicians' daily routine and then usefulness and effectiveness should be continuously validated and monitored: proof of effectiveness, transparency, medical education and consumer protection for the applied methods and the medical recommendations for individual intervention.

- The measurements of insulin sensitivity, endothelial function and intima media thickness reflect the first steps toward glucose intolerance and atherogenesis in clinical practice. The sonographic assessment of these vascular parameters may enhance the understanding for the individual risk profile and facilitate lifestyle changes.

- The integration of data from family history, degree of insulin sensitivity, vascular reactivity and intima media thickness in traditional risk factor scoring algorithms may represent a comprehensive strategy for a more precise prediction of individual risk for diabetes mellitus Type 2 and cardiovascular diseases.

- A clearly defined procedure with exactly defined information about the goals of all efforts undertaken in future for preventing disease is the first key step for successful preventive care with a high degree of acceptance by a population. Health-care should overcome social and economic impediments in a community.

References

1. U.S. Preventive Services Task Force. Screening for Type 2 diabetes mellitus in adults: recommendations and rationale. *Ann Intern Med* 2003; **138**: 212–214.
2. Stamler J, Wentworth D and Neaton JD. Is the relationship between serum cholesterol and risk of premature death from coronary heart disease continous and graded? Findings in 356,222 primary screenees of the Multiple Risk Factor Intervention Trial (MRFIT). *JAMA* 1986; **256**: 2823–2828.
3. American Diabetes Association and National Institute of Diabetes, Digestive and Kidney Diseases: the prevention or delay of Type 2 diabetes. *Diabetes Care* 2002; **25**: 742–749.
4. Assmann G, Cullen P and Schulte H. Simple scoring scheme for calculating the risk of acute coronary events based on the 10-year follow-up of the prospective cardiovascular Münster (PROCAM) Study. *Circulation* 2002; **105**: 310–315.
5. Becker DM and Levine DM. Risk perception, knowledge, and lifestyles in siblings of people with premature coronary disease. *Am J Prev Med* 1987; **3**: 45–50.
6. Bell IR, Caspi O and Schwartz GER *et al.* Integrative medicine and systemic outcomes research. Issues in the emergence of a new model for primary health care. *Arch Intern Med* 2002; **162**: 133–140.
7. Bloomgarden ZT. Prevention of obesity and diabetes. *Diabetes Care* 2003; **26**: 3172–3178.
8. Bonetti PO, Lerman LO and Lerman A. Endothelial dysfunction a marker of atherosclerotic risk. *Arterioscler Thromb Vasc Biol* 2003; **23**: 168–175.
9. Bonora E, Formentini G and Calcaterra F *et al.* HOMA-estimated insulin resistance is an independent predictor of cardiovascular disease in Type 2 diabetic subjects. *Diabetes Care* 2002; **25**: 1135–1141.
10. Brindle P, Emberson J and Lampe F *et al.* Predictive accuracy of the Framingham coronary risk score in British men: a prospective cohort study. *BMJ* 2003; **327**: 1–6.
11. Brindle P and Fahey T. Primary prevention of coronary heart disease. *BMJ* 2002; **325**: 56–57.
12. Calles-Escandon J and Cipolla M. Diabetes and endothelial dysfunction: a clinical perspective. *Endocrine Rev* 2001; **22**: 36–52.
13. Cavaghan MK, Ehrmann DA and Polonsky KS. Interactions between insulin resistance and secretion in the development of glucose intolerance. *J Clin Invest* 2000; **106**: 329–333.
14. Clarkson P, Celermajer DS and Powe AJ *et al.* Endothelium-dependent dilatation is impaired in young healthy subjects with family history of premature coronary disease. *Circulation* 1997; **96**: 3378–3383.
15. Cleeman J. Executive summary of the third report of the National Cholesterol Education Program (NCEP) expert panel on detection, evaluation and treatment of high blood cholesterol in adults (Adult Treatment panel III). *JAMA* 2001; **285**: 2486–2497.
16. Corretti MC, Anderson TJ and Benjamin EJ, *et al.* Guidelines for the ultrasound assessment of endothelial-dependent flow-mediated vasodilation of the brachial artery. A report of the International Brachial Artery Reactivity Task Force. *J Am Coll Cardiol* 2002; **39**: 257–265.
17. Doshi SN, Lewis MS and Goddfellow J. Improving endothelial vasomotor function may reduce cardiovascular risk, but the current evidence is circumstantial. *BMJ* 2001; **323**: 352–353.
18. Drexler H and Hornig B. Endothelial dysfunction in human disease. *J Mol Cell Cardiol* 1999; **31**: 51–60.
19. Ebbeling CB, Pawlak DB and Ludwig DS. Childhood obesity: public health crisis, common sense. *Lancet* 2002; **360**: 473–482.
20. Eckel RH, Wassef M and Chait A *et al.* Prevention Conference VI. Diabetes and cardiovascular disease. *Circulation* 2002; **105**: e138–e143.

21. Elisaf M. The treatment of coronary heart disease: an update. Part 1: An overview of the risk factors for cardiovascular disease. *Curr Med Res Opin* 2001; **17**: 18–26.
22. Fayad ZA, Fuster V and Nikolaou K *et al.* Computed tomography and magnetic resonance imaging for noninvasive coronary angiography and plaque imaging current and potential future concepts. *Circulation* 2002; **106**: 2026–2034.
23. Ferrannini E, Natali A and Capaldo B *et al.* and European Group for the Study of Insulin Resistance (EGIR). Insulin resistance, hyperinsulinemia, and blood pressure. *Hypertension* 1997; **30**: 1144–1149.
24. Festa A, D'Agostino R and Mykkänen L *et al.* Relative contribution of insulin and its precursors to fibrinogen and PAI-1 in a large population with different states of glucose tolerance. The Insulin Resistance Atherosclerosis Study (IRAS). *Arterioscler Thromb Vasc Biol* 1999; **19**: 562–568.
25. Forsyth JS, Willatts P and Agostoni C *et al.* Long chain polyunsaturated fatty acid supplementation in infant formula and blood pressure in later childhood: follow up of a randomised controlled trial. *BMJ* 2003; **326**: 953–958.
26. Freeman DJ, Norrie J and Sattar N *et al.* Pravastatin and the development of diabetes mellitus: evidence for a protective treatment effect in the West of Scotland Coronary Prevention Study. *Circulation* 2001; **103**: 357–362.
27. Freemantle N. Medicalisation, limits to medicine or never enough money to go around? Spending on preventive treatments that help a few is unaffordable. *BMJ* 2002; **324**: 864–865.
28. Füllert S, Schneider F and Haak E *et al.* Effects of pioglitazone in non-diabetic patients with arterial hypertension: a double-blind, placebo-controlled study. *JCEM* 2002; **87**: 5503–5506.
29. Ginsberg HN. Insulin resistance and cardiovascular disease. *J Clin Invest* 2000; **106**: 453–458.
30. Glowinska B, Urban M and Koput A. Cardiovascular risk factors in children with obesity, hypertension and diabetes: lipoprotein(a) levels and body mass index correlate with family history of cardiovascular disease. *Eur J Pediatr* 2002; **161**: 511–518.
31. Golden SH, Folsom AR and Coresh J *et al.* Risk factor groupings related to insulin resistance and their synergistic effects on subclinical atherosclerosis. The Atherosclerosis Risk in Communities Study. *Diabetes* 2002; **51**: 3069–3076.
32. Greenland P, Grundy S and Pasternak RC *et al.* Problems on the pathway from risk assessment to risk reduction. *Circulation* 1998; **97**: 1761–1762.
33. Greenland P, Smith SC and Grundy SM. Improving coronary heart disease risk assessment in asymptomatic people. *Circulation* 2001; **104**: 1863–1867.
34. Grover SA, Lowensteyn I and Esrey KL *et al.* Do doctors accurately assess coronary risk in their patients? Preliminary results of the coronary health assessment study. *BMJ* 1995; **310**: 975–978.
35. Grundy SM. Primary prevention of coronary heart disease. Integration risk assessment with intervention. *Circulation* 1999; **100**: 988–998.
36. Grundy SM, Balady GJ and Criqui MH *et al.* Primary prevention of coronary heart disease: guidance from Framingham. A statement for healthcare professionals from the AHA task force on risk reduction. *Circulation* 1998; **97**: 1876–1887.
37. Grundy SM, Bazzarre T and Cleeman J *et al.* Prevention conference V. Beyond secondary prevention: identifying the high-risk patient for primary prevention. Medical office assessment. *Circulation* 2000; **101**: e3–e11.
38. Grundy SM, Benjamin IJ and Burke GL *et al.* Diabetes and cardiovascular disease. A statement for healthcare professionals from the American Heart Association. *Circulation* 1999; **100**: 1134–1146.
39. Grundy SM, D' Agostino, RB and Mosca L *et al.* Cardiovascular risk assessment based on US cohort studies. Findings from a national heart, lung and blood institute workshop. *Circulation* 2001; **104**: 491–496.

40. Grundy SM, Garber A and Goldberg R *et al.* Prevention Conference VI. Diabetes and cardiovascular disease. Lifestyle and medical management of risk factors. *Circulation* 2002; **105**: e153–e158.
41. Grundy SM, Pasternak RC and Greenland P *et al.* Assessment of cardiovascular risk by use of multiple-risk-factor assessment equations. *Circulation* 1999; **100**: 1481–1492.
42. Haffner SM. Insulin resistance, inflammation and the prediabetic state. *Am J Cardiol* 2003; **92**: 18J–26J.
43. Haffner SM, Mykkänen L and Festa A *et al.* Insulin-resistant prediabetic subjects have more atherogenetic risk factors than insulin-sensitive prediabetic subjects. Implications for preventing coronary heart disease during the prediabetic state. *Circulation* 2000; **101**: 975–980.
44. Harris R, Konahue K and Rathore SS *et al.* Screening adults for Type 2 diabetes: a review of the evidence for the U.S. Preventive Services Task Force. *Ann Intern Med* 2003; **138**: 215–229.
45. Hayden MR and Tyagi SC. Is Type 2 diabetes mellitus a vascular disease (atheroscleropathy) with hyperglycemia a late manifestation? The role of NOS, NO and redox stress. *Cardiovasc Diabetol* 2003; **2**: 1–10.
46. Howard BV, Rodriguez BL and Bennet PH *et al.* Prevention Conference VI. Diabetes and cardiovascular disease – Writing group I: Epidemiology. *Circulation* 2002; **105**: e132–e137.
47. Hsueh WA. Introduction: new insight into understanding the relation of Type 2 diabetes mellitus, insulin resistance and cardiovascular disease. *Am J Cardiol* 2003; **92**: 1J–2J.
48. Hsueh WA and Quinones MJ. Role of endothelial dysfunction in insulin resistance. *Am J Cardiol* 2003; **92**: 10J–17J.
49. Hu FB, Stampfer MJ and Haffner SM *et al.* Elevated risk of cardiovascular disease prior to clinical diagnosis of Type 2 diabetes. *Diabetes Care* 2002; **25**: 1129–1134.
50. Hunt K, Davison C and Emslie C *et al.* Are perception of a family history of heart disease related to health-related attitudes and behaviour? *Health Educ Res Theory Pract* 1987; **15**: 131–143.
51. Ikezaki A, Hosoda H and Ito K *et al.* Fasting plasma Ghrelin levels are negatively correlated with insulin resistance and PAI-1, but not with leptin in obese children and adolescents. *Diabetes* 2002; **51**: 3408–3411.
52. Iozzo P, Chareonthaitawee P and Dutka D *et al.* Independent association of Type 2 diabetes and coronary artery disease with myocardial insulin resistance. *Diabetes* 2002; **51**: 3020–3024.
53. Ishizaka N, Ishizaka Y and Takahashi E *et al.* Atherosclerosis and lipoproteins: association between insulin resistance and carotid arteriosclerosis in subjects with normal fasting glucose and normal glucose tolerance. *Arterioscler Thromb Vasc Biol* 2003; **23**: 295.
54. Jarvisalo MJ, Jartti L and Toikka JO *et al.* Noninvasive assessment of brachial artery endothelial function with digital ultrasound and 13-MHz scanning frequency: feasibility of measuring the true inner luminal diameter using the intima–lumen interface. *Ultrasound Med Biol* 2000; **26**: 1257–1260.
55. Järvisalo MJ, Jartti L and Näntö-Salonen K *et al.* Increased aortic intima-media thickness. A marker of preclinical atherosclerosis in high-risk children. *Circulation* 2001; **104**: 2943–2947.
56. Kaprio J. Genetic epidemiology. *BMJ* 2000; **320**: 1257–1259.
57. Khan A, Lasker SS and Chowdhury TA. Are spouses of patients with Type 2 diabetes at increased risk of development diabetes? *Diabetes Care* 2003; **26**: 710–712.
58. Konrad T, Vicini P and Kusterer K *et al.* α-lipoic acid treatment decreases serum lactate and pyruvate concentrations and improves glucose effectiveness in lean and obese patients with Type 2 diabetes. *Diabetes Care* 1999; **22**: 280–287.
59. Larkin M. Can cities be designed to fight obesity? *The Lancet* 2003; **362**: 1046–1047.

60. Lee S, Colditz GA and Berkman LF *et al.* Caregiving and risk of coronary heart disease in U.S. women. A prospective study. *Am J Prev Med* 2003; **24**: 113–119.
61. Lerman C, Hughes C and Croyle RT *et al.* Prophylactic surgery and surveillance practices one year following BRCA1/2 genetic testing. *Prev Med* 2000; **1**: 75–80.
62. Lim PO. Yee KM. Overlap analysis of the West of Scotland Coronary Prevention Study (WOSCOPS). *Circulation* 1999; **100**: 685–688.
63. Lindström J and Tuomilehto J. The diabetes risk score: a practical tool to predict Type 2 diabetes risk. *Diabetes Care* 2003; **26**: 725–731.
64. Marteau TM and Kinmonth AL. Screening for cardiovascular risk: public health imperative or matter for individual informed choice? *BMJ* 2002; **325**: 78–80.
65. Marteau TM and Lerman C. Genetic risk and behavioural change. *BMJ* 2001; **322**: 1056–1059.
66. McCarthy HD, Ellis SM and Cole TJ. Central overweight and obesity in British youth aged 11–16 years: cross sectional surveys of waist circumference. *BMJ* 2003; **326**: 624.
67. McManus RJ, Mant J and Meulendijks CFM *et al.* Comparison of estimates and calculations of risk of coronary heart disease by doctors and nurses using different calculations tools in general practice: cross sectional study. *BMJ* 2002; **324**: 459–464.
68. Moran A, Jacobs DR and Steinberger J *et al.* Insulin resistance during puberty. Results from clamp studies in 357 children. *Diabetes* 1999; **48**: 2039–2044.
69. Murtaugh MA, Jacobs DR and Moran A *et al.* Relation of birth weight to fasting insulin, insulin resistance, and body size in adolescence. *Diabetes Care* 2003; **26**: 187–192.
70. Narayan KMV, Boyle JP and Thompson TJ *et al.* Lifetime risk for diabetes mellitus in the United States. *JAMA* 2003; **290**: 1884–1890.
71. O'Leary DH, Polak JF and Kronmal RA *et al.* Carotid-artery intima and media thickness as a risk factor for myocardial infarction and stroke in older adults. *N Engl J Med* 1999; **340**: 14–22.
72. Padwal R, Straus SE and McAlister FA. Cardiovascular risk factors and their effects on the decision to treat hypertension: evidence based review. *BMJ* 2001; **322**: 977–980.
73. Pahor M, Elam MB and Garrison RJ *et al.* Emerging noninvasive biochemical measures to predict cardiovascular risk. *Arch Intern Med* 1999; **159**: 237–245.
74. Pearson TA. New tools for coronary risk assessment. What are their advantages and limitations? *Circulation* 2002; **105**: 886–892.
75. Pearson TA, Blair SN and Daniels SR *et al.* AHA Guidelines for primary prevention of cardiovascular disease and stroke: 2002 update. Consensus panel guide to comprehensive risk reduction for adult patients without coronary or other atherosclerotic vascular diseases. *Circulation* 2002; **106**: 388–391.
76. Perticone F, Ceravolo R and Candigliota M *et al.* Obesity and body fat distribution induce endothelial dysfunction by oxidative stress. Protective effect of vitamin C. *Diabetes* 2001; **50**: 159–165.
77. Pfützner A, Kunt T, Hohberg C, Mondok A, Pahler S, Konrad T, Lübben G and Forst T. Fasting intact proinsulin is a highly specific predictor of insulin resistance in Type 2 diabetes. *Diabetes Care* 2004; **27**: 682–687.
78. PricewaterhouseCoopers: Health Cast 2010. *HealthCast 2010* 1999; 1–52.
79. Raitakari OT, Juonala M and Kahonen M *et al.* Cardiovascular risk factors in childhood and carotid artery intima-media thickness in adulthood. The Cardiovascular Risk in Young Finns Study. *JAMA* 2003; **290**: 2277–2283.
80. Rembold KE, Ayers CR and Wills MB *et al.* Usefulness of carotid intimal medial thickness and flow-mediated dilation in a preventive cardiovascular practice. *Am J Cardiol* 2003; **91**: 1475–1477.

81. Ridker PM. C-reactive protein: a simple test to help predict risk of heart attack and stroke. *Circulation* 2003; **108**: e81–e85.
82. Schrader J and Lüders S. Preventing stroke. High risk patients should receive ramipril irrespective of their blood pressure. *BMJ* 2002; **324**: 687–688.
83. Schwartz LM, Ellner A and Woloshin S. Making sense of risk information on the web. *BMJ* 2003; **327**: 695–696.
84. Semenza GL. Tissue ischemia: pathophysiology and therapeutics. *J Clin Invest* 2000; **106**: 613–614.
85. Shah P, Vella A and Basu A *et al.* Effects of free fatty acids and glycerol on splanchnic glucose metabolism and insulin extraction in nondiabetic humans. *Diabetes* 2002; **51**: 301–310.
86. Sing CF, Haviland MB and Reilly SL. Genetic architecture of common multifactorial diseases. In *Variation in Human Genome* Chadwick D and Cardew G (eds). 1996. New York: Wiley, pp. 211–232.
87. Singhal A, Farooqi IS and Cole TJ *et al.* Influence of leptin on arterial distensibility: a novel link between obesity and cardiovascular disease? *Circulation* 2002; **106**: 1919–1924.
88. Sorof J and Daniels S. Obesity hypertension in children. *Hypertension* 2002; **40**: 441–447.
89. Steinberg HO, Chaker H and Leaming R *et al.* Obesity/insulin resistance is associated with endothelial dysfunction. *J Clin Invest* 1996; **97**: 2601–2610.
90. Stern MP, Williams K, Fatehi P and Haffner SM. Predicting future cardiovascular disease. *Diabetes Care* 2002; **25**: 1851–1856.
91. Stumvoll M, Mitrakou A and Pimenta W *et al.* Use of the oral glucose tolerance test to assess insulin release and insulin sensitivity. *Diabetes Care* 2000; **23**: 295–301.
92. Uwaifo GI, Fallon EM and Chin J *et al.* Indices of insulin action, disposal and secretion derived from fasting samples and clamps in normal glucose-tolerant black and white children. *Diabetes Care* 2002; **25**: 2081–2087.
93. van Maarle MC, Stouthard MEA and Marang-van de PJ *et al.* Follow up after a family based genetic screening programme for familial hypercholesterolaemia: is screening alone enough? *BMJ* 2002; **324**: 1367–1368.
94. Verma S and Anderson TJ. Fundamentals of endothelial function for the clinical cardiologist. *Circulation* 2002; **105**: 546–549.
95. Visser M, Bouter LM and McQuillan GM *et al.* Low-grade systemic inflammation in overweight children. *Pediatrics* 2001; **107**: 1–6.
96. Weck M and Fischer S. Volkskrankheit Adipositas: Hier rollt eine Lawine auf uns zu! *MMW* 2002; **40**: 23–24.
97. Wilson PWF, D'Agostino RB and Levy D *et al.* Prediction of coronary heart disease using risk factor categories. *Circulation* 1998; **97**: 1837–1847.
98. Winkler K, Konrad T and Füllert S *et al.* Pioglitazone reduces atherogenic dense LDL particles in nondiabetic patients with arterial hypertension. *Diabetes Care* 2003; **26**: 2588–2594.
99. Wylie G, Hungin APS and Neely J. Impaired glucose tolerance: qualitative and quantitative study of general practitioners' knowledge and perceptions. *BMJ* 2002; **324**: 1–6.

12

Prevention of Obesity and Lipid Disorders

Hermann Liebermeister

The concept that obesity can, and the challenge that it should, be prevented are rather new developments in medicine. The word 'prevention' does not appear – for example – on the agendas of the first, fourth and fifth International congresses on obesity in 1974, 1983 and 1986 respectively.[1–3] However, recognition has increased: the eighth international congress on obesity[4] had a special section (XV) on prevention.

Reasons for Prevention

There are several good reasons for the late recognition of obesity as an illness sui generis and for recognizing the need for its prevention.

Reason no. 1: the importance of obesity and its concomitant diseases for public health have been underestimated for a long time

'The most common disease in the USA was treated with scorn, contempt and indifference.'

I will try to substantiate this statement from my own professional experience.

When I entered internal medicine in the mid-1960s, moderate degrees of overweight were considered a cosmetic defect. Reports to the contrary were not

Prevention of Type 2 Diabetes Edited by Manfred Ganz
 ISBN: 0-470-85733-1

taken into account.[5] Pronounced obesity, which had been very rare in post-war Germany, developed at an astonishing rate in the wake of the so called 'Fress-Welle'. These patients were sent to our outpatient department at the Medizinische Universitäts-Poliklinik in Düsseldorf mostly with diagnoses such as hypothyroidism or Cushing's syndrome. These suspicions turned out to be justified in a very small percentage of cases only – as we all might have expected 40 years later – however, in order to avoid sending these people home very disappointed, an obesity out-patient clinic was founded. In charge: myself, being the youngest doctor, just returned from 3 years in the USA.

Fatness is a burden not just for Germany though, but for many industrialized countries and also for the affluent city populations in developing countries which are on the verge of abundance.

Obesity concerns more than 100 million people worldwide, with a sharply growing trend. The tendency is especially strong in countries and regions that have suffered from a lack of nutrition until comparatively recently and where – e.g. among the Australian aborigines – the chance of 'survival of the fattest' was especially pronounced.

TABLE 12.1 The global epidemic of obesity (BMI $>$ 30, in %, modified from WHO, 1997)

Country	Year	Age	Men	Women
England	1980	16–64	6	8
	1986/87		7	12
	1991/92		13	15
	1995		15	16.5
Eastern Germany	1989	25–65	13	21
	1992		21	27
USA	1973	20–74	11.6	16.1
	1978		12.0	14.8
	1991		19.7	24.7
Brazil	1975	25–64	3.1	8.2
	1989		5.9	13.3
Japan	1982	20+	0.9	2.6
	1987		1.3	2.8
	1993		1.8	2.6
China	1989	20–45	0.29	0.89
	1991		0.36	0.86
	1992		1.20	1.64
Western Samoa				
urban	1978	25–69	38.8	59.1
	1991		58.4	76.8
rural	1978		17.7	37.0
	1991		41.5	59.2

TABLE 12.2 Health status of contemporary Australian aborigines[6]

'Traditional' lifestyle	'Western' lifestyle
Slim (BMI < 20)	Abdominal obesity
Low blood pressure	Hypertension
Body weight and blood pressure do not increase with age	Age-dependent increase of body weight and blood pressure
Low fasting blood sugar	Emergence of Type 2 diabetes
Low cholesterol	Hypertriglyceridaemia, low HDL-cholesterol
Diabetes and coronary heart disease unknown	Frequent coronary heart disease
Physical fitness	Insulin resistance

It has also become clear that for many people their genetic heritage, which developed in a mostly hunger-stricken past, has led to a 'survival of the fattest' at the root of their weight problems.[7]

We have lived – at least for two generations and in the industrialized countries – in a world of food surplus and too little physical movement (*Schlaraffenland*), to which we are not adjusted. Apparently, there has been no genetic adaptation to this superabundance.

In the meantime, obesity has been rightly declared by the WHO as the greatest chronic health problem worldwide,[9] and this WHO report carries the fitting subtitle '*Preventing* and managing the global epidemic'. McGinnis and Foege[10] have reported that in the USA obesity and its dire consequences are (after cigarette-smoking and ahead of infectious diseases, alcohol, fire-arms, car accidents and drug abuse) the second leading cause of mortality.

Type 2 diabetes is a well known consequence of obesity and its prevalence is frightful (see Chapter 1 and Figure 12.1).[11]

We assume nowadays that the metabolic derangements leading to diabetes by the chain of lipid deposition in muscle, insulin resistance and obesity originate in lipid rather than in carbohydrate metabolism. As a consequence, Shafrir and Raz[12] have even proposed changing the disease's name to 'diabetes lipidus' instead of 'mellitus'.

Reason no. 2: the expectations of conservative obesity treatment and its long-term results have not been fulfilled

Back to my past in the obesity clinic: I was an enthusiastic believer in the equation

energy uptake minus energy consumption equals weight gain or weight loss

which in the meantime has rightfully been replaced by the dynamic equation.[13] This modern formula takes into account that our organism has developed powerful

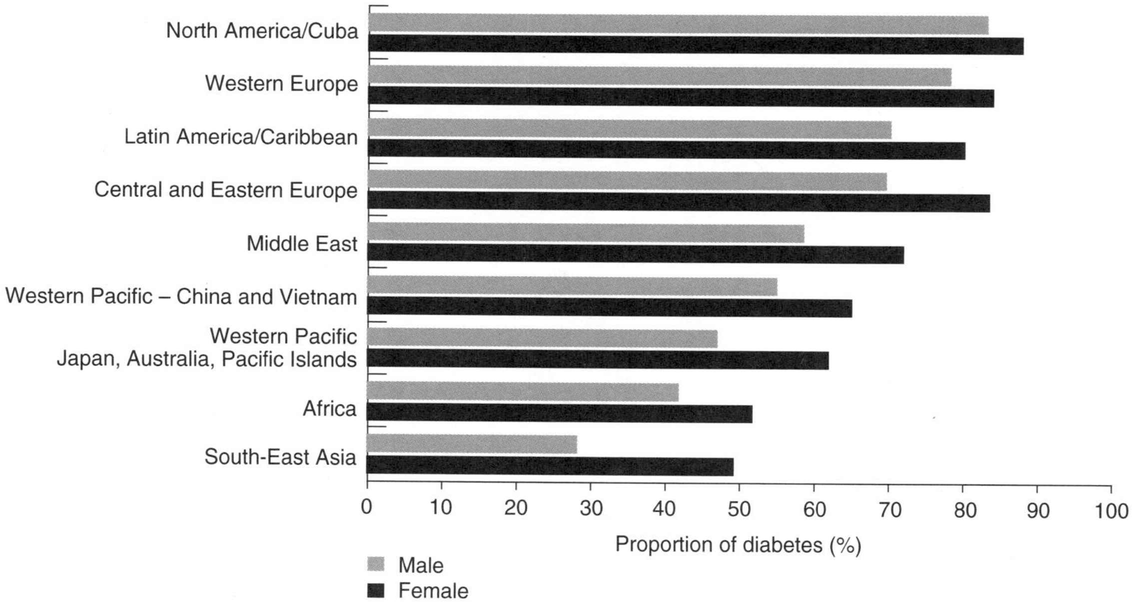

Source: *Diabetes Atlas* second edition, ©International Obesity Task Force, 2003

FIGURE 12.1 Proportion of diabetes attributable to weight gain by region (30+ years) (IOTF)

TABLE 12.3 Hunger periods and nutrition crises adapted from reference 7

3700 BC: Deluge in Mesopotamia
1140 BC: Grain-price explosion in Egypt (seven meagre years)
750 BC: Famine among farmers in Greece
Old Testament: Dry spells and drought in Israel
146 BC: Dispossession of peasants in Rome
164–180: Inflation and plague in Rome
257–310: Financial catastrophe in Rome
395: Penury and fighting in Rome
542–600: Plague in Europe
857–14th century: *fire of Anthony*, ergotism in France
1315–1317: Bad harvests in Europe
1348–1350: Deterioration of climate in Europe
1433–1438: Freezing destroys harvests in Europe
1600: Meat rationing in Southern Germany
1618–1648: 30 Years War in Germany
1720: Famine (people eating marl!) in Anhalt-Zerbst
1770–1772: Famine in Moravia
1816–1817: Agricultural crisis in Germany
1918–1924: Post-war crisis in Germany and neighbouring countries
1945–1948: Post-war crisis in Germany and neighbouring countries
Our Times: More than one billion people suffering from hunger worldwide

adaptations to weight loss and to a lesser degree to weight gain, because this latter condition was a bonus to health and survival in famine stricken periods in the past, which favoured the 'thrifty genotype'[14] (Table 12.3).

Treatment for me and others seemed so simple: eat and drink less, i.e. ca. 1000 calories including at least 50 g protein, and get moving. I was very surprised when, after 4 years and maximal weight losses of more than 80 kg, not one of my patients had attained his or her 'normal' weight on the then Broca scale.[15] This sad fact is now common knowledge.[16] Long-term weight loss after conservative treatment on average is less than 5 kg.[17] Therefore, results of conservative treatment – even after the development of combined therapies and of evidence-based guidelines[18,19] – leave much to be desired.

To a lesser degree, the same applies to *bariatric surgery*, where the surgical treatment of extreme obesity has better long-term outcomes.[20,21] Husemann[22] observed that in 682 super-obese cases, 5 years after vertical gastroplasty, their weight had descended from 140.2 (+/−25.7) to 87.1 (+/− 21.3) and their BMI respectively from 49.2 (+/−7.5) to 30.7 (+/− 5.7). Besides this large and persistent weight loss after surgery, there is considerable improvement in diabetes control, hypertension, obstructive sleep apnoea, lipid profile, endocrine disorders, and joint-related pain after surgery.[23] The Scandinavian Obesity Study[24] has shown significant decreases in depression and anxiety, as well as greater pleasure in shopping for clothes, swimming in public and even eating at restaurants in the operated upon group of the super-obese.

But sadly, if we consider only the results and exclude even therapy costs etc., *individual treatment – be it conservative or operative – is not a promising solution for this world-wide dilemma.*

Reason no. 3: obesity is a heavy financial burden on the health economy

Being a mass phenomenon, obesity engenders tremendous costs worldwide. These are of a triple nature: *direct* costs for the health systems, *indirect* costs, mostly by diminished production due to illness, early retirement and premature death, and *intangible* costs such as pain, discrimination and social dependency.[25] Colditz estimates that in the USA obesity in 1990 induced direct costs of $70 billion ($10^9$) alone, i.e. 5.7 per cent of the total spending on health. Comparable figures are in 1996 for Germany[26] 5–10 billion DM (2.5–5 billion Euro) and 2–5 per cent of health-system spending, and in 1992 for France[27] 12 billion Francs (2 billion Euro) and two per cent of health spending. From the Netherlands and Australia comparable data have also been reported.[26] Data vary though, since there are several methods of calculating the expenses arising from concomitant diseases (attributable costs). An old yiddish saying puts it this way: 'Woss a grober bojch kosst, wolt ich gewolt farmogn; woss er ist wert, soln meine ssjonem farmogn', i.e. I would be glad to have kept all the expenses for my belly; its value should go to my enemies.[28]

In summary, such arguments must lead us to discuss to what extent prevention could be used to reduce this huge financial burden on society. Standl[29] comes to the conclusion 'The impending restructuring of the social systems in Germany can succeed in the long run only if the rolling epidemic of diabetes (due to overweight) and its consequences are included in any of the recommendations with their full impact'.

The German health ministery (Bundesministerium für Gesundheit und soziale Sicherung) together with 27 partners from the health sector and public life has founded a forum: 'health targets' (www.gesundheitsziele.de). It is supposed to register and possibly coordinate – maybe even to assist financially – prevention initiatives concerning in the first line obesity, diabetes mellitus and breast carcinoma.

Reason no. 4: we now have an internationally accepted classification scheme (BMI) for overweight and its precursors and sequels

Not only comparative epidemiological studies on overweight, but also classification for diagnosis and therapy, have become much easier since the BMI system

TABLE 12.4 WHO classification of overweight in adults (reference 9, p. 9)

Classification	BMI (kg/m²)	Risk for concomitant diseases
Underweight	<18.5	Low, but risk for other clinical problems increased
Normal range	18.5–24.9	Average
Overweight	>25	
Pre-obese	25–29.9	Increased
Obese class I	30.0–34.9	Moderate
Obese class II	35.0–39.9	Severe
Obese class III	>40	very severe

(Quetelet's index of body surface, Lambert Adolphe Jaques Quetelet, Belgian astronomer and anthropologist 1796–1874) was introduced.

The WHO BMI classification (Table 12.4) has replaced Broca, Fogarty and many other systems. The famous Build and Pressure Study[30] for example based its calculations on the average weight of US applicants for life insurance, who are not really a representative sample population and a valid parameter for international application.

However, this internationally accepted BMI scheme has several, unavoidable ('terrible simplification') drawbacks:

- it does not consider age or sex,
- it does not take into account the populations of slim build (e.g. in the Far East),
- its calibration is rough and mostly follows steps of 5,
- to obtain height in metres squared, most of us need a calculator;
- however, at least this difficulty has been proven not to be so necessary as Sjöström[31] *has demonstrated that the simple expression w/h correlates better with the amount of dangerous intraabdominal fat than does* w/h^2*!*

Reason no. 5: lifestyle changes can prolong life and help avoid complications

Paffenbarger *et al.*[32] have demonstrated that giving up smoking can prolong life by 1.46 years and that adding more sport to this change will extend life-span by 2.49 years (confidence limits (1.27–3.72, $p < 0.001$)). Keeping BMI below 26 adds another 0.65 (−0.16–1.47) years to life-span.

A recent synopsis by Biermann[33] has shown that lifestyle changes can help delay the manifestation of diabetes mellitus Type 2 with striking efficiency (see Table 12.5).

TABLE 12.5 Lifestyle changes can be more effective than drug therapy[33]

Type of intervention	NNT by period	NNT/year	Endpoint	Study
Rigorous lowering of blood pressure	18 for 8.4 years	151	death by diabetes	UKPDS 38
Statin therapy	20 for 5 years	100	severe vascular complications	HPS
Multifactorial RR, blood-sugar, fats	5 for 7.8 years	39	"	Steno–2
Lifestyle change	6.9 for 3 years	20	diabetes manifestation	several studies from USA and Finland

NNT, numbers needed to treat to obtain specific endpoint in one patient.

This comparison is based on work by MRC/MBF:HPS,[34] UKPDS[35] and Gaede *et al.*[36]

The importance of weight gain prevention is underlined by the fact that once Type 2 diabetes mellitus, due to overweight, manifests itself or is discovered many of its complications are already present. One-quarter of newly detected diabetics show a microalbuminuria as an early sign of endothelial damage.[37] The DEMAND Study included 32, 248 patients with Type 2 diabetes in 34 countries. It showed that treatment by better management of the accompanying hypertension and blood-sugar reduction can effectively reduce and slow the development of the manifest diabetic nephropathy with its final need for expensive treatments such as dialysis and renal transplantation, but only if it is instituted early – i.e. during the period of microalbuminuria. In Germany – and elsewhere – diabetes is typically discovered 5–10 years too late,[38] and this fact also underlines the enduring importance of the old saying ‘Principiis obsta’: ‘fight against the beginning’; that is, prevent obesity in the first place!

Reason no. 6: lifestyle changes have no chemical side-effects and work on many levels

Practically every medical textbook recommends changes in life– and working-style as primary and remedial action for a number of pathological conditions. This holds true for obesity, Type 2 diabetes, hypertension, dyslipidaemia, arteriovascular diseases, arthrosis, gout and many others.

Such changes can be recommended to people who fear side-effects of drug therapy. They lead to positive effects on many different levels and improve many pathological metabolic changes,[39] whilst drugs in general have more specific and thereby limited effects: antihypertensives on blood pressure, insulin on blood sugar, CSE-blocking agents on cholesterol.

TABLE 12.6 Weight loss increases, fat loss decreases total mortality[41]

- Two cohort studies with measurements of skin-fold thickness as a parameter for fat depots
- Tecumseh Community Health Study: 1890 participants, 321 deaths during a 16 year observation period
- Framingham Heart Study: 2731 participants, 507 deaths during an 8 year observation period
- One standard deviation for weight loss (Tecumseh Study: 4.6 kg) increased the risk by 29% (95% confidence range: +14 to +47%)
- And in the Framingham Study SD 6.7 kg, risk +39%, (95% confidence range, CR: +25 to +54%)
- Vice versa, one standard deviation in skin-fold thickness (Tecumseh: 10.0 mm) lowered the risk by 15% (CR: −4 to −25%)
- And in the Framingham Study SD 4.8 mm, risk −17% (CR: −8 to −25%)

Conclusion: at least in overweight and only slightly obese persons (BMI < 34) only the reduction of fat depots can prolong life; loss of fat free body mass is risky.

A *meta-analysis of 23 studies* on 599 volunteers[40] has demonstrated that weight reduction diminishes in the first line the abdominal fat depots with their dire consequences on the metabolism of carbohydrates and lipids. It thereby hits the target of our therapeutic endeavours, and we can observe that it has a favourable effect on obesity-linked diseases.[39] The close connection between intra-abdominal fat depots and increased overall mortality rate,[41] increased risk of coronary heart disease, hypertension, hyperinsulinaemia and insulin-resistance, as well as frank diabetes, risk of stroke, dyslipidaemia and gallbladder disease was demonstrated some years ago.[42]

It has taken a long time for the expected prolongation of life span by weight reduction to be proven. One condition for this success was that research had to differentiate between voluntary weight reduction and loss of weight for other reasons (e.g. non-diagnosed malignancies). However, finally it has been demonstrated in two cohort studies that weight loss increases, but fat loss decreases, all-cause mortality[41] (see Table 12.6).

Reason no. 7: duration and degree of overweight complicate its treatment

It is advisable to prevent this condition rather than to treat its established state.[43] Once complications of obesity have developed, they are frequently not entirely reversible even after considerable weight-loss.[42] Moreover, the increasing prevalence of obesity in most industrialized nations places demands on financial resources that even these well-off countries cannot afford.[44]

This is especially true for Type 2 diabetes, with its enormous costs and complications.[45] During 2001 direct costs caused by diabetes in Germany were estimated at above 20 billion Euro. If we draw parallels from the costs induced by obesity, the indirect cost for diabetes should be at least twice as high. The Deutsche Diabetes Union (DDU), which unites under one roof associations of doctors, patients and medical assistants, has produced a brochure outlining the inherent dangers to our own and worldwide health systems and possible ways of prevention.[47] New studies have demonstrated that once manifest diabetes is discovered, one-quarter of these patients already show a microalbuminuria, which is an early and ominous indicator of existing endothelial damage in small and large arteries and capillaries.[48] In Germany alone with its approximately 80 million inhabitants and in spite of the recommendations and efforts since the St. Vincent Declaration in 1989 to reduce the complications of diabetes, we still have 27 900 amputations, 6000 patients becoming blind, 8300 going onto dialysis because of renal failure, 27 000 myocardial infarcts and 44 400 cases of stroke due to diabetes per year.[49]

All these arguments speak convincingly in favour of early and vigorous preventative action against overweight and its dire complications.

Problems in Prevention

On the other hand, efforts to prevent obesity have to cope with a great number of difficulties.

Problem no. 1: in conditions such as overweight and obesity there is no clear cut-off point as in myocardial infarction; treatment and prevention cannot be separated easily, not to mention primary and secondary – or even tertiary – prevention[50]

Primary prevention tries to lower the number of new cases (incidence), secondary prevention aims at decreasing the rate of established cases in the community (prevalence) and tertiary prevention works on stabilizing or reducing the amount of disability associated with the disorder.

In its memorandum,[9] WHO therefore proposes a three-tiered 'bull's eye' obesity prevention approach.

The innermost tier is called 'targeted prevention' and aims at prevention of weight gain in already obese patients and tries to prevent or at least manage the co-morbidities of this condition. The middle tier, called 'selective prevention', focuses on persons at a higher risk of becoming obese. The outermost, third tier is called 'universal prevention' and focuses on obesity prevention at large, regardless of the risk factor status of the total population.

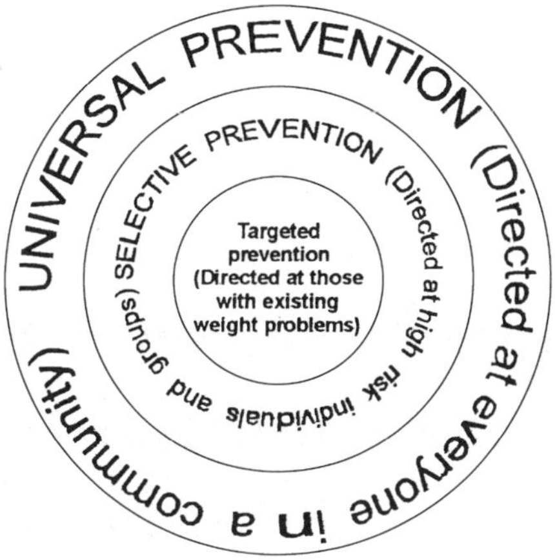
UNIVERSAL PREVENTION (Directed at everyone in a community)
SELECTIVE PREVENTION (Directed at high risk individuals and groups)
Targeted prevention (Directed at those with existing weight problems)

FIGURE 12.2 Levels of prevention measures (WHO)[175]

Problem no. 2: prevention of obesity calls for distinct and all-over changes in modern lifestyle

It took more than 200 years from the introduction of Jenner's vaccination against small-pox until the world could be declared free from this evil.[51] Yet this disease did not have any positive side-effects. Now, think of the pleasures eating and drinking can confer and consider the fact that at least drinking is one of the very first things we learn in life. Thus, low compliance is to be expected if anyone tries to change this important part of our very personal and long-established life-style, and compliance will decrease even more if this endeavour aims at activating people who – sometimes forcibly and for medical reasons – prefer the couch to the running-track.[52] But this activation is important, since the continuing increase in average body weight is probably more due to a persisting lowering of our activity levels than to specific mistakes in our nutrition.[53,54]

Problem no. 3: difficulties in motivation

Cato sen. (234–149 BC) said 'It is difficult to talk to the belly, since it has no ears'. This characterizes one of the main problems in obesity prevention: the way we eat and drink has little to do with concepts about nutrition, fats and calories; other things such as tradition, local habits, taste and well-being have much more influence.

Konrad Lorenz[55] stated[56]

- 'said is not heard,
- heard is not understood,

- understanding is not consenting,
- consenting is not implementing
- and implementing is far away from continuing'.

Modern strategies of 'empowerment' try to circumvent these problems and to enable the patient to make his choices for himself after considering their advantages and drawbacks for his personal situation.[57] Diabetic patients should continue the treatment proposed because they are convinced it does facilitate their personal every-day situation. The principle of empowerment has been characterized by Antoine de St. Exupéry (1900–1944), the famous French pilot and poet:

'If you want to build a ship, don't convoke men to get wood, to prepare tools, to delegate tasks and to distribute the work, but teach the men the longing for the vast and boundless sea!'.

However, prevention and also treatment of obesity suffer from the dilemma between present feeling and possible future good or bad outcomes, characterized by the saying

'A match in your hand has more warmth to it than a furnace at the horizon'.

Problem no. 4: (financial) advantages of prevention are not well proven

Group programs such as Optifast® may lower at least expenses for medication of concomitant diseases such as diabetes mellitus, hypertension and dyslipidaemia considerably, i.e. by about one-half 1 year after the end of acute treatment.[58,59] On the other hand, as will be shown later, community-based efforts at weight reduction have not been very successful, and I know of no studies that prove that such preventative measures have led to impressive lowering of costs induced by obesity. This is one of the reasons why health-care providers are not very interested in financing outcome studies in this area.

The chances are that a well organized and cost-effective intervention in diabetes prevention could cut expenses on this disease, if one considers that its indirect costs are at least twice, maybe five times, as high as the direct costs for diabetes treatment of more than 20 billion Euro in Germany in 2001.[45]

The *Diabetes Prevention Program*[60] provides us with some data about cost/effectiveness of diabetes prevention over a 3 year period in patients with impaired glucose tolerance (IGT). This rather stringent intervention cost ca. $24 000 for each diabetes case prevented or retarded by lifestyle intervention, whilst the corresponding expenses for the participants in the metformin group amounted to $34 500 per case prevented. Expenses per quality adjusted life-year (QUALY) gained reached $51 600 (lifestyle) or $99 200 (metformin). The author estimated that by applying the intervention principles in clinical practice these costs could be lowered to $13 200 (lifestyle) or $14 300 (metformin) per case prevented. Under these conditions, they calculated the expenses per QUALY as $27 100 or $35 000. These figures are still much lower than those for invasive cardiovascular interventions, but with the number of high-risk patients with signs of IGT, costs to society would reach a level that must motivate us to look for more effective and low-cost prevention strategies during childhood and youth.

Problem no. 5: our organism has powerful means to avoid weight loss

Since our bellies have no ears (Cato sen.), we cannot tell them that our weight reduction cure is for their own good. Moreover, since for millions of years lack of nutrition was a deadly menace, they can activate powerful counter-measures:[61]

- increased appetite
- drastic reduction of basal metabolism[62,63] leading to freezing during hunger periods (personal experience in 1946 and 1947)
- increase of insulin sensitivity; this is what we hope for in our diabetic patients, but it also promotes fat (re-)accumulation
- lipoprotein lipase, the key enzyme for lipogenesis, is expressed much more efficiently and this also favours fat deposition.[64]

These mechanisms explain part of the well known 'yoyo' effect, whose fanciful denomination has impressed and discouraged many of our obese patients considerably. They should be told that in the long run weight loss does not differ between persons with a continuous loss of body weight and others – especially women – whose weight curve shows the well known 'saw-tooth-pattern', in part due to water accumulation during pre-menorrhoea.[65]

Problem no. 6: the medical profession treats individual patients and is not used to prevention on a larger scale

In 1854, John Snow, a London physician, stopped a cholera epidemic which had already killed thousands of people by removing the handle of the Broad Street water pump and thereby saving many lives.[66] Nowadays, such easy triumphs have become much rarer and our medical education is committed more to the treatment of individual sick patients.[51]

Unlike our medical great-grandfathers,[67] who had to fight for better sanitation, vaccination, improvement in water quality, habitation and working conditions, we, the contemporary doctors, rarely develop a preventative approach in thinking and acting, and in so doing we consider only secondary or tertiary prevention. Physicians are not used to creating a safe and physically active environment, where this activity is fun, even in school. We do not think enough about buildings and streets to walk and to climb and about regulations to promote healthier nutrition and lifestyle, and we have not realized that, by one estimate, two-thirds of all deaths and years of lost life before age 65 are attributable to lifestyle choices that could have been prevented.[173]

Problem no. 7: literature on prevention is plentiful, but not of a very high standard

In 1997 Glenny *et al.* identified and reviewed 97 articles on this subject, but only 10 of them explained their method of randomization.[68] With the exception of the community-based interventions, the sample sizes were generally very small; two-thirds had fewer than 30 participants in each group.

Community-Based Prevention Studies

Having listed seven reasons for and seven problems with the prevention of obesity (and dyslipidaemia), I shall try to discuss some community-based studies in more detail (see Table 12.7).

As can be seen, the overall effects of these education programmes on long-term weight loss were disappointing.

The experts responsible for the Minnesota Heart Health Program[75] list the following possible reasons for this failure.

TABLE 12.7 Community-based prevention studies[8]

Study	Intervention	Level of activity	Results on obesity
Stanford Five-City Project,[69] USA	Teaching programme ending with activation	slightly elevated	BMI increased somewhat less
Heartbeat Wales Programme,[70] UK	Teaching programme	2–3% more active participants	obesity *increased* by 2%
Minnesota Heart Health US Programme[71]	Opinion leaders, point of purchase education	transient elevation	no difference in BMI
CINDI-Project Germany[72]	Teaching programme in doctors' offices	not tested	no change in prevalence of BMI above 25
Bootheel Heart Health Project,[73] USA	Teaching programme, jogging trail	1% less inactive participants	overweight *increased*
German Cardiovascular Prevention Study[74]	Teaching programme, activation	transient elevation	BMI 26.14 instead of 26.17

- mass media effects can be markedly reduced by widespread opposing messages
- maybe the environment was already saturated with such programmes
- the messages were sometimes conflicting (e.g. smoking cessation leads to weight gain, food rich in salt can be poor in calories)
- education per se has limited success.

As we have learned in treating diabetic patients and trying to modify their lifestyles, we need 'empowerment'; see Problem No. 3. Education is not enough.

In general, these programmes are aimed at several disorders that play a role in the development of cardiovascular disease, and they achieve better results in improving these other parameters than in lowering overweight.[76] During the German Cardiovascular Prevention Study for example, which included 13 947 participants from seven German towns and lasted 7 years, systolic and diastolic blood pressure decreased by two per cent, total cholesterol by 1.8 per cent, and the percentage of smokers fell by 6.7 per cent, but it did not influence BMI (26.14 instead of 26.17).

Thus, lifestyle changes can be effective for some endpoints besides weight change, and in outcome studies the numbers needed to treat (NNT) in lifestyle change are low compared with drug therapy (Table 12.5).

On the other hand, it is possible that trying to target too many factors at once (cholesterol lowering, blood pressure control, physical activation and smoking cessation) leads to conflicting messages and explains part of the failed weight reduction.[77]

Improving physical fitness seems to play a key role in obesity prevention or – as we would better call it – slowing of weight gain.[78]

The data demonstrate that in this community-based activation study to prevent weight gain only those few participants who achieved a state of fitness that could be changed from unfit to fit lost a little more than 1 kg of weight in 7.5 years,[78] whereas the large majority continued to gain (men 0.61 +/− 5.29 kg; women 1.51 +/− 4.67 kg). The authors conclude 'Thus, an active life-style should be promoted

TABLE 12.8 Fitness change leads to weight change[78]

After 1.8 years		After 7.5 years			
Fitness change		men		women	
First	Second examination	n	Weight change	n	Weight change (kg)
unfit	unfit	96	−0.16 +/−0.5	15	+0.35+/−1.2
unfit	fit	204	−1.43+/−0.4	23	−0.22+/−1.0
fit	unfit	69	+2.02+/−0.6	69	+3.42+/−0.6
fit	fit	4230	+0.70+/−0.1	617	+1.39+/−0.2

unfit, quintile 1 of the age-specific fitness distribution; fit, quintile 2–5 (maximal treadmill time).

early and maintained through adulthood to prevent substantial weight gain and obesity with age'.

Promoting Physical Activity

It has been known for a long time that most obese people are not very prone to voluntary or even involuntary movement.[79,52]

Moreover, it has been shown that inactivity contributes more to obesity in modern times than overnutrition.[53,54,80,81]

Therefore, physical activity plays an important role in prevention of obesity and related disorders.

There are several good reasons for this claim.

- Exercise training enhances fat-free mass preservation during weight reduction.[82]

- However, these beneficial changes result only if the training effort is continued for a long time,[83] and long-term (2½ years) adherence to prescribed moderate exercise can be poor.[84] Thus, long-term health benefits require long-term behavioural changes, or 'Sport pays no long-term interest'.

- It has a favourable effect on inflammation parameters leading to atherogenicity.[85,86]

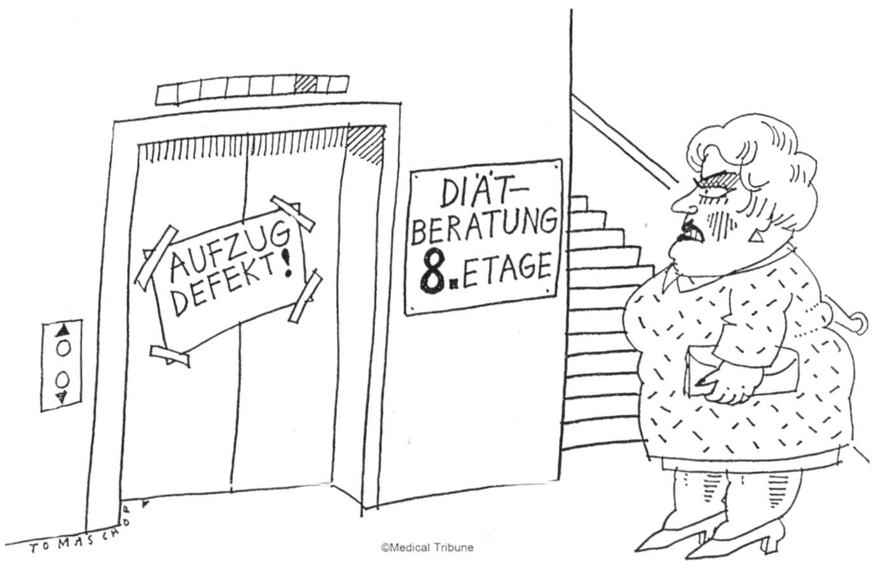

FIGURE 12.3 Not inclined towards activity (Medical Tribune caricature)

- Physical activity improves glucose and insulin metabolism in men.[87,88]

- Intensive treadmill training enhances oxidation of carbohydrates (balance +31 to –98 g/day, but – too bad – not of fat (balance −26 to +38 g/day). In triathletes and cyclists, carbohydrate oxidation increased even more (balance −103 g/day with a low-fat diet, and −185 g/day with a diet rich in fats).[89]

- Normal-weight (BMI 19–25) physically fit persons had a 2.3 times lower risk of total mortality than unfit normal-weight men. There was no risk difference of overweight (BMI > 27.8), but physically fit men compared with fit individuals of normal weight.[90] The life-prolonging effect of physical activity is especially pronounced (RR = 0.29!) in obese (BMI > 30), but moderately to highly fit, men compared with their obese peers with low fitness.[91]

- For sedentary overweight women – only 22 per cent of Americans are regularly active – a diet combined with a lifestyle programme of gradual and moderate physical activity can enhance weight management as efficiently as a diet plus structured aerobic activity.[92]

- Strength training in a fitness centre is accepted rather well and maintained for half a year. After 39 weeks, fat-free mass increased by 0.89 kg; 0.98 kg of fat were lost, 1.63 per cent more than in the control group, but there was no significant weight loss or waist circumference attenuation.[93]

Social class also seems to play a role in the outcome of prevention actions.[94] In the *Pound of Prevention Study*, they noticed after over 1 year that participating women with high incomes gained less weight than women with low incomes in comparison with a control and men (Table 12.9). The programme centred on recommendations: weekly weighing, a 'five-a-day principle' (five portions of vegetables or fruits, www.wcrf.org) for nutrition, reducing fat intake and walking for at least 20 min three times a week. Participants were sent a newsletter once per month with a stamped, addressed postcard asking about weighing, walking and the 'five-a-day' incentive. People who returned their postcards regularly were allowed to participate in a monthly lottery ($100).

We also have to consider that improvements of other concomitant pathological changes in the framework of the metabolic syndrome[9,39] (see Table 12.10) are

TABLE 12.9 Income plays a role in (kg) weight change[94]

Intervention	Men	High-income women	Low-income women
Control	+0.88	+0.63	+0.59
Education	+0.33	+0.47	+0.96
Education plus lottery	+0.10	+0.23	+1.47

TABLE 12.10 Definition of the metabolic syndrome[9]

Diabetes mellitus	Obesity (BMI > 30) or WHR > 0.90 (M), 0.85 (F)
Fasting blood sugar > 126 mg/dl	Hypertension RR > 160/90 mm Hg or antihypertensive therapy
or	
Impaired glucose tolerance 2 h blood sugar > 140 mg/dl	Dyslipidaemia: TG > 150 mg/dl, HDL < 35 mg/dl (M), 39 mg/dl (F)
	Microalbuminuria >20 pg/min overnight

observed after a *long-term weight loss of at least five per cent of the starting weight*. This minimal target is proposed in most guidelines for the prevention and treatment of obesity.[18] Over a 2 year perspective, treatment with Xenical has shown that a maintained weight reduction of 4–5 per cent is not enough in this respect, whilst eight per cent seems to be sufficient.[95]

Worksite Interventions in Adults

Worksite intervention has a number of advantages:

- existing networks,
- a large group of people can be reached,
- low barriers to reach the intervention site,
- worksite cafeterias as a natural laboratory to change adult eating habits.[50]

There have been more interventions of this type than community- or school-based trials. However, they generally did not specifically focus on weight gain prevention in overweight or on obese adults or on adults at high risk of developing obesity.[96] The main target was a beneficial change in nutrition habits. The authors list 11 such trials at worksite or college or university cafeterias. After reviewing the literature, they concluded that the worksite remains an interesting setting for obesity prevention in adults. Particular care should be taken to reduce sedentary behaviour besides efforts to influence eating (and drinking) patterns.

Specific Weight Gain Prevention Trials in Adults

There seem to be only three such interventions aimed at the general population.[50]

The first of these is the Pound of Prevention Study.[97] It included 1226 community volunteers addressed by monthly newsletters about weight gain prevention and opportunities for no-cost or low-cost intervention activities. After 3 years and increasing weight in all groups, the intervention group demonstrated a 10 per cent lower weight gain, but this difference was not statistically significant. The interest of participants had been sustained for 3 years and the dropout rate reached only 34 per cent.

The *Women's Healthy Lifestyle Project (WHLP)*,[98] a 5 year randomized control study, included 535 premenopausal women and tried to prevent weight gain and increases in LDL-cholesterol. The intervention focused on low-fat eating and increasing physical activity. It started with almost weekly meetings during the first 3 months and in the final phase contact was maintained by post or phone calls every 2–3 months. Menopausal weight gain was successfully prevented: treatment group −0.18 kg, control group +2.4 kg, $p < 0.01$!

The third study[99] compared three methods for weight-gain prevention in 102 normal-weight women, aged 25–34 years for a rather short period of 10 weeks. The three treatment formats were weekly group meetings centred on mild dietary and activity changes, a weekly correspondence course with similar content and a lifestyle brochure (considered as no-treatment control group). The correpondence course was the most popular with participants. 55 women were weighed after 10 weeks with the following results: weekly group meetings, −1.9 +/− 1.18 kg; correspondence course, −1.1 +/− 2.1 kg; lifestyle brochure, −0.2 +/− 1.3 kg. At the 6 month follow-up (n = 50) there was no statistically significant difference in weight change, since both the meeting and correspondence groups had gained weight.

The authors of the successful WHLP Project conclude that their model has only limited value for dissemination to the general public because of its behavioural and financial costs.

They also state that these trials have demonstrated that future studies should focus on creating a balance between acceptability and efficacy – hopefully by using electronic communication technologies for a minimal-contact education. This method was preferred to face-to-face class formats by the participants.

Mass media campaigns[100] seem to have little effectiveness in promoting behaviour changes, but they may raise awareness, convey information, help to set up agendas and change attitudes. Until now, they have mostly focused on promoting low-fat milk purchases, high-fibre cereal consumption or walking.[50] They reached their goal for periods of 1 year, but 1 year later participants in one study reported for example that they walked as little as before.[101]

In Germany, Ellrott and Pudel[102] started the 'Pfundkur' in Baden-Württemberg and Saxony. 30 000 people with a mean BMI of 31 were contacted by a multimedia approach, business channels and local conferences. Participants were informed and could – if they wanted – get more intensive management at the offices of the local Allgemeine Ortskrankenkasse (AOK). First evaluations hope to achieve a mean weight reduction of 3–5 kg.

Prevention of Diabetes and Obesity

A number of interventions to prevent or retard the manifestation of Type 2 diabetes have been reported. (See Markus Hanefeld in Chapter 4.)

In general the proposed lifestyle changes were the following:

- weight loss (hopefully 5–7 per cent)
- 2–3 hours more of physical activity per week
- 15 g of bulk material per 1000 calories intake
- at most 30 per cent fat in daily consumption and
- less than 10 per cent saturated fatty acids.

These recommendations have been proven to be effective in preventing or retarding diabetes manifestation, but the nutritional proposals could – at least in my opinion – be simplified and better explained to the public by the 'five-a-day' slogan. This says five portions (mostly a handful) of vegetables or fruits per day. This provides enough bulky matter, vitamins, phytochemicals and phytoestrogens, lowers consumption of saturated fatty acids and promotes saturation by better and slower gastric filling (www.5aday.com, www.wcrf-de.org). One word of caution: the successes of the 'five-a-day' principle in prevention of malignomas and arteriosclerosis have been proven,[103] but its probable effect on diabetes prevention has not yet been established.

I shall limit myself to discussing the effect of these efforts on *obesity prevention*.

The *Diabetes Program Research Group*[104] studied 3234 non-diabetic mostly obese (mean BMI 34.0) individuals with IGT. In 27 centres, they were randomly assigned to three interventions: standard lifestyle recommendations plus 850 mg metformin twice daily (1073), standard lifestyle recommendations plus placebo (1082) or an intensive programme of lifestyle modification (1079). Efforts centred on a weight reduction of at least seven per cent through a healthy low-calorie, low-fat diet and increased physical activity such as brisk walking for at least 150 minutes per week. A 16-lesson curriculum was taught by case managers on a one-to-one basis and followed by monthly individual reinforcement sessions. After a mean follow-up of 2.8 years, diabetes incidence was lowered by 58 per cent in the lifestyle-intervention group, and by 38 per cent in the metformin group ($p < 0.001$). Crude incidence was 11.0, 7.8 and 4.8 cases per 100 person-years for the placebo, metformin and lifestyle-intervention groups.

Weight changes are only shown in Figure 1 of their paper and amount to about 0.5 kg in the control group, ca. 2 kg with metformin treatment and 4 kg with lifestyle changes.

Tuomilehto *et al.*[105] have randomized 522 women and men with a mean BMI of 31 and IGT to an intervention and to a control group. By comparing individual counselling with lifestyle modification they observed the following weight losses:

- after one year: intervention group 4.2 +/− 5.1 kg, control group 0.8 +/− 3.7 kg
- after two years: 3.5 +/− 5.5 kg in the intervention group, controls 0.8 +/− 4.4 kg.

Interestingly enough, in their study, lowering of diabetes manifestation by lifestyle intervention after 4 years corresponded to the results of the DPR Group with a decrease by 58 per cent in comparison with the control group (11 per cent instead of 23 per cent).

The *Da Quing IGT and Diabetes Study Group* in Northern China[106] reported similar successes in diabetes prevention by diet and exercise in lean and obese participants.

Over 6 years, 577 people with impaired glucose tolerance (IGT) had been randomly assigned to either a control group or three treatment groups: diet only, exercise only or diet plus exercise. The diet proposed to participants with a BMI < 25 (39.2 per cent of total participants) contained 25 to 30 kcal/kg body weight, 55–60 per cent carbohydrate, 10–15 per cent protein and 25–30 per cent fat. Subjects were encouraged to consume more vegetables, less alcohol and less simple sugars. Participants with BMI > 25 were proposed to gradually lose weight at a rate of 0.5 to 1.0 kg per month with a target weight corresponding to a BMI of 23.

Participants in the exercise group were taught and encouraged to increase the amount of their daily leisure physical exercise by at least one unit, and by two units if under 50 years of age and free of cardiovascular or athritic diseases. Typical examples of these units were 30 min of housecleaning, 20 min of fast walking or cycling, 10 min of slow running or disco-dancing, 5 min of playing basketball or swimming.

The weight changes shown in Table 12.11 were oberved in the overweight subgroups.

TABLE 12.11 Changes in weight and diabetes incidence[106]

	Control (83)	Diet (75)	Exercise (84)	Diet + Exercise (80)
BMI at baseline	28.5 +/− 2.9	28.3 +/− 2.2	27.9 +/− 2.2	29.5 +/− 2.7
BMI after 6 years	27.5 +/− 2.4	27.1 +/− 2.7	27.0 +/− 2.4	27.0 +/− 2.7
Change in BMI	−0.9 +/− 2.9	−1.1 +/− 2.0	−0.9 +/− 1.6	−1.6 +/− 1.6
Diabetes incidence (100 person-years)	17.2	11.5	10.8	11.4
Confidence limits	13.3–21.3	8.0–15.0	7.8–13.8	8.1–14.6

The decrease in diabetes manifestation was significant ($p < 0.05$) in all three treatment groups, but similar for lean and overweight participants. 'Those who developed diabetes lost weight, and the change was significant in the lean and obese groups'.

This latter study demonstrates that weight loss is not an absolute prerequisite to diabetes prevention.

Obesity prevention by commercial groups

To mention just some of the oldest and probably the best known programmes:[66]

- TOPS: Take Off Pounds Sensibly
- Overeaters Anonymous
- Weight Watchers.

TOPS was founded in 1948 by a Milwaukee housewife and is based on her understanding of Alcoholics Anonymous. Its working principles have been studied.[107] Long-term members are reported to have lost an average of about 10 kg, but slowly regained it, even though they remained in TOPS.[66]

Overeaters Anonymous adheres even more firmly to the principles of Alcoholics Anonymous. Therefore, evaluation of its outcome is very difficult and firm data are lacking because of data protection.

Weight Watchers® (www.weightwatchers.de) – also founded in 1961 by a housewife – base their work on inspirational lectures given by successful members. They also offer a carefully designed nutritional programme and a behaviour therapy. In Germany alone it has enrolled 3.5 million – mostly temporary members – since its introduction in 1970. It addresses participants with an average BMI of 27.[108] It can therefore also be considered as a preventive measure, and has reported its long-term results.[109] 97 per cent of lifetime members, especially sucessful participants, are reported to maintain their weight goals with a variation within 2 kg after 1 year, whilst after 5–12 years only 35 per cent of these motivated people can maintain this success. Comparing 212 obese individuals randomly assigned to a self-help group and 211 assigned to Weight Watchers regular meetings demonstrated after 2 years a significant ($p < 0.01$) difference in a rather small weight loss (2.9 +/− 0.5 to 0.2 +/− 0.4 kg) in favour of the commercial group.[110] Regular and successful Weight Watchers participants – who no longer have to pay – showed a long-term weight loss of 5 kg.

Other commercial groups, to mention only two with which I have personal experience, are Optifast® (www.optifast.de) and Bodymed®. (www.bodymed.de). However, they treat really obese patients, mostly with a BMI above 32, and for this reason cannot be discussed at length in this chapter dealing with prevention of obesity. Their long-term results can be impressive though.[111,112]

The *Xendos Study,*[113] which included 3304 participants, has demonstrated that lifestyle change plus an anti-obesity drug (orlistat) can further lower the incidence of clinical diabetes. Compared with placebo plus change in lifestyle, this combination lowered diabetes manifestation after 4 years from 9.0 to 6.2 per cent ($p < 0.0032$), whilst weight loss was also significantly larger ($p < 0.01$) (6.9 versus 4.1 kg) due to the addition of this drug, which interferes with fat absorption in the gut.

Another, this time anti-diabetic, drug, *metformin,* was less effective compared with lifestyle changes.[114] The drug improved weight loss compared with placebo by 2.0 kg, whilst lifestyle change resulted in an improvement of 5.5 kg. In preventing diabetes manifestation (3234 participants, diabetes incidence after 2.8 years placebo 11.0 per cent, metformin 7.8 per cent and lifestyle change 4.8 per cent), the lifestyle intervention also demonstrated its greater effectiveness.

In a another prevention trial *(STOP-NIDDM),*[115] *acarbose*, which inhibits uptake of disaccharides in the gut, lowered weight by only 1.1 kg instead of 0.8 kg ($p < 0.042$, 1429 participants), but decreased diabetes incidence after 3.3 years from 41.5 to 32.4 per cent. An analysis of covariance demonstrated no relation between this small weight loss and diminution of diabetes incidence.

Prevention of obesity in children and adolescents

Overweight and obesity are increasing with economic development, with the US also leading in this respect, followed by Europe (Figure 12.4).

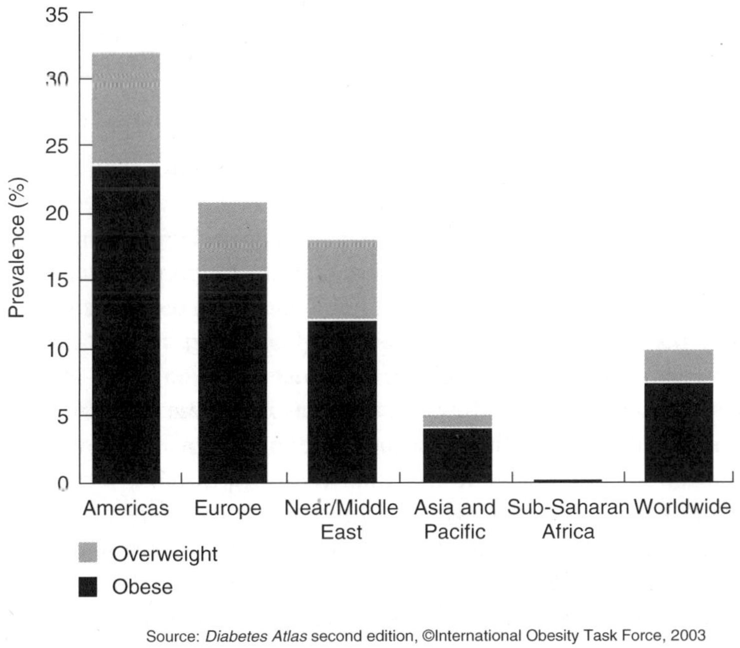

FIGURE 12.4 Overweight and obesity among school-age children[117]

Life-quality of these children is severely ($p < 0.01$) reduced to a total score of 67 +/− 16.3 instead of 83 +/− 14.8 in healthy children[118] and was found by these authors to be comparable to data observed in children suffering from a malignancy. Their educators estimated their risk of developing psychosocial curtailments at a factor of 13(!) compared with normal-weight children. Thus, juvenile obesity is a risk[119] and a stigma at the same time. For example, in the United Kingdom, the first cases of Type 2 diabetes have been described in overweight children.[120]

Overweight, obesity and their complications[121] are frequently carried over into adulthood. This – among much else – has been demonstrated in a 55 year follow-up of the Harvard Growth Study from 1922 to 1935.[122] Viewed from the perspective of childhood, 25–50 per cent of individuals who are obese in adolescence remain so as adults[123,124]

Predisposing to this development are parental fatness, social factors, a high birth weight, early maturation, low physical activity, television addiction,[125] dietary factors (soft drinks[126]) and other behavioural and psychological factors (reference 127 – a systematic review of these problems).

Treatment of childhood obesity should therefore be considered of prime importance alongside selective prevention strategies aimed at high-risk groups of children.[128] It also is an important part of a universal approach to the community-wide prevention of childhood obesity.[9]

In a very intensive and probably expensive effort, Epstein *et al.*[129] have demonstrated in four studies on 158 children at high risk of adulthood obesity, suffering from 40–50 per cent overweight that after 10 years six out of nine actively treated groups showed a net reduction in percentage overweight of between 10 per cent and 20 per cent. In a meta-analysis of 13 studies using physical exercise as treatment of childhood obesity,[130] these authors also demonstrated that the development of an active lifestyle in obese children has the potential for multiple benefits for obesity, comorbid physical and psychological problems and life quality. Very important is the inclusion and cooperation of the parents.[131] Their one-year randomized prospective study comparing the parents and the 60 obese (20 per cent overweight above ideal) children (6–11 years) themselves as agents of change in behaviour found significant differences in the exposure to food stimuli and changes in eating habits (eating while standing, watching TV, reading or doing homework, eating following stress and eating between meals). Both groups showed significant ($p < 0.01$) decreases in overweight, but the change was greater in the experimental (parent) intervention group, with 14.6 per cent compared with 8.4 per cent after one year. In general, we have fewer reports on long-term outcomes of obesity management in children than in adults.[132,8]

Guidelines for obesity treatment and prevention in children and adolescents[133] have been developed (reference 134, www.a-g-a.de) which follow these principles. A European Childhood Obesity Group (ECOG) (www.childhoodobesity.net) has been founded as well as an investigative task force of the European Association for the Study of Obesity (EASO).[174]

Treatment in children is facilitated by their natural desire to move and by the fact that they have the chance to grow and thus normalize their present overweight, if they can avoid gaining more pounds, but we must consider also the risks of obesity management in this age-group: the temptation to use dangerous procedures for weight loss such as using laxatives and vomiting or – even worse – developing a bulimia or an anorexia nervosa.[135,136]

Prevention of Lipid Disorders

The *Multiple Risk Intervention Trial (MRFIT)*[137] in a 12 year follow-up confirmed older assumptions[138] on the role of serum cholesterol as an important coronary risk factor. The *NCEP*[139] has proposed targets for lipid management reflecting existing clinical trials.[140]

The dangerous elevation of LDL-cholesterol must be considered in its combination with risk factors that cannot be changed, age, sex and family history, and others that can be modified such as plasma lipids, blood pressure, smoking, diabetes Type 1 or 2, overweight and elevated plasma fibrinogen.[141]

This combination of factors is amenable to lifestyle modification addressing most of these issues. This desired change includes the following:[140]

- a healthy balanced diet (less saturated fat, salt, refined sugar, alcohol and calories, more fibre, fruit and vegetables; www.5aday.com)
- regular physical activity
- smoking cessation
- sustained weight loss in the overweight
- lowering blood pressure ($<$140/90 mm Hg).

Dietary measures

The Dietary Approach to Stop Hypertension (*DASH*[142]) working on the 'five-a-day' principle plus low-fat dairy products and decreased consumption of total fat and cholesterol reported a net reduction of LDL-cholesterol levels by nine per cent. In 112 Italian diabetic patients, lifestyle intervention in a 4 year randomized controlled clinical trial increased the 'protective' HDL-C from 49 to 55 mg/dl with a significant difference ($p < 0.001$) compared with 51 to 53 mg/dl parallel to a significant decrease in BMI from 29.9 +/− 4.5 to 28.7 +/− 4.0.[143] In another follow-up study of long-term weight control,[43] after 4 years (10 weeks after the end of treatment) HDL had increased by 15 per cent compared with baseline levels, the ratio between total cholesterol and HDL-C was decreased by

25 per cent, and triglyceride levels by 16 per cent, whilst total cholesterol levels and LDL-C showed less dramatic changes. Another randomized trial[92] demonstrated that their programme of diet plus lifestyle activity can induce significant beneficial changes of total cholesterol, as well as LDL-C and HDL-C in week 16, but that these metabolic ameliorations – with the exception of total cholesterol lowering – do not persist into week 68.

These beneficial changes – among others – in lipid pattern find their expression in a reduction of CHD mortality, for example in the high-risk *North Karelia* region.[144] *Restricting meat intake* may also have beneficial effects: mortality from ischaemic heart disease in people who eat meat only occasionally or who eat fish but no meat are lower by 20, and 34 per cent respectively compared with regular meat eaters.[145] A comparable reduction in CVD mortality by 24 per cent is seen in *vegetarians* compared with non-vegetarians.[145]

However, simply lowering fat intake is not enough! A meta-analysis of 27 reports by the *Cochrane Collaboration*[146] has confirmed once more that a diet reduced in fat can lower cardiovascular mortality significantly, but only if the intake of ω-3-fatty acids from sea fish is increased for at least 2 years.

The *Mediterranean diet*[147] has also been demonstrated to be associated with a low CVD mortality, probably because its principal source of fat (olive oil) contains many monounsaturated fatty acids.[148]

Physical activitiy

In the working rat-heart model[149] and *in vitro* and *in vivo* studies of human skeletal muscle,[150] it has been demonstrated that activity can improve insulin sensitivity and glucose transport dramatically.

A randomized trial of lifestyle activity versus aerobic exercise during 16 weeks in 40 obese women[92] demonstrated highly significant decreases in triglycerides, total and LDL-cholesterol levels immediately after the intervention, but which did not last until the follow-up at week 68. This finding seems to underline once more the saying 'Sport accumulates no long-term interest'.

At least the decrease in LDL depends on the duration and intensity of activation.[151] In their study, 111 overweight men and women with mild to moderate dyslipidaemia were randomized to a treatment group with 32 km jogging equivalents per week, and to two others with 19.2 jogging equivalents or 10 km walking per week for 8 months and a fourth control group. LDL decrease was dependent on training duration, but also on its intensity. Weight loss had no influence on LDL levels, but all training groups had superior results to controls, and physical activation reduces blood pressure, a further advantage of physical activity.[152] It is a mainstay of preventive effort.[153]

TABLE 12.12 Changes in lipid levels by diet + lifestyle changes or diet + aerobic exercise during 16 weeks and at 1 year follow-up[92]

	Baseline	Week 16	p	Week 68	p
Triglycerides (mg/dl)					
Diet + aerobic	113 (50)	89 (33)	<0.001	94 (5.1)	<0.31
Diet + lifestyle	100 (49)	82 (45)		105 (63)	
Cholesterol (mg/dl)					
Diet + aerobic	208 (45)	186 (32)	<0.001	201 (30)	<0.01
Diet + lifestyle	207 (44)	184 (39)		202 (32)	
LDL – C (mg/dl)					
Diet + aerobic	134 (32)	122 (25)	<0.001	128 (21)	<0.27
Diet + lifestyle	134 (41)	119 (37)		128 (35)	
HDL – C (mg/dl)					
Diet + aerobic	51 (13)	46 (9)	<0.001	55 (16)	<0.11
Diet + lifestyle	53 (12)	48 (13)		55 (16)	

Mean (SD).

Prevention using drugs

The *UK-Heart Protection Study (HPS)* published in 2002 studied 20 536 high-risk individuals between 40 and 80 years of age. In a double-blind arrangement, they were treated for 5 years with either 40 mg simvastatin or placebo. Compared with controls, LDL levels were about 1 mmol = 38.8 mg/dl lower and total mortality decreased to 12.9 per cent versus 14.7 per cent in the placebo group (1328/1507 deaths). In respect to coronary events + stroke + revascularization, the simvastatin group fared better by a relative risk reduction of 24 per cent (19.8/25.2 per cent). Numbers needed to treat were 25 in diabetics and nearly 20 in the total group. *No positive effect could be demonstrated for a substitution with 600 mg vitamin E + 250 mg vitamin C + 20 mg β-carotene, 10 269 persons, versus placebo, 10 267 persons.* However, these at first sight striking improvements of LDL levels and relative risk by statins, cholestyramine, gemfibrozil or clofibrate can be seen only in high-risk patients, and to a much lesser degree in the general population.[140] In 2001, costs per life-year saved by statin treatment have been estimated to between $8000 and 18 000 in secondary prevention of high-risk patients and between $115 000 and 230 000 in primary prevention.[154] This correponds to roughly 210 000 up to 350 000 DM for one prevented death and to NNT 162–264[155] in secondary prevention and 940 000 DM and NNT 528–679 in

TABLE 12.13 NNT per year for myocardial infarction in three drug and five lifestyle studies[155]

Study	NNT to prevent one myocardial infarction per year
Prosper Study (pravastatin)	143
HPS Study (simvastatin)	156
Hope Study (ramipril)	200
Lifestyle Heart Trial	40
STRIP Study (diet including sitosterin)	112
Stress management	70
Indo-Med. Diet Heart Study	38
Lyon Heart Study	46

primary prevention.[156] Even in secondary prevention, this is 65–100 times the amount needed for prevention with ASS (NNT 187; 3200 DM).[156]

Comparing numbers needed to treat (NNTs) per year at least for the endpoint myocardial infarction shows a definite superiority of lifestyle modification compared with prevention with drugs (see Table 12.13).

However, on the other hand, in secondary prevention diabetics patients and other high-risk individuals should be given the chance to profit from a statin treatment. In Germany alone, with its 6–8 million diabetics, we could save 30–40 000 of these persons per year by an appropriate statin treatment, i.e. 40 mg simvastatin or an equivalent dose of some other statin per day.[157]

Sitosterin offers another possibility for dyslipidaemia prevention.[158] A diet margarine (Becel plus®) containing sitosterol, a plant sterol ester competitively inhibiting cholesterol absorption in the human gut, lowers LDL-C levels by 14 per cent, and in combination with simvastatin by up to 44 per cent.[159]

Perspectives of Obesity and Dyslipidaemia Prevention

A further *meta-analysis of the Cochrane Library*[160] has analysed 7193 abstracts and 99 full versions on the subject of obesity treatment. The authors arrived at the following conclusion: ‘Given the limited resources available for health care, cost-effective interventions to promote effective management of obesity need to be developed’.

This sobering statement stands in contrast to our rising need to treat even more endangered persons and to treat them even earlier, since we now recognize the progressive complications of diabetes and of the metabolic syndrome, which develop very early on. The ‘common soil’ hypothesis discussed at the 18th IDF congress[117] considers myocardial infarction and stroke not so much as consequences of elevated blood-sugar levels, but as due to the parallel development of complex metabolic disorders, which include Type 2 diabetes among others.

We must also take into account *that the different risk-factors obey the rule of multiplication rather than that of addition*. This explains why our therapeutic targets in correcting metabolic deviations have become stricter. Thus, whilst the *European NIDDM Policy Group* in 1989[161] defined a well controlled Type 2 diabetes by fasting blood glucose 80–120 mg/dl, HbA_1 (not HbA_{1c}!) < 8.5 per cent, triglycerides < 150 mg/dl and blood pressure $< 140/90$ mm Hg, today, Eberhard Standl,[162] president of the Deutsche Diabetes Union, proposes the formula :'6.5 and three times 100', i.e. $HbA_{1c} < 6.5$ per cent, fasting blood sugar < 100 mg/dl, LDL-cholesterol < 100 mg/dl and mean blood pressure < 100 mm Hg for the same situation. This reminds me of the old military idea of 'Asking for the impossible to get the possible'.

In our work for these possibilities with rather limited financial resources, prophylaxis of obesity and dyslipidaemia by lifestyle intervention recommends itself by its comparably low NNT (see Table 12.12). But we know that its long-term results are far from satisfying.[8] Moreover, treatment costs of fully developed obesity are high: between \$2.50 and 23 per kg weight lost by commercial outpatient weight-loss programmes in the early 1990s[9] and 616 DM (\$354) per kg weight lost during inpatient treatment even in 1980.[163]

Experts and practitioners involved in this work have come to recognize that classic individual treatment and primary prevention in a certain way represent a fight against the 'normal' situation in our time. Thus, we have to ask for a *certain degree of asceticism* and for more physical exertion in a time of cars, school buses and labour-saving devices. Lifestyle intervention programmes based on the principles of personal education and behaviour change are not likely to succeed in an environment that induces us to engage in opposing behaviours that lead to a chronic positive energy imbalance.[164]

The odds are not in our favour. Obesity is not due to one genetic abnormality or one behaviour-related abnormality. It is a by-product of modern lifestyle with many different roots.[9,165] *(see Figure 12.5)*.

In our prevention strategies, we must consider these different levels, address them and include the responsible authorities in our work.

These intervention strategies[166,9] are directed at

- improving the knowledge and skills of the community
- reducing population exposure to obesity-promoting environments
- increasing physical activity
- improving the quality of nutrition.

Building on the suggestions of Gill,[167] the WHO[9] proposes the strategies shown in Table 12.14.

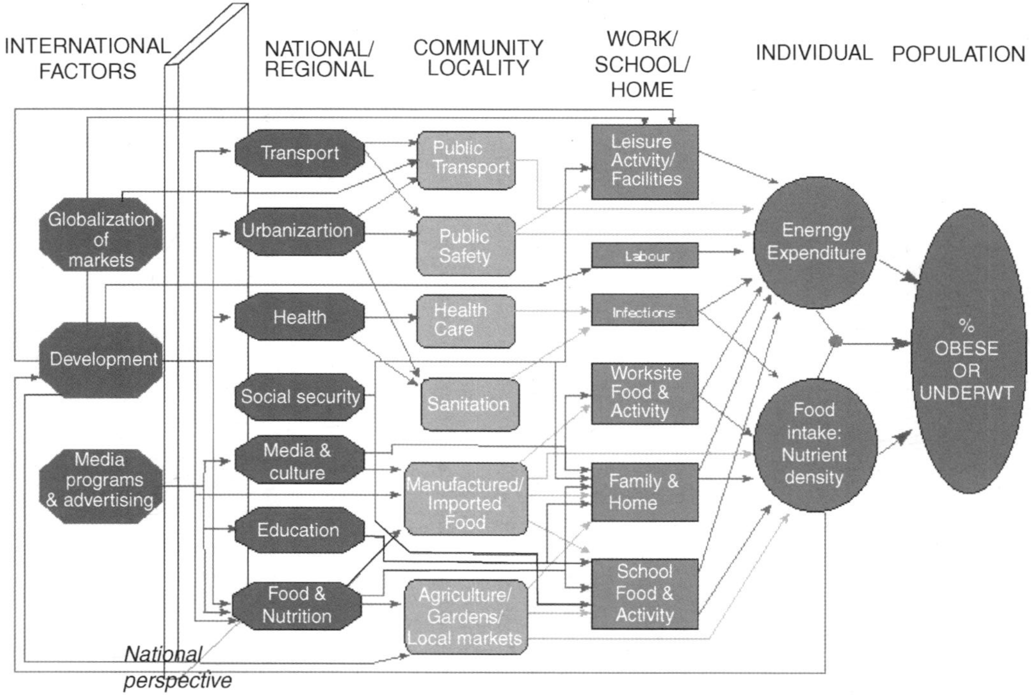

Modified from Ritenbaugh C, Kunaryika S, Morabia A, Jeffery R, Antipatis V.IOTF website 1999:

FIGURE 12.5 Many divergent factors determine obesity or underweight[165]

TABLE 12.14 Potential environmental strategies to control obesity[9,47]

Area for action	Example of possible strategies
Urban design and transportation policies	Create pedestrian zones in city centres
	Construct safe walkways and cycle paths
	Encourage use of peripheral car parks (park and ride)
	Provide affordable facilities for securing bikes in public areas
	Open public roads for biking and skating on holidays[47]
	Improve public transport
	Improve street lighting for safety
	Calm traffic to improve safety for children walking or playing
	Allocate resources to build and manage community recreation centres
	Provide half pipes for skating and playing fields for basketball and football[47]
	Modify building design to encourage use of stairs
	Reduce circulation of school buses[47]
Laws and regulations	Improve labelling of food products
	Limit and regulate advertising to children
	Parallel to measures against killers such as nicotine and alcohol, advertisment for obesity-promoting foodstuffs should be limited[47]
Economic incentives	Introduce subsidies for low-energy-density food (five a day)
	Reduce car tax for those who take public transport to work. Introduce tax breaks for companies that provide exercise and changing facilities for employees
School curricula	Provide adequate sport and activity areas and facilities, including changing and showering areas
	Ensure sufficient allocation of curriculum time to physical activity education
	Ensure training in the preparation of basic foodstuffs for all children
	Encourage well accepted sports such as inline skating and breakdance instead of gymnastics, which requires apparatus and is less popular among children[47]
	Introduce ice water taps instead of cola[47]
	Serve fruit and whole-grain products instead of cake and chocolate[47] at school shops
Food and catering standards	Develop nutritional standards and guidelines for institutionalized food services and catering (school meals and worksite catering)
	Indicate caloric content of portions on food wrappers
Promotion and education	Promote from an early age a knowledge of food and nutrition, food preparation and healthy diets and lifestyles through curricula for schoolchildren, teachers, health professionals and farmers and growers. Promote www.5aday.com[47]
	Limit TV viewing by children
	Use the media to promote positive behavioural change
	Educate the public, especially in areas where food is purchased, on appropriate behaviour change to reduce risk of weight gain
	Educate the public on the need for collective action to encourage an environment that promotes rather than inhibits improved exercise and good dietary habits
	Educate the public about important factors in the development of obesity so that victimization of the obese is reduced
	Discourage the 'slimness folly' in modelling[47]
	Incentives e.g. by newspapers to gain new clients by proposals of other clients should offer bonus points for fitness centres, swimming pools, tennis courts or golf courses instead of the usual hampers or coffee percolators[47]

TABLE 12.15 Number of centenarians increases in Germany[168]

Year	Number	Year	Number	Year	Number	Year	Number
1938	4 (!)	1991	1745	1995	2333	1999	2843
1975	146	1992	1627	1996	2515	2000	3098
1985	1142	1993	1959	1997	2756	2001	3483
1990	1416	1994	2164	1998	2948	2002	3883

This endeavour will be difficult and will take a lot of time, but we can be encouraged by the fact that medical – in line with other progress – has already prolonged – and is still prolonging – human lifetime expectation in developed countries to a large extent.

This is dramatically demonstrated by the growing number of *centenarians* in Germany,[168] for which we have exact figures as our Bundespräsident sends out anniversary congratulations to these seniors (see Table 12.15).

For the Netherlands Knook[169] has published comparable figures illustrating this sometimes mixed blessing:

1960, 63; 1970, 133; 1985, 583; 1990, 818 Dutch centenarians.

The level of *HDL-C* seems to be dramatically increased in 40 per cent of the offspring of centenarians and seems to correlate with their cognitive functioning.[170]

However, we still have a long way to go in this direction, since McDonald's, the favourite caterer of our kids for their birthday parties, at present offers only two salads and many more meals of the type 'Hamburger Royal TS economy menu with ketchup, a medium size portion of french (freedom) fries and a medium size cola' containing 60.605 g of fat and 1321.19 calories.[171] And our task is not facilitated by an ad of my favourite German carmaker proclaiming 'One movement too much is an extra too little'!

In conclusion I want to cite two statements on obesity prevention, an old and a modern one.

The experienced clinician *Herman Boerhave* (1668–1738) claimed[8] 'There are overly greedy savants who dare to eat the same meals as farmers, but they are not able to digest these foods: they must choose, either they have to abstain from their studies or change the order of their life; if not a long and terrible constipation will be the fruit of their thoughtlessness'.

And *GA Colditz*[172] wrote 'Programs aimed at avoiding weight gain in middle and later life, as well as preventing obesity in childhood, are important approaches to containing the rapidly rising health care costs in the United States as well as improving the quality of life.'

Acknowledgement

I want to thank Mr. David Jones, Holywell UK, for helping me with the translation and in developing my alpine skiing skills.

References

1. Howard A (ed.) *Recent Advances in Obesity Research I* 1975; London: Newman.
2. Hirsch J. and van Itallie TB (ed.) *Recent Advances in Obesity Research IV* 1985; London: Libbey.
3. Berry EM, Blondheim SH, Eliahou HE and Shafrir E (eds). *Recent Advances in Obesity Research* V. 1987. London: Libbey.
4. Guy-Grand B and Ailhaud G (eds). *Progress in Obesity Research: 8.* 1999; London: Libbey.
5. Bouchardat A. *De la Glycosurie ou Diabète Sucré* 1875; Paris: Germer-Baillière.
6. O'Dea K. Diabetes in Australian Aborigines: impact of Western diet and lifestyle. *J Intern. Med* 1991; **232**: 103–117.
7. Fußgänger RD. Die Geschichte des Fastens. In *Das modifizierte Fasten,* Ditschuneit H, Wechsler JG (eds). 1981; Baden-Baden: Witzstrock, pp. 3–34.
8. Liebermeister H. *Adipositas – Ursachen, Diagnostik, moderne Therapieoptionen.* 2002; Köln: Deutscher Ärzteberlag.
9. WHO Report (1998) of a Consultation on Obesity (3–5 June 1997) (WHO/NUT/NCD/ 98.1). Geneva.
10. McGinnis JM and Foege WH. Actual causes of death in the United States. *J Am Med Assoc* 1993; **270**: 2207–2212.
11. International Diabetes Federation (IDF). *Diabetes Atlas, Second Edition Executive Summary* 2003; Brussels: IDF (www.idf.org).
12. Shafrir E and Raz I. For debate. Diabetes: mellitus or lipidus. *Diabetologia* 2003; **46**: 433–440.
13. Alpert S. Growth, thermogenesis and hyperphagia. *Am J Clin Nutr* 1990; **52**: 784–792.
14. Neel JV. Diabetes mellitus: a 'thrifty' genotype rendered detrimental by 'progress'? *Am J Hum Genet* 1962; **14**: 353–357.
15. Liebermeister H, Voss HJ, Englhardt A, Probst G and Jahnke K. Initial– und Spätergebnisse der Diätbehandlung bei Fettsucht. *Dtsch Med Wschr* 1968; **93**: 2149–2155.
16. Ohno M, Arai K, Tsukahara S, Miura I, Yokohama J and Ikeda Y. Long-term effectiveness of combined therapy by behaviour modification and VLCD: a three year follow-up. In *Progress in Obesity Research* 1990; Oumura Y et al. (eds). London: Libbey. pp. 523–529.
17. McGuire MT, Wing RR, Klem ML, Seagle HM and Hill JO. Long-term maintenance of weight loss: do people who lose weight through various weight loss methods use different behaviors to maintain their weight? *Int J Obes* 1998; **22**: 572–577.
18. Hauner H (ed.) Deutsche Adipositas Gesellschaft, Deutsche Diabetes Gesellschaft, Deutsche Gesellschaft für Ernährung: Prävention und Therapie der Adipositas. 2003; www.awmf-leitlinien.de.
19. European Project for Primary Care. 2002; www.iotf.org/oonet/easo.
20. Kral J, Wadden TA and van Itallie TB (eds). Surgical treatment of obesity. In *Treatment of the Seriously Obese Patient,* 1995; New York: Guilford: pp. 496–506.
21. Husemann B. Zukunft der Adipositaschirurgie. *Dtsch. Ärzteblatt* 2003; **100**: C1061–C1067.
22. Husemann B. Die chirurgische Therapie der extremen Adipositas. Adipositas-Mitteilungen 2000; **20/2000**: 10–21.
23. Latifi R, Kellum JM, De Maria EJ and Sugerman HJ. Surgical treatment of obesity. In *Handbook of Obesity Treatment.* Wadden TA, Stunkard AJ (eds). 2002; New York: Guilford, pp. 339–356.
24. Sjöström D, Lissner L and Sjöström L. Relationships between body composition and changes in cardiovascular risk factors: the SOS-intervention study. *Obes Res* 1997; **5**: 519–530.

25. Colditz GA. Economic costs of obesity and inactivity. *Medicine and Science in Sports and Exercise, American College of Sports Medicine* 1999; S663–S667.
26. Schneider R. *Relevanz und Kosten der Adipositas in Deutschland. Ernährungsumschau* 1996; **43**: 369–374.
27. Lévy E, Lévy P, LePen C and Basdevant A. The economic cost of obesity: the French situation. *Int J Obes* 1995; **19**: 788–792.
28. Landmann S. *Jüdische Anekdoten und Sprichwörter, 6th edn.* 1972; München: dtv, p. 205.
29. Standl E. *Preface to the Deutscher Gesundheitsbericht Diabetes* 2003; Mainz: DDU–Kirchheim, p. 9.
30. *Build Study.* 1979. Society of Actuaries and Association of Life Insurance Medical Directors of America. Boston, MA: Recording and Statistical Corporation. 1980.
31. Sjöström L. Impacts of body weight, body composition and adipose tissue distribution on morbidity and mortality. In *Obesity: Theory and Therapy* Stunkard AJ, Wadden TA (eds), 2nd edn. 1993; New York: Raven, pp. 13–42.
32. Paffenbarger RS, Hyde RT, Wing AL, I-Min Lee, Jung DL and Kampert JB. The association of changes in physical activity and other lifestyle characteristics with mortality among men. *N Engl J Med* 1993; **328**: 538–545.
33. Biermann E. Wichtige Diabetes Begleiterkrankungen. In *Deutscher Gesundheitsbericht Diabetes 2003,* Standl E. (ed.) for the Deutsche Diabetes Union. 2003; Mainz: Kirchheim, pp. 22–26.
34. MRC/MBF. Heart Protection Study (HPS). *Lancet* 2002; **361**: 2005–2013.
35. UKPDS Study Group. Tight blood pressure control and risk of macrovascular and microvascular complications in Type 2 diabetes. *BMJ* 1998; **317**: 703–713.
36. Gaede P, Vedel P, Larsen N, Jensen GV, Parvina HH and Pedersen O. Multifactorial intervention and cardiovascular disease in patients with Type 2 diabetes. *N Engl J Med* 2003; **348**: 383–393.
37. Lewis J, Parving HH, Ravid M and Remuzzi G. DEMAND-Study (Developing Education on Microalbuminuria for Awareness of renal and cardiovascualr risk in Diabetes). *36th Annual Conference of the American Society of Nephrology*, San Diego, 2003.
38. Rathmann W, Haastert, Icks A, Löwel H, Meisinger C, Holle R and Giani G. High prevalence of undiagnosed diabetes mellitus in southern Germany: target populations for efficient screening. *The KORA survey 2000. Diabetologia* 2003; **46**: 182–189.
39. Liebermeister H. *Effects of Weight Reduction on Obesity-Associated Diseases.* 2003; www.egms.de/en/gms/2003–1/000004.shtml.
40. Smith SR and Zachwieja JJ. Visceral adipose tissue: a critical review of intervention strategies. *Int J Obes Relat Metab Disord* 1999; **23**: 329–335.
41. Allison DB, Zannolli R, Faith MS, Heo M, Pietrobello A and Van Itallie DB *et al.* Weight loss increases and fat loss decreases all-cause mortality rates: results from two independent cohort studies. *Int J Obes* 1999; **23**: 603–611.
42. Pi-Sunyer FX. Medical hazards of obesity. *Ann Intern Med* 1993; **119**: 655–660.
43. Weintraub M, Sundaresan PR, Madan M, Schuster B, Balder A and Lasagna L. Long-term weight control study. I–VII. *Clin Pharmacol Ther* 1992; **51**: 634–641.
44. WHO. *Obesity: Preventing and Managing the Global Epidemic*, WHO Technical Report Series 894. 2000; Geneva.
45. Hillenbrand H and Standl E. Diabetes und gesundheitsökonomische Aspekte. In *Deutsche Diabetes Union,* Standl E. (ed.). *Deutscher Gesundheitsbericht Diabetes 2003.* 2003; Mainz: Kirchheim, 62–67.
46. Colditz GA. Economic costs of obesity. *Am J Clin Nutr* 1992; **55**: S503–S507.
47. Liebermeister H. Lifestyle-Faktoren: treibende Kraft der Epidemie. In *Deutscher Gesundheitsbericht Diabetes 2003,* Standl E. for the DDU (ed.). 2003; Mainz: Kirchheim, pp. 12–16.

48. Demand-Study. International Diabetes Federation (IDF): presented at the 36th Annual Meeting of the American Society of Nephrology, San Diego, 2003.
49. Grüneklee D. Zahlen und Fakten im Überblick, Deutsche Diabetes Stiftung, Ausgabe 2003, Paderborn.
50. Schmitz KH and Jeffery RW. Prevention of obesity. In *Handbook of Obesity Treatment*, Wadden TA and Stunkard AJ (eds). 2002; New York: Guilford, pp. 556–593.
51. Rössner S. Prevention of obesity – highlights from the Stockholm meeting 26–28 August 1998. In *Progress in Obesity Research: 8* Guy-Grand B and Ailhaud G (eds). 1999; London: Libbey, pp. 825–828.
52. Stern JS. (ed.). *Weighing the Options*. Institute of Medicine. 1995; Washington, DC: National Academic, pp. 112–115.
53. Bloom WL and Eidex MF. *Inactivity as a major factor in adult obesity* 1967; Metabolism **16**: pp. 679–684.
54. Wing RR. Changing diet and exercise behaviors in individuals at risk of weight gain. *Obes Res* 1995; **3**: (Suppl. 2): S277−S282.
55. Lorenz K. *Über menschliches und tierisches Verhalten* 1965; München: Piper R.
56. Berger M et al. *Schulungsmaterial für Typ-II−Diabetiker, die nicht Insulin spritzen.* 1991; Köln: Deutscher Ärzteberlag.
57. Frank M. Schulungskonzepte bei Diabetikern im stationären und ambulanten Bereich. *Der Internist* 2001; **42**: (Suppl. 1): S55–S61.
58. Collins RW and Anderson JW. Medication cost savings associated with weight loss for obese non-insulin-dependent diabetic men and women. *Preventive Med* 1995; **24**: 369–374.
59. Lenthe-Schäfer K. *Medikamenteneinsparung durch Gewichtsreduktion.* 1999; Medizinische Dissertation, Homburg-Saar.
60. DPP Group.Within-trial cost-effectiveness of lifestyle intervention or metformin for the primary prevention of Type 2 diabetes. *Diabetes Care* 2003; **26**: 2518–2523.
61. Hauner H. Personal communication. 1999.
62. Apfelbaum M and Bostsarron J. Le bilan d'énergie de l'obèse soumis à un régime restrictif. *Presse Médicale* 1969; **77**: 1941–1943.
63. Leibel RL, Rosenbaum M and Hirsch J. Changes in energy expenditure resulting from altered body weight. *N Engl J Med* 1995; **332**: 621–628.
64. Kern PA, Ong JM, Saffari B and Carty J. The effects of weight loss on activity and the expression of adipose-tissue protein lipase in very obese humans. *N Engl J Med* 1990; **322**: 1053–1059.
65. National Task Force (US) on the Prevention and Treatment of Obesity. *J Am Med Assoc* 1994; **272**: 1196–1202.
66. Taylor CB and Stunkard AJ. Public health approaches to weight control in *Obesity – Theory and Therapy*, Stunkard AJ and Wadden TA (eds). 2nd edn, 1993; New York: Raven, 335.
67. Liebermeister C. Verbreitung des Abdominaltyphus durch Trinkwasser. *Dtsch Archiv für Klin Med* 1870; **VII**: 155–182.
68. Glenny AM, O'Meara S, Melville A, Sheldon TA and Wilson C. The treatment and prevention of obesity: a systematic review of the literature. *Int J Obes* 1997; **21**: 715–737.
69. Taylor CB, Fortman SP, Flora J, Kayman S, Barrett DC, Jatulis D and Farquhar JW. Effect of long-term community health education on body mass-index, the Stanford Five City Project. *Am J Epidemiol* 1991; **134**: 235–249
70. Tudor-Smith C, Nutbeam D, Moore L and Catford J. Effects of the Heartbeat Wales programme over five years on behavioural risks for cardiovascular disease, quasi experimental comparison of results from Wales and a matched reference area. *BMJ* 1998; **316**: 818–822.

71. French SA, Jeffery RW and Murray D. Is dieting good for you?: prevalence, duration and associated weight and behaviour changes for specific weight-loss strategies over four years in US-adults. *Int J Obes* 1999; **23**: 320–327.
72. Wiesemann A, Metz J, Nuessel E, Scheidt R and Scheurermann W. Four years of practice-based and exercise-supported behavioural medicine in one community of the German CINDI-area: countrywide integrated non-communicable disease intervention. *Int J Sports Med* 1997; **18**: 308–315.
73. Brownson RC, Smith CA and Pratt M *et al.* Preventing cardiovascular disease through community-based risk reduction: the Bootheel Heart Health Project. *J Publ Health* 1996; **86**: 206–213.
74. Hoffmeister H, Mensink GBM, Stolzenberg H, Hoeltz J, Kreuter H and Laaser U *et al.* Reduction of coronary heart disease risk factors in the German Cardiovascular Prevention Study. *Prevent Med* 1996; **25**: 135–145.
75. Jeffery JW, Gray CW, French SA, Hellerstedt WL, Murray D, Luepker RV and Blackburn H. Evaluation of weight reduction in a community intervention for cardiovascular disease risk: change in body-mass index in the Minnesota Heart Health Program. *Int J Obes* 1995; **19**: 30–39.
76. Hoffmeister H, Mensink GBM and Stolzenberg H *et al.* Reduction of coronary heart disease risk factor in the German Cardiovascular Prevention Study. *Prevent Med* 1996; **25**: 135–145.
77. Wirth A. Community programmes for weight prevention: are they effective? *Int Monitor Obes Metab Weight Control* 1997; **6** (1): 9–10.
78. DiPietro L, Kohl HW III, Barlow CE and Blair SN. Improvements in cardiorespiratory fitness attenuate age-related weight-gain in healthy men and women: The Aerobic Center Longitudinal Study. *Int J Obes* 1998; **22**: 55–62.
79. Bullen BA, Reed RB and Mayer J. Physical activity of obese and nonobese adolescent girls appraised by motion picture sampling. *Am J Clin Nutr* 1964; **14**: 211–223.
80. Prentice AM and Jebb SA. Obesity in Britain: gluttony or sloth?. *BMJ* 1995; **311**: 437–439.
81. Martinez-Gonzalez MA, Martinez JA, Hu FB, Gibney MJ and Kearney J. Physical inactivity, sedentary lifestyle and obesity in the European Union. *Int J Obes* 1999; **23**: 1192–1201.
82. Baller DL and Poehlman ET. Exercise-training enhances fat-free mass preservation during diet-induced weight loss: a meta-analytical finding. *Int J Obes* 1994; **18**: 35–40.
83. Wilmore JH, Despres JP, Stanford PR, Mandel S, Gagnon J, Leon AS, Rao DC, Skinner JS and Bouchard C. Alterations in body weight and composition in 20 wk of endurance training: the Heritage Family Study. *Am J Clin Nutr* 1999; **70**: 346–352.
84. Borg P, Kukkonen-Harjula K, Fogelholm M and Pasanen M. Effects of walking or resistance training on weight loss maintenance in obese, middle-aged men: a randomized trial. *Int J Obes* 2002; **26**: 676–683.
85. Ford ES. Does exercise reduce inflammation? Physical activity and C-reactive protein among U.S. adults. *Epidemiology* 2002; **13**: 561–569.
86. Berg A. Körperliche Aktivität und Übergewicht – was können Sport und Bewegung leisten? *Aktuelle Ernährungsmedizin* 2003; **28**: 292–299.
87. Byberg L, Zethelius B, McKeigue PM and Lithell HO. Changes in physical activity are associated with changes in metabolic cardiovascular risk factors. *Diabetologia* 2001; **44**: 2134–2139.
88. Short KR, Vittone JL, Bigelow ML, Proctor DN, Rizza RA, Coenen-Schimke JM and Nair KS. Influence of aerobic exercise training on age-related changes in insulin sensitivity and muscle oxidative capacity. *Diabetes* 2003; **52**: 2304–2314.

89. Pasman WJ, Westerp-Platenga MS and Saris WHM. The effect of body weight changes and endurance training on 24 h substrate oxidation. *Int J Obes* 1999; **23**: 1223–1232.
90. Lee CD, Jackson AS and Blair SN. US weight guidelines: is it also important to consider cardiorespiratory fitness? *Int J Obes* 1998; **22** (Suppl. 2): 2–7.
91. Barlo CE, Kohl HW, Gibbons LW and Blair SN. Physical fitness, mortality and obesity. *Int J Obes* 1995; **19** (Suppl. 4): S41–S44.
92. Andersen RE, Wadden TA, Bartlett SJ, Zemel B, Verde TJ and Franckowiak SC. Effects of lifestyle activity vs structured aerobic exercise in obese women. *J Am Med Assoc* 1999; **261**: 335–340.
93. Schmitz KH, Jensen MD, Kugler KC, Jeffery BW and Leon AS. Strength training for obesity prevention in midlife women. *Int J Obes* 2003; **27**: 326–333.
94. Jeffery RW and French SA. Preventing weight gain in adults: design, methods and one-year results from the Pound of Prevention Study. *Int J Obes* 1997; **21**: 457–464.
95. Sjöström L. What should be primary treatment: obesity or obesity complications? *Int J Obes* 1998; **22** (Suppl. 3): S3.
96. Hennrikus DJ and Jeffery RW. Worksite interventions for weight control: a review of the literature. *Am J Health Promotion* 1996; **10** (6): 471–498.
97. Jeffery JW and French SA. Preventing weight gain in adults: the Pound of Prevention Study. *Am J Publ Health* 1999; **89** (5): 747–751.
98. Simkin-Silverman L, Wing RR, Boraz MA, Meilahn EM and Kuller LH. Maintenance of cardiovascular risk factor changes among middle-aged women in a lifestyle-intervention trial. *Women's Health* 1998; **4** (3): 255–271.
99. Klem ML, Viteri JE and Wing RR. Primary prevention of weight gain for women aged 25–34: the acceptability of treatment formats. *Int J Obes* 2000; **24**: 219–225.
100. Cavill N. National campaigns to promote physical activity: can they make a difference? *Int J Obes* 1998; **22** (Suppl. 2): S48–S51.
101. Owen N, Bowman A, Booth M, Oldenburg B and Magnus P. Serial mass-media campaigns to promote physical activity: reinforcing or redundant? *Am J Publ Health* 1995; **85** (2): 244–248.
102. Ellrott T and Pudel V. Pfundskur – Multimediale Prävention in Baden-Württemberg und Sachsen. *Ernährungs-Umschau* 2003; **50**: B5–B8.
103. Trichopoulos A, Costacou T, Bamia C and Trichopoulos D. Adherence to a Mediterranean diet and survival in a Greek population. *New Engl J Med* 2003; **348**: 2599–2608.
104. Knowler WC for the DPP Group. Reduction in the incidence of Type 2 diabetes with lifestyle intervention or metformin. *N Engl J Med* 2002; **346**: 393–403.
105. Tuomilehto J. For the Finnish Diabetes Prevention Study Group. Prevention of Type 2 diabetes mellitus by changes in lifestyle among subjects with impaired glucose tolerance. *N Engl J Med* 2001; **344**: 1343–1350.
106. Pan XR *et al.* Effects of diet and exercise in preventing NIDDM in people with impaired glucose tolerance. The Da Quing IGT and Diabetes Study. *Diabetes Care* 1997; **20** (4), 537–544.
107. Garb JR and Stunkard AJ. Effectiveness of a self-help group in obesity control: a further assessment. *Arch Intern Med* 1971; **134**: 716–720.
108. Wirth A. *Adipositas*. 1997, Heidelberg: Springer.
109. Christakis G and Miller-Kovach K. Maintenance of weight goal among Weight Watchers lifetime members. *Nutrition Today* 1996; **31**: 29–31.
110. Heshka S, Anderson JW, Atkinson RL, Greenway FL, Hill JO, Phinney SD, Kolotkin RL, Miller-Kovach K and PiSunyer FX. Weight loss with self-help compared with a structured commercial program. A randomized trial. *J Am Med Assoc* 2003; **289**: 1792–1798.

111. Olschewski P, Ellrott T, Jakanen J, Pudel V, Scholten T, Heisterkamp F and Siebeneick S. Langzeiterfolg eines multidisziplinären Gewichtsmanagement-Programms. *Müchener Med Wochenschrift* 1997; **139**: 245–250.
112. Walle B and Walle H. Diät mit Zusatz-Eiweiß verhindert Jojo-Effekt. *Ärztezeitung* 5 November 2003: **15**.
113. Sjöstöm L, Torgerson JS, Hauptman J and Boldrin M. XENDOS: Xenical for diabetes prevention in overweight persons. Poster-Presentation, 9th. Congress ICO Sao Paulo, 2002, update April 2003 for 1st. Arbeitstagung der AG Prävention des Typ–2-Diabetes der DDG, Dresden, 2003.
114. Diabetes Prevention Program Research Group (DPPRG). Reduction in the incidence of type 2 diabetes with life style intervention or metformin. *N Engl J Med* 2002; **346**: 393–403.
115. Chiasson JL, Josse RG, Gomis R, Hanefeld M, Karasik A, Laakso M for the STOP-NIDDM Trial Research Group. Acarbose for prevention of Type 2 diabetes mellitus: the STOP-NIDDM randomised trial. *Lancet* 2002; **359**, 2072–2077.
116. Löllgen H. Primärprävention kardialer Erkrankungen. *Dtsch Ärzteblatt* 2003; **100** (15): C773–C779.
117. *IDF Congress.* 2003; Paris.
118. Schwimmer JB, Burwinkle TM and Varni JW. Health-related quality of life of severely obese children and adolescents. *J Am Med Assoc* 2003; **289**: 1813–1819.
119. Must W and Strauss RS. Risks and consequences of childhood and adolescent obesity. *Int J Obes* 1999; **23** (Suppl. 2): S2–S11.
120. Ehtisham S, Barrett TG and Shaw NJ. Type 2 diabetes mellitus in UK children – an emerging problem. *Diabetic Med* 2000; **17**: 867–871.
121. Power C, Lake JK and Cole TJ. Measurement and long-term health risks of child and adolescent fatness. *Int J* Obes 1997; **21**: 507–526.
122. Must A, Jacques PF, Dallal GE, Bajema CJ and Dieth WH. Long-term morbidity and mortality of overweight adolescents. A follow-up of the Harvard Growth Study of 1922 to 1935. *N Engl J Med* 1992; **327**: 1350–1355.
123. Charney E, Goodman HC, McBride M, Lyon B and Pratt R. Childhood antecedents of adult obesity (do chubby infants become obese adults?) *N Engl J Med* 1976; **295**: 6–9.
124. Garn SM. Continuities and changes in fatness from infancy through adulthood. *Curr Probl Pediatr* 1985; **15**: 2–47.
125. Robinson TM, Hammer LD, Killen JD, Kraemer HC, Wilson DM, Hayward C and Taylor CB. Does television viewing increase obesity and reduce physical activity? Cross-sectional and longitudinal analyses among adolescent girls. *Pediatrics* 1993; **91**: 273–280.
126. Ludwig DS, Peterson KE and Gortmaker SL. Relation between consumption of sugar-sweetened drinks and childhood obesity: a prospective, observational analysis. *Lancet* 2001; **357**: 505–508.
127. Parsons TJ, Power C, Logan S and Summerbell CD. Childhood predictors of adult obesity: a systematic review. *Int J Obes* 1999; **23** (Suppl. 8): S1–S107.
128. Lissner L and Eiben G. Is it possible to prevent obesity in SOS-offspring? Pilot data from the Health Hunters Program. *Progress in Obesity Research 8*, Guy-Grand B, Ailhaud G (eds.) 1999; London: Libbey, pp. 845–851.
129. Epstein LH, Valoski A, Wing RR and McCurley J. Ten-year follow-up of behavioral family-based treatment for obese children. *J Am Med Assoc* 1990; **264**: 2519–2523.
130. Epstein LH and Goldfield GS. Physical activity in the treatment of childhood overweight and obesity: current evidence and research issues. *Medicine and Science in Sports and Exercise* 1990; **31** (Suppl. 11): S553–S559.

131. Golan M, Fainaru M and Weizman A. Role of behaviour modification in the treatment of childhood obesity with the parents as the exclusive agents of change. *Int J Obes* 1998; **22**: 1217–1224.
132. Kanders BS. Pediatric obesity. In *Weighing the Options*, Paul IT (ed.). 1995; Washington, DC: Institute of Medicine, National Academy Press; pp. 210–233.
133. Korsten-Reck U, Wolfarth J, Bonk K, Keul B and Berg A. Therapie von übergewichtigen Kindern – Behandlungskonzepte und Erfahrungen. *Zschr Ärztl Fortb Qual Sich* 2000; **94**: 677–681.
134. Barlow SE and Dietz WH. Obesity evaluation and treatment. Expert committee recommendations. *Pediatrics* 1998; **102** (3): e 29.
135. Fairburn CG and Cooper Z. New perspectives on the dietary and behavioural treatment for obesity. *Int J Obes* 1996; **20** (Suppl. 1): S9–S13.
136. Vialettes B. La prise du poids à l'adolescence. *Equilibre* 2001; **223**: 27–30.
137. Neaton JD, Blackburn H and Jacobs D *et al.* Serum cholesterol levels and mortality findings for men screened in the Multiple Risk Factor Intervention Trial. *Arch Intern Med* 1992; **152**: 1490–1500.
138. Pooling Project Research Group. Results of blood pressure, serum cholesterol, smoking habit, relative weight and ECG-abnormalities to incidence of major coronary events: final report of the Pooling Project. *J Chron Dis* 1978; **31**: 201–306.
139. National Cholesterol Education Program (NCEP). Expert panel on detection, evaluation, and treatment of high blood cholesterol in adults. Executive summary of the third report of the NCEP expert panel (Adult Treatment Panel III). *J Am Med Assoc* 2001; **285**: 2486–2497.
140. Schwandt P. The importance of reaching lipid targets: statins and the prevention of atherosclerosis. *IJCP* 2003; **57**: 396–404.
141. European Atherosclerosis Society. Prevention of coronary heart disease: scientific background and new clinical guidelines. *Nutr Metab Cardiovasc Dis* 1992; **2**: 113–156.
142. Obarzanek E, Sacks FM and Vollmer WM *et al.* effects of blood pressure-lowering diet: the Dietary Approaches to Stop Hypertension (DASH) Trial. *Am J Clin Nutr* 2001; **74**: 80–89.
143. Tremo M, Passera P, Bajardi M, Tomalino M, Grassi G, Borgo E, Donnola C, Cavallo F, Bondonio P and Porta M. Lifestyle intervention by group care prevents deterioration of Type 2 diabetes: a 4-year randomized controlled clinical trial. *Diabetologia* 2002; **45**: 1231–1239.
144. Pietinen P, Lahti-Koski M, Vartiainen E and Puska P. Nutrition and cardiovascular disease in Finland since the early 1970's: a success story. *J Nutr Health Aging* 2001; **5**:150–154.
145. Key TJ, Fraser GE and Thorogood M *et al.* Mortality in vegetarians and non-vegetarians: detailed findings from a collaborative analysis of five prospective studies. *Am J Clin Nutr* 1999; **70** (Suppl. 3): S516–S524.
146. Hooper L, Summerbell CD, Higgins JPT, Thompson RL, Clements G, Capps N, Davey Smith G, Riemersma RA and Ebrahim S. Reduced or modified dietary fat for prevention of cardiovascular disease. *Cochrane Library Document* 2000; Oxford, pp. 1–81.
147. World Cancer Research Fund (WCR). *Food, Nutrition and the Prevention of Cancer: a Global Perspective* 1997; Washington, DC: American Institute for Cancer Research, pp. 31–32.
148. Visioli F and Galli C. Antiatherogenic components of olive oil. *Curr Atheroscl Rep* 2001; **3**: 64–67.
149. Neely JR, Liebermeister H and Morgan HE. Effect of pressure development on membrane transport of glucose in isolated rat heart. *Am J Physiol* 1967; **212**: 815–822.
150. Zierath JR, Krook A and Wallberg-Henrikson H. Insulin action and insulin resistance in human skeletal muscle. *Diabetologia* 2000; **43**: 821–835.

151. Kraus W, Houmard JA, Duscha BD, Knetzger KJ and Wharton MB *et al.* Effects of the amount and intensity of exercise on plasma lipoprotein. *N Engl J Med* 2002; **347**: 1483–1492.
152. Kostka T, Lacour JR and Bonnefoy M. Response of blood lipids to physical exercise in elderly subjects. *Prev Cardiol* 2001; **4**: 122–125.
153. Després JP, Lamarche B, Bouchard C, Tremblay A and Prud'homme D. Exercise and the prevention of dyslipidemia and coronary heart disease. *Int J Obes* 1995; **19** (Suppl. 4): S45–S51.
154. Kübler W. Was kostet ein Lebensjahr? 27. Jahrestagung Deutsche Gesellschaft für Prävention und Rehabilitation von Herz-Kreislauf–Erkrankungen, *Berlin Med Tribune* 2001; **36** (6): 10.
155. Arzneimittelbrief, N.N. Bewertung von Studien zur Modifikation des Lebensstils mit Hilfe der Number Needed to Treat. 2003; **37** (8): 63–64.
156. Berufsverband Deutscher Internisten (BDI) N.N. CSE-Hemmer (Statin-Studien) im Vergleich: Patienten, Sterblichkeit, Risikoreduktion (bezogen auf kardiovaskuläre und Gesamtmortalität) sowie Kosten. *BDI-Rundschreiben* 2001; **5–2001**: 44–45.
157. Füchtenbusch M and Schnell O. Die UK-Medical Research Council (MRC/British Heart Foundation (BHF) Heart Protection Study (HPS)). *Diabetes Stoffwechsel* 2003; **12**: 129–134.
158. Westrate JA and Meijer GW. Plant sterol-enriched margarines and reduction of plasma total– and LDL-cholesterol concentrations in normocholesterolaemic and mildly hypercholesterolaemic subjects. *Eur J Clin Nutr* 1998; **52**, 334–343.
159. Richter WO. Sicherheit der Behandlung mit CSE-Hemmern. *VitaMinSpur* 2001; **16**: 183–187.
160. Harvey EL, Glenny A, Kirk SFL and Summerbell CD. Improving health professional's management and the organisation of care for overweight and obese people. *Cochrane Library Document* 1998.
161. European NIDDM Policy Group. *A Desktop Guide for the Management of Non-Insulin-Dependent Diabetes Mellitus (NIDDM)* 1989; Brussels.
162. Standl E. Presentation. *Deutscher Gesundheitsbericht Diabetes* 2003; Berlin.
163. Oelschlägel G and Liebermeister H. Vergleich von totalem und modifiziertem Fasten in bezug auf: Effizienz, Laborparameter und Kosten. Akt. Endokr. *Stoffw* 1983; **4**: 189–195.
164. Jeffery JW. Public health approaches to the managment of obesity. In *Eating disorders and Obesity: a Comprehensive Handbook*, Brownell KD, Fairburn CG (eds). 1995; London: Guildford, pp. 558–563.
165. International Obesity Task Force: Ritenbaugh C, Kunaryika S, Morabia A and Jeffery R. www.iotf.org/groups/phapo/causal.htm. 1999.
166. James WPT. A public health approach to the problem of obesity. *Int J Obes* 1995; **19** (Suppl. 3): S37–S45.
167. Gill TP. Key issues in the prevention of obesity. *Br Med Bull* 1997; **53**: 359–388.
168. Bundespräsidialamt 2003; Berlin.
169. Knook DL. Wie alt kann ein Mensch werden? *Der Bayerische Internist* 1993; **13**: 26–28.
170. Evert J, Lawler E, Bogan H and Perls T. Morbidity profiles of centenarians: survivors, delayers and escapers. *J Gerontol Med Sci* 2003; **58A** (3): 232–237.
171. Kaiser T. McDonald's will kein Dickmacher mehr sein. *Welt am Sonntag* 16 November 2003; **33**.
172. Colditz GA. The costs of obesity: medical and socioeconomic aspects. *Medicographia* 1994; **16** (3): 43–45.
173. Amler RW and Dull HB (eds). *Closing the Gap: the Burden of Unnecessary Illness* 1987; New York: Oxford University Press.

174. European Association for the Study of Obesity. www.iotf.org/oonet/easo. 2002;
175. Hu G, Qiao Q, Silventoinen K, Eriksson JG, Jousilahti P, Lindstöm J, Valle TT, Nissinen A and Tuomilehto J. Occupational, commuting, and leisure-time physical activity in relation to risk for Type 2 diabetes in middle-aged Finnish men and women. *Diabetologia* 2003; **46**: 322–329.

13

Renal Dysfunction and Hypertension, Focus on Type 2 Diabetes

Carl Erik Mogensen

Introduction

Nephropathy in Type 2 diabetes has emerged as a severe clinical problem and diabetes of this type is now more frequently seen than advanced renal disease in Type 1 diabetes.[4,9,93] However, in the 1970s and 1980s, renal complications due to Type 2 diabetes seemed to be rare in the clinic so this new development is surprising. Today, most patients in dialysis units are Type 2 diabetic patients.[23,94,120] You may thus ask why and how Type 2 diabetes lost its 'renal innocence'.[91]

There is probably not one single factor that is responsible for this new problem. In all likelihood, there are more frequent referrals of old severely ill patients with terminal renal failure than earlier. It is also clear that there is a dramatically rising prevalence of Type 2 diabetes in the general population. This is partly due to the adoption of new and 'less healthy' lifestyles. However, an even more important factor in this context is that survival of patients with Type 2 diabetes is much better now simply because of better treatment of hypertension and coronary heart disease, conditions that previously were quite common in these patients, and which could not be or were not treated.

There is thus a change in life pattern of these patients – they often live long enough to develop renal disease and even renal failure. The increase in number of patients is also a result of medical progress[21,66] where cardiovascular mortality to some extent has been replaced by end-stage renal disease (ESRD) as the terminal fate of these patients. It should be noted that the strict classification of Type 1 and

Prevention of Type 2 Diabetes Edited by Manfred Ganz
 ISBN: 0-470-85733-1

Type 2 diabetes may by no means be completely relevant because there are many patients in whom classification is problematic and besides the pathogenesis and treatment strategy is very similar. Thus, new studies suggest that the clinical course of renal disease is very much the same in the two types of diabetes,[10,46,92,93] but further studies are clearly needed.[49]

Type 2 diabetes is probably a polygenic condition that acts in a complicated interplay of lifestyle and environment. Ironically, our improved living conditions, with more abundant food and less hard physical work, have re-appeared as a boomerang, creating new degenerative diseases, which are not due to physical burdens or hard work, as discussed elsewhere in this volume.

Historical Aspects

Going back to the pre-insulin era, patients who developed complications related to diabetes would be Type 2 diabetic patients because Type 1 patients would simply not survive long enough. As early as the 19th century, it was recognised that urine of diabetic patients contained abnormal amounts of coagulable matters, likely to be proteins.[35,98]

The French physician Rayer[89] also described the characteristic renal hypertrophy that was rediscovered only in the 1970s, and German physicians identified renal involvement in diabetes; when glucosuria disappeared due to a severe decrease in renal function, patients would quite often have heavy proteinuria and be oedematous.[91]

Pathologists were also aware of the typical diabetic kidney and quite often Arman Epstein lesions were identified because of lack of treatment.[26] The understanding of the disease was completely changed by the observation in 1936 by Kimmelstiel and Wilson,[52] who found glomerular lesions in eight patients, all of whom were likely to be Type 2 diabetic patients. Kimmelstiel and Wilson clearly understood that the disease was due to diabetes. However, for many years to come, renal complications were still considered rare in Type 2 diabetes and the clinical course was not considered malignant ('benign diabetes').[34]

In the last few years, there has been a change in treatment strategy, partly because of the UKPDS study that clearly negated the concept that glycaemic treatment, especially with sulfonylurea agents, but also with metformin and even insulin, could be deleterious.[44,102,106–108] The opposite is rather the case, although with some reservations.[33] In the US, it has been a prevalent concept that especially sulfonylurea agents could be harmful to patients with diabetes due to the influence on cardiac function, and this debate seems not to be completely closed as special doctors still argue that certain oral agents could be harmful to diabetic patients.

Evaluation of Diabetic Renal Disease and Classification

It is now widely accepted that patients with Type 1 diabetes exhibit a very characteristic evolution of renal changes (Table 13.1). Initially, there may be

TABLE 13.1 Characteristics in the development of renal dysfunction and nephropathy in Type 2 diabetes

Stage 1: at the clinical diagnosis without pre-diagnostic diabetes	Normal serum creatinine and somewhat elevated GFR (but not to the same extent as in Type 1 diabetes). Some patients may have microalbuminuria at clinical diagnosis due to so far undiagnosed diabetes. Blood pressure may be elevated since essential hypertension may be related to the metabolic syndrome, and Type 2 diabetes.
Stage 2: 'Silent stage'	After the diagnosis and treatment of hyperglycaemia abnormal albuminuria is usually not found (or is reduced if initially increased). GFR may decrease slightly with better glycaemic control. Blood pressure has a tendency to increase over years.
Stage 3:	Microalbuminuria typically develops from normoalbuminuria after some years with diabetes related to blood pressure elevation and glycaemic control. Hypertension is quite common in such patients. GFR may be normal, but tend to decrease.
Stage 4: overt diabetic nephropathy	Proteinuria typically after 10–20 years with diabetes. GFR declines variably related to metabolic control and blood pressure. The risk factors hyperglycaemia and especially hypertension, even borderline, should be aggressively treated. Blood pressure should be reduced to values as low as possible. Cardiovascular disease is common. On biopsy, these patients typically have lesions, but a few percentages do not show any changes or non-diabetic lesions. Biopsy is, however, generally not indicated. Retinopathy is quite often found, but not obligatory.
Stage 5:	The late stage, just before or with renal insufficiency.

hyperfiltration and renal hypertrophy, but there is normal albumin excretion rate unless patients are badly controlled with respect to glycaemia. Blood pressure is normal in Type 1 diabetes, but often elevated in Type 2 diabetes. Several Type 2 diabetic patients may have undiagnosed diabetes for years and thus present with proteinuria due to long diabetes duration.

In contrast to Type 1, patients with Type 2 diabetes quite often have hypertension related to abnormalities of the metabolic syndrome and obesity.[39] They may also exhibit signs of loss of renal autoregulation, meaning that a high blood pressure is inflicted on the glomeruli.[73] In Type 1 diabetes, the next stage is the situation where there are usually neither symptoms nor laboratory signs. However, over the years, there is an increasing thickening of the basement membrane and expansion of the mesangium. GFR is quite often high because of glycaemic dysregulation.[111]

The same may be the case in patients with Type 2 diabetes, but again there may be more unspecific renal changes due to long-standing hypertension and therefore it is not uncommon that many patients have microalbuminuria early on.

The typical finding in Type 1 and 2 diabetes with incipient nephropathy is microalbuminuria, generally found after 5–15 years' duration of diabetes

TABLE 13.2 Albumin excretion in microalbuminuria

Range short-term collections	20–200 μg/min
24 h urines	30–300 mg/24 h
Albumin–creatinine ratio[85]	Men: 2.5–25 mg/mmol creatinine
(morning or spot urine)	Women: 3.5–35 mg/mmol creatinine

Below is normoalbuminuria, higher proteinuria or microalbuminuria.

(Table 13.2). The renal excretion of albumin is clearly elevated and patients with Type 1 diabetes start to exhibit elevated blood pressure, but quite often in the so-called normal range of blood pressure.

Regarding Type 2 diabetes, arterial hypertension is very common, and when a patient with microalbuminuria is followed for many years s/he is at an increased risk of overt renal disease and importantly also of cardiovascular mortality.[43,109,118,119] This observation was made in Europe many years ago and it has now been confirmed in a number of subsequent studies. Persistent microalbuminuria is a clear ominous sign of both renal involvement and cardiovascular disease and also an indicator for treatment, as discussed later in this chapter.

The next stage is the well known situation with proteinuria, diagnosed by means of old-fashioned methods. If biopsies are performed, clear changes are found in Type 1 diabetes. GFR starts to fall and correlates with the level of blood pressure and glycaemia, but without treatment the fall rate is about 10 ml/min/year.[43] Proteinuria increases, correlated again to glycaemia and perhaps dyslipidaemia.

High blood pressure is common in Type 1 and even more so in Type 2 diabetes. As shown in two large trials as well as other studies, the decline in GFR in Type 2 diabetes is quite rapid.[11,57] Thus, patients with proteinuria and Type 2 diabetes have a very poor prognosis, not only due to renal disease and lurking end-stage-renal disease, but also due to the increase in risk of cardiovascular mortality that currently may be better controlled by new agents that control the risk elements,[61,114] such as beta blockers controlling dysrhythmia, diuretics controlling fluid overload and, ACE inhibition controlling increased pressure in the glomeruli and cardiac abnormalities (Table 13.3).

There has been some discussion about the significance of nondiabetic renal disease in diabetic patients. In my experience this is quite rare, but selected studies in nephrology departments show that the problem may be more common and it is now generally accepted that nondiabetic renal disease is not more common in

TABLE 13.3 Optimal blood pressure level in diabetic patients[3,32]

Without nephropathy	$<130/80$
With nephropathy	Somewhat lower

diabetic patients than in the background population. It has taken many years to reach this understanding.[77]

The understanding of diabetic renal disease has been hazardously distorted by the following hypotheses.

(a) It has been claimed that high blood pressure would be essential to maintain renal function – a prevailing concept in the US for many years.[62]

(b) It has also been alleged that hyperglycaemia is not important in the genesis of diabetic renal disease – clearly an unsound and faulty statement.

(c) It has also been claimed that genetic factors are decisive in determining renal disease – this has never been adequately substantiated.[8]

(d) The idea that nondiabetic renal disease such as glomerulonephritis was important also disturbed the situation for many years.[63,77]

It is now clear that normalizing or even 'sub-normalizing' blood pressure is essential.[1,116,119] It is also clear that hyperglycaemia is a main risk factor in the genesis of diabetic renal disease. Genetic factors have not been identified and there is no reason to believe that genetic factors are decisive although they may modulate the development. This is, however, not proven. Combining the effect of high blood pressure and hyperglycaemia is very likely sufficient to explain the development of renal disease.

Diagnostic Procedures

It is imperative to ensure the correct diagnosis of diabetic renal disease in patients with Type 2 diabetes and, fortunately, the procedures to obtain this are usually very simple.

First of all, it should be ensured that the patients actually have diabetes. This is not difficult based upon the patients' medical history, treatment, blood glucose measurements and HbA_{1c} levels. On this background, the diagnosis is usually certain. There may of course be cases that are not quite obvious, for instance a patient who has had diabetes, but who has become euglycemic by weight loss; he may still have renal lesions from diabetes. In this case, a biopsy may be needed unless the patient's medical history is known.

In the presence of diabetes, it is always indicated to examine the patient for other diabetic lesions, such as retinopathy and heart disease. It is perhaps surprising, but retinopathy is not always found in Type 2 diabetic patients with microalbuminuria or even proteinuria.[66,77]

Measurements of albuminuria are essential and usually it is necessary to do two or three tests at intervals of some weeks or months to be on solid ground.[45,85,86] Normally, early morning urine is used and albumin–creatinine ratio is measured in this specimen. It is a very simple and reliable test. If the test is positive, two more tests should be taken to be sure of the degree of renal involvement. One should ensure that glycaemic control is satisfactory since there may be a fall in albuminuria levels with better glycaemic control. There are several simple tests for measuring albumin concentrations that are also quite easy and reliable to use, such as nephelometry, radio-immuno assays or sensitive dipstick tests. All patients should be followed longitudinally in the out-patient clinic.[87,88]

It should be noted that some patients may already have signs of renal disease at the time of diagnosis and maybe even retinopathy.[76] This is due to the fact that some patients may not have been aware of their diabetes because sometimes symptoms are mild or even nonexistent. Measurement or examination of urine sediment may be useful to differentiate from other renal diseases, but it may not always be needed.

Regarding measurements of renal function, it is usually sufficient in the clinical setting to measure serum creatinine although exact measurements of GFR may be warranted in some cases, e.g. determined as EDTA clearance, or creatinine clearance.

In rare situations, renal biopsy may be indicated, in particular if the disease has developed very rapidly, but even so, in most cases typical diabetic lesions are found.[77] In some situations, the renal biopsy may not show specific diabetic abnormalities, which is by no means a sign of nondiabetic renal disease such as minimal change disease. Structural lesion could also be explained by hypertension.[95,112] Obviously, screening for urinary tract infection that may be more common in diabetic patients due to cystopathy is a very reasonable procedure. Quite often, blood pressure is moderately elevated in these patients so careful measurements of blood pressure are always warranted. This is sometimes related to sodium retention.[24] Therefore, careful clinical examination regarding oedema is important as well as control of dietary sodium.

However, the conclusion is that in the daily clinic and in the follow-up of diabetic patients the diagnosis is not difficult. Usually, patients are followed longitudinally and it is possible to observe the slow increase in albuminuria in these patients, 5–20 per cent per year[74] as well as change in S-creatinine. These increases are related to glycaemic control and blood pressure, and in patients with high blood pressure and poor glycaemic control there is often a rapid rate of progression.

Measurements of serum lipid levels are also warranted, although this parameter is not decisive in determining the renal treatment for these patients.[54,75,104] Most patients should be prescribed statin because of evolving cardiovascular disease. There may be other clinicians who are more inclined to renal biopsies, but in my opinion this is not necessary. Usually, the treatment strategy is exactly the same, with or without biopsy, and it is extremely rare that the treatment strategy is altered due to a biopsy.

Careful cardiac and vascular examination is also part of the general examination strategy because cardiovascular disease is so common in these patients and strongly related to microalbuminuria.[66]

Prevention

It has been suggested that there may be a genetic background for the development of renal disease in Type 2 diabetes,[8] but so far this has not been clearly defined. There may be a higher risk in certain patients, and some patients may be critically exposed due to clustering of risk factors, but there are no genetic markers either for hypertension or for adiposity. Risk factors/markers are indicated in Tables 13.4 and 13.5. Dietary strategy may be important in prevention of Type 2 diabetes itself.[110]

TABLE 13.4 Risk factors/markers for development of diabetic renal disease in Type 2 patients

Normoalbuminuria (above median)	+
Microalbuminuria	+
Sex	M > F
Familial clustering	+
Predisposition to arterial hypertension	+
Ethnic conditions	+
Glycaemic control	+
Prorenin	?
Smoking	? (+)
S-cholesterol	+
Presence of retinopathy	+
Protein intake	not documented

+ = present; ? = scanty or no relevant information.

TABLE 13.5 Pathogenesis of diabetic nephropathy

Familial/genetic pathways
Metabolic pathways
Glucose itself
Non-enzymatic glycosylation
Increased PKC activity
Abnormal polyol metabolism
Biochemical abnormalities of extracellular matrix
Haemodynamic pathways
Cytokines and growth factors
Endothelial dysfunction

It is quite clear, both from experimental studies and human studies, although intervention studies may not be so clear cut, that glucose toxicity is an important factor in the genesis of diabetic renal disease.[84] The mechanistic background for glucose toxicity is not completely clear, but it may well be that advanced glycation end-products play an important role along with the activation of the polyol pathway. Activation of protein kinase C and growth factors are of potential interest, but a detailed discussion of these pathogenetic factors is outside the scope of this chapter. All studies show that the duration of diabetes is of importance, but, as mentioned earlier, lesions may be present even at the clinical diagnosis of diabetes due to the fact that some patients live in complete unawareness of their diabetes for years.

Obviously, the UKPDS study was important in this respect as in particular it verified the effectiveness of sulfonylurea agents, insulin and metformin. Combination therapy is quite often used and there is no reason to believe that any of these treatment strategies should be problematic. Unfortunately, the difference between the well treated and the less well treated group in the UKPDS was not dramatic: HbA_{1c} levels 7.0 versus 7.9. With larger differences the results may have been more impressive.

Besides optimal glycaemic control, it is also clear that antihypertensive treatment is of top priority, as documented in the UKPDS where both beta blockers and ACE inhibitors together with other types of antihypertensive therapy were effective in preventing albuminuria. The UKPDS showed that the lower the blood pressure, the better the outcome, and therefore the usual goals for antihypertensive treatment may be lower in diabetic patients: 140/90 in nondiabetic and 130/80 in diabetic patients. Some studies indicate that ARBs are to be preferred in Type 2 diabetes but this is in contrast to a newly published important study.[8,11,57]

One should however be careful regarding patients who may be at risk for renal arteriostenosis and therefore frequent follow-up in such patients is needed. Patients who are generally arteriosclerotic should be followed even more carefully, including patients who are smokers.[78]

Treatment Strategy

The first sign of diabetic renal disease in the clinical setting is the presence of microalbuminuria. The genesis of microalbuminuria is perhaps complex, being related not only to long-standing diabetes, but also to blood pressure elevation, which is quite common in these patients (Figures 13.1 and 13.2). Interestingly, the BENEDICT study (NESM in press) showed that development of microalbuminuria can be reduced by ACE-inhibition as also shown by Ravid.[88] Loss of renal autoregulation may also be important due to lesions in the vasculature of the kidney and therefore the systemic blood pressure may be transferred unhindered to glomeruli in these patients.[17,73] Still, the best possible glycaemic control is

- Non-pharmacological measures (particularly weight loss and reduction in salt intake) should be encouraged in all patients with Type 2 diabetes, independently of the existing blood pressure. These measures may suffice to normalize blood pressure in patients with high normal or grade 1 hypertension and can be expected to facilitate blood pressure control by antihypertensive agents.
- The goal blood pressure to aim at during behavioural or pharmacological therapy is below 130/80 mm Hg.
- To reach this goal, most often combination therapy will be required.
- It is recommended that all effective and well-tolerated antihypertensive agents be used, generally in combination.
- Available evidence indicates that renoprotection benefits from the regular inclusion in these combinations of an ACE inhibitor in Type 1 diabetes and of an angiotensin receptor antagonist in Type 2 diabetes.
- In Type 2 diabetic patients with high normal blood pressure who may sometimes achieve blood pressure goal by monotherapy, the first drug to be tested should be a blocker of the renin-angiotensin system.
- The finding of microalbuminuria in Type 1 or Type 2 diabetic patients is an indication for antihypertensive treatment, especially by a blocker of the renin-angiotensin system, irrespective of the blood pressure values.

2003 European Guidelines for Management of Hypertension[32]

FIGURE 13.1 Position statement: antihypertensive therapy in diabetics

important in patients with microalbuminuria just as in the prevention situation. However, antihypertensive treatment is a key feature in these patients and blood pressure should probably be much lower in patients with microalbuminuria and overt renal disease, perhaps around 125/80. Several studies show that ACE inhibitors or angiotensin receptor blockers are effective in the treatment of these patients,[8] but obviously other agents may be used if the goal for antihypertensive treatment is not reached[18,30,38,53,59,61,64,87,88] (Table 13.10; Figures 13.3 and 13.4).

According to the newly published CALM study,[65] it is possible to combine ACE inhibitors with receptor blockers. It should be mentioned that small doses of ACE inhibitors[22] are usually not sufficient. Increasing the dose of the agent that blocks the RAS system is important.[5,8]

When inhibiting, the renal angiotensin system is not adequate; diuretic treatment should be added, and it is almost obligatory in patients with diabetes because of the tendency to sodium retention.

Beta blockers also have a strong case and overriding hypoglycaemic unawareness is extremely rare, so the counter-indication for beta blockers is not present in most patients. On the contrary, many patients need beta blockers for cardiac

Routine tests

- Plasma glucose (preferably fasting)
- Serum total cholesterol
- Serum highdensity lipoprotein (HDL) - cholesterol
- Fasting serum triglycerides
- Serum uric acid
- Serum creatinine
- Serum potassium
- Haemoglobin and haematocrit
- Urinanalysis (dipstick test complemented by urinary sediment examination)
- Electrocardiogram

Recommended tests

- Echocardiogram
- Carotid (and femoral) ultrasound
- C-reactive protein
- Microalbuminuria (essential test in diabetics)
- Quantitative proteinuria (if dipstick test positive)
- Fundoscopy (in severe hypertension)

Extended evaluation (domain of the specialist)

- Complicated hypertension: tests of cerebral, cardiac and renal function
- Search for secondary hypertension: measurement of renin, aldosterone, corticosteroids, catecholamines, arteriography, renal and adrenal ultrasound; computer-assisted tomography (CAT), brain magnetic resonance imaging.

2003 European Guidelines for Management of Hypertension

FIGURE 13.2 Laboratory investigation in hypertension

A	Angiotensin blockade (ARB and/or ACE I) (Possibly aldosteron-blockade)
B	Beta blockers
C	Calcium-blockers
D	Diuretics
E	Eating more healthily and less – exercise more
F	Find out what to do ('resistance' to treatment) Compliance e.g. PCO (polycystic ovarian syndrome)

FIGURE 13.3 Antihypertensive treatment

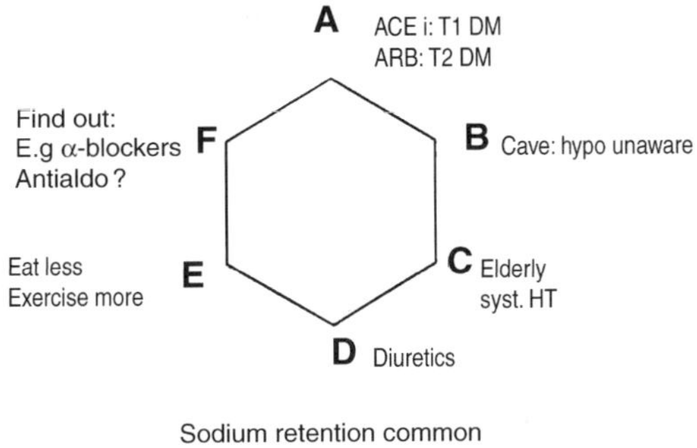

FIGURE 13.4 The treament hexagon for hypertension

protection against dysrhythmia and heart insufficiency. Combination therapy with calcium channel blockers is also useful, but most physicians do not start treatment with these agents alone and instead they use them as a supplement.

The goal regarding antihypertensive treatment is stable serum creatinine, decline in albuminuria, and decline in blood pressure. There seems to be no lower limit regarding blood pressure, and if patients can manage a level of 120/75 this may be very useful in renal protection. So far, there is no evidence of a so-called J-shaped curve in these patients.[1]

There are few studies that use low-protein diets in diabetic patients. Studies so far performed are not positive in patients with Type 2 diabetes.[48,82,83] Regarding the dietary approach, a low-protein diet may not be warranted, but rather it may be useful to use a low-sodium diet, especially if the patient does not respond to ordinary therapy. In some cases, restriction of sodium may be useful in achieving the goal for antihypertensive treatment.[24]

There is little evidence that treatment of dyslipidaemia will protect renal function and the few studies that do exist are somewhat conflicting. Obviously, treatment of hyperlipidaemia is more important for the prevention of cardiac and vascular disease.

Cigarette smoking is also considered a risk factor and all patients should be given advice regarding smoking cessation.[78]

Treatment in Overt Diabetic Renal Disease

The treatment strategy is essentially the same throughout the course of diabetic renal disease, from incipient to overt.[64] Two studies, the RENAAL and the irbesartan studies, show that treatment with angiotensin receptor blockers can postpone end-stage renal disease and help proteinuric patients with Type 2 diabetes. Both studies showed that there is a significant, but limited, effect in these patients. However, prognosis unfortunately remains poor[11,57,100] (Tables 13.6 and 13.7).

TABLE 13.6 RENAAL & IDNT trial comparison cohort baseline characteristics

RENAAL	IDNT
Age: 60 ± 7.5 years	Age: 59 ± 8 years
sCr: 19.9 ± 0.5 mg/dl	sCr: 17 ± 0.6 mg/dl
BP: 152/82 ± 19/10 mm Hg	BP: 156/85 ± 18/11 mm Hg
HbA_{1c}: 8.5 ± 1.6%	HbA_{1c}: 8.1 ± 1.7%
UA/Cr 1867 ± 2701 mg/g (~3.9 g/24 h)	UPE: 4.2 ± 4.1 g/24 h

The RENAAL study[11] showed a significant effect on all pre-defined end-points considered together, namely end-stage renal disease, doubling of serum creatinine and mortality. Mortality in itself was not significant,[100] but mortality along with end-stage renal disease was positively affected by the treatment. This study may be a little more encouraging than the IDNT study,[57] but in principle the two studies of similar design gave the same results. The IDNT study also included patients who were treated with a calcium channel blocker and indeed the angiotensive receptor blocker was more successful in preventing or postponing the course of renal disease. The RENAAL study also showed a beneficial effect on hospitalization for cardiac insufficiency, which is indeed a noteworthy result.

Another study, the IRMA-II,[80] showed a positive effect on patients with microalbuminuria regarding reduction in albuminuria, but not in preventing a fall in GFR. From a more theoretical point of view, it may be more advantageous to treat the patient with microalbuminuria early on and perhaps even before the onset of microalbuminuria. There is evidence that suggests that renal disease in

TABLE 13.7 RENAAL & IDNT trial results. Comparison of primary endpoint and components[100]

Composite and components	Losartan vs pbo RR%	Irbesartan vs pbo RR%	Irbesartan vs amlo RR%	Amlodipine vs pbo RR%
DsCr, ESRD, death	16 $p = 0.024$	20 $p = 0.024$	23 $p = 0.006$	−4 NS
Doubling of SCr	25 $p = 0.006$	33 $p = 0.003$	37 $p = 0.001$	−6 NS
ESRD	28 $p = 0.002$	23 NS	23 NS	0 NS
Death	NS	NS	NS	NS
ESRD or death	20 $p = 0.010$	?	?	?

RR = risk reduction; NS = not significant.

diabetes is a self-perpetuating process and with more advanced disease there may be less autoregulation and more transmission of systemic blood pressure to glomeruli.[81]

It is clear that anti-lipidaemic treatment could also be of importance to these patients although there is no clinical trial regarding renal end-points. Obviously, cardiovascular disease is important and this may well be positively affected by a lipid-lowering agent, especially statins.

Recent Treatment Guidelines for Patients with Diabetes Mellitus with Focus on Hypertension

Several guidelines have emerged over the years, focusing on hypertension as a modifiable risk factor, especially in the presence of other risk factors.[3,4,15,16,32,117,118] The dividing line between normotension and hypertension is somewhat arbitrary and clearly new definitions may be needed for hypertension. Other papers have focused particularly on diabetic patients with incipient or overt renal disease.[66]

The cardiovascular risk factors favouring early treatment can be divided into those that are modifiable (elevated blood pressure, smoking, dyslipidaemia, cardiovascular hypertrophy, obesity, sedentary lifestyle, and diabetes, especially when associated with microalbuminuria or renal disease) and those that are not modifiable (age, gender, family history of premature cardiovascular disease and previous cardiovascular events).

Several risk factors may be modified by reducing blood pressure. Aggressive antihypertensive treatment does not appear to impose a further risk in patients obtaining low blood pressure (the so-called J-shaped curve),[1] but care should be taken that blood pressure is not reduced too rapidly. Risk of serious cardiovascular disease varies greatly among persons with mild hypertension, depending a great deal on the presence of additional risk factors. Patients without additional risk factors show evidence of so-called white coat hypertension. Treatment of hypertension is usually lifelong so careful evaluation of patients is needed before treatment is started.[32]

The Dual- or Triple- Jeopardy Concept[67]

Diabetes and hypertension are frequent concomitant diseases with microalbuminuria acting as the early triple indicator of increased risk.[66] Diabetic patients with microalbuminuria and proteinuria have a particularly poor prognosis, especially when accompanied by renal disease. Evidence suggests that lowering of high (or even normal) blood pressure reduces microalbuminuria and slows the decline in glomerular filtration rate. Therefore, the presence of diabetes, both insulin-dependent diabetes mellitus (Type 1 diabetes) and non-insulin-dependent diabetes mellitus (Type 2 diabetes), in patients with mild hypertension is an indication to begin antihypertensive treatment. In these patients, particular attention should be paid to glucose levels and accompanying disorders of lipid metabolism.[32]

Goals for Blood Pressure

The goal is to reduce the pressure to at least 130/80 mm Hg in diabetic patients, but maybe up to 140/90 mm Hg in old patients. Still, this level especially of systolic blood pressure is very difficult to achieve.[60] In patients with isolated systolic hypertension, the treatment goal should be to achieve a systolic blood pressure of at least 140 mm Hg if this is well tolerated. Therefore, careful evaluation is needed not only before, but also during, treatment to ensure that the blood pressure goal is reached without subjective or metabolic side effects. In the US, diuretics are recommended as first-line antihypertensive, effective, as well as inexpensive drugs.[15] Angiotensin-converting enzyme inhibitors are proposed to diabetic patients as the first agent both in Europe and in the US[32,15] (see Figure 13.1). The drugs should be used in as low doses as possible (often in combination) and agents should be selected that do not cause glucose intolerance or dyslipidaemia which may be the case with diuretics and beta blockers. In particular, diuretic agents are very valuable as ancillary treatment to enhance the effectiveness of many other antihypertensive drugs. Diuretics and angiotensin-converting enzyme inhibitors are effective in combination and do not usually disturb potassium metabolism. Nevertheless, careful monitoring of serum creatinine and serum potassium is needed.

Old and Very New Guidelines

Personally, I have witnessed the appearance of many clinical guidelines, especially within the area of essential hypertension and the area of diabetes; initially, there were no guidelines in 1967 when I graduated. Indeed, these two main diseases or risk factors often come together in the guidelines; this is also the case for the new major guidelines that have just appeared.[32,15]

The main American guideline is the JNC 7, published in *JAMA*,[15,16] with a backing group that is mainly NIH, Bethesda. One month later, we see the European guidelines endorsed by the European Society of Hypertension and the European Society of Cardiology, and also by the International Society of Hypertension. These European guidelines are published in the *Journal of Hypertension*.[32] See Figures 13.1 and 13.2.

The purpose of both guidelines is, of course, to guide all those involved in the management of hypertension where there is a need for new, clear and concise guidelines since many new studies have been published on the natural history of hypertension and, indeed, many important trials have also been finished.

Regarding classification, JNC 7 now talks about pre-hypertension; maybe it is an odd terminology. Rather, it may be relevant to use the European ideas of optimal, normal, high–normal, and grade 1–3 hypertension. Still, the border for defining hypertension is a clinically measured blood pressure of more than 140/80 or 140/90 mm Hg. However, it is clear that high–normal is indeed a risk factor for cardiovascular complications. Essential hypertension is a risk factor and also a disease; the higher the blood pressure, the higher the risk. It is usually not a strict entity, which is easily and genetically determined. Table 13.8 shows an extensive list of guidelines published in the last few years.

Regarding organ damage/risk, the traditional factors are included and both guidelines, as in the new concept, also introduce microalbuminuria and low GFR, especially in those with diabetes. Otherwise, the ordinary clinical laboratory tests and examinations are carefully discussed in a very similar manner (Figure 13.2). Obviously, secondary hypertension is also discussed, maybe more carefully and profoundly in the European guidelines.

A new important element is that lifestyle intervention with exercise and diet, including a low salt intake, is clearly emphasized and should be used in borderline cases and obviously also in those with hypertension.

There are important differences in the treatment strategies since the JNC 7 recommends thiazide diuretic as initial treatment, but nevertheless JNC 7 also suggests that combination therapy is quite often needed, which is also a paradigm in the European guidelines.

However, the European guidelines leave the choice of treatment more to the clinicians' discretion since there may be many elements in the treatment strategy that are important. The European guidelines include an important hexagon in the treatment strategy with many combinations. The many drugs can be combined in several ways and an important combination, especially for diabetes, is agents that block the renin-angiotensin system along with diuretics. Calcium blockers or beta blockers may be used as the next choice.

Generally speaking, the two sets of guidelines are rather similar and clearly stress the case for early treatment, including lifestyle intervention. Combination therapy is clearly needed in most situations. Everybody interested in hypertension and its treatment should carefully read these guidelines. Microalbuminuria is included as an important marker, also for treatment. My own 'treatment hexagon' is shown in Figures 13.3 and 13.4 (A, B, C, D, E, F). Goals for blood pressure are shown in Table 13.9.

Screening for Microalbuminuria

Several guidelines on microalbuminuria and prevention of diabetic nephropathy emphasize the importance of early treatment before the glomerular filtration rate declines. Therefore, early screening for microalbuminuria using the

TABLE 13.8 2004: How many guidelines and related papers? (relevant to Type 2 diabetes and cardiovascular and renal disease)

(A) Focus on prevention of T2 DM (ADA)
Difficult. *Diabetes Care* 2004; **27** (1): S47–S54[2]

(B) Focus on glycaemic control (ADA)
Diabetes Care 2004; **27** (Suppl. 1)
Diabetes Care 2003; **26** (Suppl. 1)
Can J Diabetes 2003; **27** (Suppl. 2)[12]
NICE 2002[69–72]
General (focus on A_{1C} and end-point)

• Insulin }	similar effect on end-point
• SU }	
• Metformin	save lives
• Glitazones (TZD)	no end-point studies terminated
• Combinations	

(C) Focus on lipid control (ADA, HPS)
- Statins
- Other agents
- Cardiology (AHA): *Circulation* 2003; **108**: 1527–1532[19]

(D) Combined diabetes and blood pressure
(a) ADA: *Diabetes Care* 2004; **27**; (Suppl. 1): 65–67; 79–83
(b) JNC VII: *Hypertension* 2003; **42**: 1206–1252[16]
(c) ESH/ESC: *J Hypertens* 2003; **21**: 1011–1053[32]
(d) IDF (Europe): *Diabetic Med* 2003; **20**: 972–987[50]
(e) WHO/ISH: *J Hypertens* 2003; **21**: 1983–1992[117]
(f) Sub-Saharan Africa: *J Hypertens* 2003; **21**: 1993–2000[55]
(g) Canada: *Can J Diabetes* 2003; **27** (Suppl. 2): 58–65[12]
(h) Australia: *MJA* 2003; **179**: 306–312[13]

(E) Combined diabetes and vascular disease
(a) Cardiology (AHA): *Circulation* 2003; **108**: 1527–1532[19]

(F, a) Combined diabetes and renal disease
(a) Levey AS *et al. Ann Intern Med* 2003; **139**: 137–147[56]
(b) Eknoyan G *et al. Am J Kidney Dis* 2003; **42** (4): 617–622[28]

(F, b) Microalbuminuria
(a) Mogensen CE. *J Intern Med* 2003; **254**: 45–66[66]
(b) Donnelly R *et al. J Hypertens* 2003; **21** (Suppl. 1): S7–S12[25]
(c) Gaede P *et al. N Engl J Med* 2003; **348**: 383–393[40]

(F) Combined diabetes and metabolic syndrome
(a) Sowers. *Am J Hypertens* 2003; **16**: 41S–45S[101]
(b) Isomaa B. *Life Sci* 2003; **73**: 2395–2411[51]
(c) Park YW *et al. Arch Intern Med* 2003; **163**: 427–436[79]

(G) General lifestyle (for everybody)
General: ESH/ESC: *J Hypertens* 2003; **21**: 1011–1053[32]
Salt restriction
(a) MacGregor. *Hypertension* 2003; **42**: 1093–1096[36]
Protein intake
(b) *Eur J Clin Nutr* 2002; **56**: 1200–1207[83]
(c) *Am J Clin Nutr* 2003; **78**: 671–672[27]

(H) Guidelines and cost
(a) Zanchetti A. *J Hypertens* 2003; **21**: 2207–2209[121]

(I) Guideline comments
(a) Weber M. *J Hypertens* 2003; **21**: 1977–1982[115]

TABLE 13.9 10 recommendations for goal blood pressure and initial antihypertensive therapy to reduce cardiovascular risk in patients with diabetes (2001–2004)

Organization	Goal blood pressure	Initial therapy (but multiple drugs)
NICE (2002)	140/80	ACE-i ARBs
Canadian Hypertension Recommendations (2002)	$<$130/80	ACE-i ARBs
Canadian Diabetes Working Group (2004)	$<$130/80	ACE-i ARBs
American Diabetes Association (2004)	$<$130/80	ACE-i ARBs
European Society of Hypertens. and Card. (2003)	$<$130/80	ACE-i ARBs (early)**
National Kidney Foundation (2003)	$\leq$130/80	ACE-i ARBs
IDF – Europe (2002–2003)	140/85 130/75 (microalbuminuria)	ACE-i/ARBs
WHO + ISH (2003)*	$<$130/80	ACE-i/ARBs
Seventh Report of the JNC (2003)	$<$130/80 (sparse data)	ACE-i/ARBs**

ACE = angiotensin-converting enzyme; ARBs = angiotensin II receptors.
* Michael A Weber, SUNY, New York: Yet more hypertension guidelines: what do they add?
** Often combined with diuretics and especially with abnormal albuminuria.

albumin–creatinine ratio is recommended. The best defined urine sample to use is the first morning urine. This urine sample can be brought to the clinic for measurement of albumin–creatinine ratio or can be screened for albumin with the newly developed stix. An increased albumin–creatinine ratio found on several occasions gives good evidence for abnormal albuminuria, but may be further confirmed by measuring overnight urine collection. Screening should be carried out at yearly or 6 month intervals. Note that confounding factors (such as heavy exercise, urinary tract infection, acute illness, cardiac failure or metabolic decompensation) increase microalbuminuria,[66] and patients should be screened for associated abnormalities, such as retinopathy, cardiovascular disease and dyslipidaemia.

Prevention and Intervention Related to Type 2 Diabetes

Meticulous control of hypertension, particularly with agents that prevent increases in intercapillary pressure within the kidney, is essential; many studies are now conducted in typically older patients. Studies on patients with isolated systolic hypertension seem to show a beneficial effect on nonrenal end points, such as reduction of stroke.[66] Strokes are more common in Type 2 diabetic patients and are associated with a poor prognosis. Early treatment with antihypertensive agents, using agents that reduce blood pressure efficiently without glucose intolerance, dyslipidaemia or other side-effects, is recommended.

The case for better glycaemic control has gained wide acceptance over the past few years, especially since the completion of the UKPDS. Long-term microvascular complications take several years to develop and therefore further metabolic

TABLE 13.10 Recent controlled studies with or including Type 2 diabetes mellitus (T2 DM) microalbuminuric patients

Study	Treatment	No. of patients	Duration of study	Effect on microalb./ albuminuria	Effect on BP	Additional effect parameter
HOPE, 2000[47]	Ramipril 10 mg at night versus placebo	1140 micro (many T2 DM)	4.5 years	Yes	Yes	Combined CV outcome/ positive
ABCD, 2000 (hypertensive pts)[31]	Nisoldipine versus enalapril	470	5 years	Yes	Yes	Creatinine clearance stable
Chan *et al.*, 2000[14]	Nifedipine versus enalapril (E)	102	5 years	Better with E	Yes	Renal function better with enalapril in macro
Lacourcière *et al.*, 2000[53]	Losartan versus enalapril	92	1 year	Yes	Yes	Similar effect on GFR and albuminuria
CALM, 2000[6,65]	Candesartan versus lisinopril	199	24 weeks	Yes	Yes	Better effect with dual blockade on BP
Fernandéz, 2001[37]	Verapamil versus trandolapril	103	6 months	Yes	Yes	Combination possible
Parving, 2001[80]	Irbesartan versus placebo	590	2 years	Yes	Yes	Dose–response curve
Sasso, 2002[96]	Irbesartan versus placebo	124	17 weeks	Yes	Yes	No correlation between M and BP fall
Viberti, 2002[113]	Valsartan versus amlodipine	332	24 weeks	Yes (better with valsartan)	Yes	No correlation between M and BP fall
Schrier, 2002 (normotensive pts)[99]	Intensive versus moderate BP lowering	480	5 years	Yes	Yes	Less retinopathy and less incidence of stroke with intensive treatment
PREMIER, 2003[68]	Perindopril plus indapamide (preterax) versus enalapril	481	1 year	Yes	Yes	Better effect with preterax
DETAIL, 2004[5,90]	Telmisartan versus enalapril	252	5 years	Similar effects	Similar effects	Similar GFR changes
LIFE, 2002[58]	Losartan versus atenolol	Micro?	4.7 years	Possibly	No	Effect on mortality in diabetes
Epstein, 2003[29,97]	Eplenerone and ACE-I	215	duration	Yes	Yes	Good effect of combination
Steno II, (Gaede), 2003[41]	Optimized multifactorial, including lipid lowering	120	8 years	Yes	Yes	GFR falls with progression to proteinuria. Otherwise stable
DIABHYCAR, 2003[22]	Ramipril 1.25 mg versus placebo	3627	4 years	Minor	Minor	No effect on any important end-points (contrast to HOPE)

GFR, glomerular filtration rate.

control may not be needed in very old patients. Follow-up studies from 1997 to 2002 in the UKPDS still show positive results.[105] The prognosis for Type 2 diabetes seems also to have improved in the recent years, probably as a result of now identified treatment related to the well known risk factor.[20,42,103]

Summary

Hyperglycaemia is an important contributor to complications, including nephropathy. In order to obtain the best possible glycaemic control throughout the course of diabetes, it is important to diagnose renal disease early on by screening for microalbuminuria.

Blood pressure elevation is also an important factor and normalizing blood pressure throughout the course of Type 2 diabetes is, of course, essential.

Studies show that treatment with ACE inhibitors can prevent the development of microalbuminuria (e.g. the Benedict study). Many studies also show that microalbuminuria can be reduced by antihypertensive treatment, especially with ACE inhibitors, but also with other agents. Usually ACE inhibitors are the best in the treatment process.

The effect on strong end-points in microalbuminuric patients is difficult to ascertain because of the long follow-up needed. However, the HOPE study suggested a positive effect in microalbuminuric diabetic patients on strong end-points. New studies using angiotensin receptor blockers show a positive effect in patients with proteinuria and Type 2 diabetes on the progression of renal disease.

Thus, ACE inhibitors seem to be important in preventing cardiovascular disease and mortality, and angiotensin receptor blockers (ARBs) are important in preventing or postponing ESRD. There may also be a theoretical case for using a combined blockade or a so-called dual blockade of the renin–angiotensin system. There is also a good patho-physiological rationale for such a combination. As is almost always the case, however, further studies are, needed.

Patients with diabetic renal disease need effective antihypertensive treatment on top of ACE inhibition using diuretic treatment and beta-blocker treatment as well as calcium blockers with prolonged action.

Dyslipidaemia should be treated carefully although there are no clinical studies that suggest that the renal outcome is better with statins or other lipid-lowering agents. All general risk factors should be treated and patients should be urged to stop smoking, lose weight and exercise a low-sodium diet. The role for protein reduction is less clear and it is even weak in patients with other types of renal disease.

References

1. Adler AI, Stratton IM and Neil HA *et al.* on behalf of the UK Prospective Diabetes Study Group. Association of systolic blood pressure with macrovascular and microvascular

complications of Type 2 diabetes (UKPDS 36): prospective observational study. *BMJ* 2000; **321**: 412–419.

2. American Diabetes Association. National Institute of Diabetes and Digestive and Kidney Diseases. Position statement. Prevention or delay of Type 2 diabetes. *Diabetes Care* 2004; **27** (Suppl. 1): S47–S54.
3. American Diabetes Association. Position statement. Hypertension management in adults with diabetes. *Diabetes Care* 2004; **27** (Suppl. 1): S65–S67.
4. American Diabetes Association. Position statement. Nephropathy in diabetes. *Diabetes Care* 2004; **27** (Suppl. 1): S79–S83.
5. Andersen NH, Poulsen PL and Knudsen ST *et al.* Long-term dual blockade with candesartan and lisinopril in hypertensive patients with diabetes mellitus. The CALM II study: prospective, randomised double blind study. *Diabetes Care* 2005; in press.
6. Andersen NH and Mogensen CE. Angiotensin converting enzyme inhibitors and angiotensin II receptor blockers: evidence for and against the combination in the treatment of hypertension and proteinuria. *Curr Hypertension Rep* 2002; **4**: 394–402.
7. Bain SC and Chowdhury TA. Genetics of diabetic nephropathy and microalbuminuria. *J R Soc Med* 2000; **93**: 62–66.
8. Barnett AH, Bain SC and Bouter P *et al.* Comparison of angiotensin-II-receptor blockade and angiotensin-converting enzyme inhibition in subjects with Type 2 diabetes and nephropathy. *N Eng J Med* 2004; in press.
9. Bergrem H and Leivestad T. Diabetic nephropathy and end-stage renal failure: the Norwegian story. *Adv Ren Replace Ther* 2001; **8**: 4–12.
10. Biesenbach G, Janko O and Zazgornik J. Similar rate of progression in the predialysis phase in type 1 and Type 2 diabetes mellitus. *Nephrol Dial Transplant* 1994; **9**: 1097–1102.
11. Brenner BM, Cooper ME and de Zeeuw D *et al.* For the Reduction of End-Points in NIDDM with the Angiotensin II Antagonist Losartan (RENAAL) Study Investigators. Effects of losartan on renal and cardiovascular outcomes in patients with Type 2 diabetes and nephropathy. *N Engl J Med* 2001; **345**: 861–869.
12. Canadian Diabetes Association. Clinical practice guidelines for the prevention and management of diabetes in Canada. *Can J Diabetes* 2003; **27** (Suppl. 2).
13. Chalmers JP and Arnolda LF. Clinical update. Lowering blood pressure in 2003. *MJA* 2003; **179**: 306–312.
14. Chan JCN, Ko GTC and Leung DHY *et al.* Long-term effects of angiotensin-converting enzyme inhibition and metabolic control in hypertensive Type 2 diabetic patients. *Kidney Int* 2000; **58**: 590–600.
15. Chobanian AV, Bakris GL, Black HR and Cushman WC *et al.* The Seventh Report of the Joint National Committee on Prevention, Detection, Evaluation, and Treatment of High Blood Pressure (The JNC7-Report). *JAMA* 2003; **289**: 2560–2571.
16. Chobanian AV, Bakris GL, Black HR and Cushman WC *et al.* Seventh Report of the Joint National Committee on Prevention, Detection, Evaluation, and Treatment of High Blood Pressure (The JNC7-Report – complete version). *Hypertension* 2003; **42**: 1206–1252.
17. Christensen PK, Hansen HP and Parving HH. Impaired autoregulation of GFR in hypertensive non-insulin dependent diabetic patients. *Kidney Int* 1997; **52**: 1369–1374.
18. Cooper M, McNally PG and Boner G. Antihypertensive treatment in NIDDM, with special reference to abnormal albuminuria. In *The Kidney and Hypertension in Diabetes Mellitus*, 5th edn., Mogensen CE (ed.). 2000. Boston, MA: Kluwer, pp. 441–460.
19. Creager MA, Lüscher TF, Cosentino F and Beckman JA. Diabetes and Vascular Disease. Pathophysiology, Clinical Consequences, and Medical Therapy: Part 1. *Circulation* 2003; **108**: 1527–1532.

20. De Backer G, Ambrosioni E, Borch-Johnsen K, Brotons C, Cifkova R, Dallongeville J, Ebrahim S, Faergeman O, Graham I, Mancia G, Manger Cats V, Orth-Gomer K, Perk J, Pyorala K, Rodicio JL, Sans S, Sansoy V, Sechtem U, Silber S, Thomsen T and Wood D. European guidelines on cardiovascular disease prevention in clinical practice. Third Joint Task Force of European and Other Societies on Cardiovascular Disease Prevention in Clinical Practice. *EJCPR* 2003; **10** (4): S1–S10.
21. Devereux RB and Alderman MH. Role of preclinical cardiovascular disease in the evolution from risk factor exposure to development of morbid events. *Circulation* 1993; **88**: 1444–1455.
22. Marre M, Lievre M and Chatellier C *et al.* DIABHYCAR Study Investigators. Effects of low-dose ramipril on cardiovascular and renal outcomes in patients with Type 2 diabetes and elevated excretion of urinary albumin: results of the DIABHYCAR study, a randomised, double-blind, placebo, controlled trial. *BMJ* 2004; **328**: 495–499.
23. Dikow R and Ritz E. Cardiovascular complications in the diabetic patient with renal disease; an update in 2003. *Nephrol Dial Transplant* 2003; **18**: 1993–1998.
24. Dodson PM, Beevers M and Hallworth R. Sodium restriction and blood pressure in hypertensive Type 2 diabetics: randomised blind controlled and crossover studies of moderate sodium restriction and sodium supplementation. *BMJ* 1989; **298**: 227–230.
25. Donnelly R *et al.* Microalbuminuria: a common, independent cardiovascular risk factor, especially but not exclusively in Type 2 diabetes. *J Hypertens* 2003; **21** (Suppl. 1): S7–S12.
26. Ebstein W. Weiteres über diabetes, insbesondere über die complication desselben mit typhus abdominalis. *Dtsch Arch Klin Med* 1882; **30**: 1.
27. Eckel RH. A new look at dietary protein in diabetes. *Am J Clin Nutr* 2003; **78**: 671–672.
28. Eknoyan G *et al.* Proteinuria and other markers of chronic kidney disease: a position statement of the National Kidney Foundation (NKF) and the National Institute of Diabetes and Digestive and Kidney Diseases (NIDDK). *Am J Kidney Dis* 2003; **42**: 617–622.
29. Epstein M, Buckalew V and Martinez F *et al.* Antiproteinuric efficacy of epleronone, enalapril and epleronone/enalapril combination therapy in diabetic hypertensives with microalbuminuria [Abstract]. *Am J Hypertens* 2002; **15**: 24A.
30. Esmatjes E, Flores L and Inigo P *et al.* Effect of losartan on TGF-β1 and urinary albumin excretion in patients with Type 2 diabetes mellitus and microalbuminuria. *Nephrol Dial Transplant* 2001; **16** (S1): 90–93.
31. Estacio RO, Jeffers BW, Gifford N and Schrier RW. Effect of blood pressure control on diabetic microvascular complications in patients with hypertension and Type 2 diabetes. *Diabetes Care* 2000; **23**: B54–B64.
32. European Society of Hypertension Guidelines Committee. 2003. European Society of Cardiology guidelines for the management of arterial hypertension. *J Hypertens* 2003; **21**: 1011–1053.
33. Ewart RM. The case against aggressive treatment of Type 2 diabetes: critique of the UK Prospective Diabetes Study. *BMJ* 2001; **323**: 854–858.
34. Fabre J, Balant LP and Dayer PG *et al.* The kidney in maturity onset diabetes mellitus: a clinical study of 510 patients. *Kidney Int* 1982; **27**: 167–194.
35. Fahr T. Über atypische Befunde aus den Kapiteln des Morbus Brightii nebst anhangsweisen Bemerkungen zur Hypertoniefrage. *Virchows Arch path Anat* 1924; **248**: 323.
36. Feng JH and MacGregor GA. How Far Should Salt Intake Be Reduced? *Hypertension* 2003; **42**: 1093–1096.
37. Fernandéz R, Puig JG, Rodriguez-Perez JC, Garrido J and Redon J on behalf of the TRAVEND Study Group. Effect of two antihypertensive combinations on metabolic control

in Type 2 diabetic hypertensive patients with albuminuria: a randomised, double-blind study. *J Human Hypertens* 2001; **15**: 849–856.

38. Foggensteiner L, Mulroy S and Firth J. Management of diabetic nephropathy. *J R Soc Med* 2001; **94**: 210–217.
39. Gaede P, Vedel P and Parving HH *et al.* Intensified multifactorial intervention in patients with Type 2 diabetes mellitus and microalbuminuria; the Steno Type 2 randomized study. *Lancet* 1999; **353**: 617–622.
40. Gaede P *et al.* Multifactorial intervention and cardiovascular disease in patients with Type 2 diabetes. *N Engl J Med* 2003; **348**: 383–393.
41. Gaede P, Vedel P and Larsen N *et al.* The Steno-2 Study: intensified multifactorial intervention reduces the risk of cardiovascular disease in patients with Type 2 diabetes and microalbuminuria. *N Engl J Med* 2003; **348**: 383–393.
42. Gale EA. Is there really an epidemic of Type 2 diabetes? *Lancet* 2003; **9383**: 503–504.
43. Gall MA, Hougaard P and Borch-Johnsen K *et al.* Risk factors for the development of incipient and overt diabetic nephropathy in patients with non-insulin-dependent diabetes mellitus: prospective observational study. *BMJ* 1997; **314**: 783–788.
44. Gerstein HC, Mann JFE and Qilong Y. Albuminuria and risk of cardiovascular events, death, and heart failure in diabetic and non-diabetic individuals. *JAMA* 2001; **286**: 421–426.
45. Hallan H, Romunstad S, Kvenild K and Holmen J. Microalbuminuria in diabetic and hypertensive patients and the general population. *Scand J Ural Nephrol* 2003; **37**: 151–158.
46. Hasslacher C, Ritz E and Wahl P *et al.* Similar risks of nephropathy in patients with Type 1 or Type 2 diabetes mellitus. *Nephrol Dial Transplant* 1989; **4**: 859–863.
47. Heart Outcomes Prevention Evaluation (HOPE) Study Investigators. Effects of ramipril on cardiovascular and microvascular outcomes in people with diabetes mellitus: results of the HOPE study and MICRO-HOPE substudy. *Lancet* 2000; **355**: 370–379.
48. Hermansen K. Diet, blood pressure and hypertension. *Br J Nutr* 2000; **83** (S1): S113–S119.
49. Hollenberg NK. Treatment of the patient with diabetes mellitus and risk of nephropathy. What do we know, and what do we need to learn? *Arch Intern Med* 2004; **164**: 125–130.
50. International Diabetes Federation (European Region). Hypertension in people with Type 2 diabetes: knowledge-based diabetes-specific guidelines. *Diabe Med* 2003; **20**: 972–987.
51. Isomaa B. A major health hazard: the metabolic syndrome. *Life Sci* 2003; **73**: 2395–2411.
52. Kimmelstiel P and Wilson C. Intercapillary lesions in the glomeruli of the kidney. *Am J Pathol* 1936; **12**: 83–97.
53. Lacourcière Y, Bélanger A and Godin C *et al.* Long-term comparison of losartan and enalapril on kidney function in hypertensive Type 2 diabetics with early nephropathy. *Kidney Int* 2000; **58**: 762–769.
54. Lam KSL, Cheng IKP and Janus ED *et al.* Cholesterol lowering therapy may retard the progression of diabetic nephropathy. *Diabetologia* 1995; **38**: 604–609.
55. Lemogoum D, Seedat YK, Mabadeje AF, Mendis S, Bovet P, Onwubere B, Blackett KN, Lenfant C, Kabangu JR, Block P, Belhocine M and Degaute JP on behalf of the International Forum for Hypertension Control and Prevention in Africa (IFHA). Recommendations for prevention, diagnosis and management of hypertension and cardiovascular risk factors in sub-Saharan Africa. *J Hypertens* 2003; **21**: 1993–2000.
56. Levey AS *et al.* National Kidney Foundation Practice Guidelines for Chronic Kidney Disease: Evaluation, Classification and Stratification. *Ann Intern Med.* 2003; **139**: 137–147.
57. Lewis EJ *et al.* Renoprotective effect of the angiotensin-receptor antagonist irbesartan in patients with nephropathy due to Type 2 diabetes. *N Engl J Med* 2001; **345**: 851–860.
58. Lindholm LH, Ibsen H and Dahlof B *et al.* Cardiovascular morbidity and mortality in patients with diabetes in the Losartan Intervention For Endpoint Reduction in Hypertension Study (LIFE): a randomised trial against atenolol. *Lancet* 2002; **359**: 1004–1010.
59. Lozano JV, Llisterri JL and Aznar J *et al.* Losartan reduces microalbuminuria in hypertensive microalbuminuric Type 2 diabetics. *Nephrol Dial Transplant* 2001; **16** (S1): 85–89.

60. Mancia G and Grassi G. Systolic and diastolic blood pressure control in antihypertensive drug trials. *J Hypertens* 2002; **20**: 1461–1464.
61. Mann JFE Gerstein HC and Pogue J *et al*. For the HOPE investigators. Renal insufficiency as a predictor of cardiovascular outcomes and the impact of ramipril: The HOPE randomized trial. *Ann Intern Med* 2001; **134**: 629–636.
62. Mogensen CE. Diabetic renal disease: The quest for normotension – and beyond. *Diabet Med* 1995; **12**: 756–769.
63. Mogensen CE. Microalbuminuria, blood pressure and diabetic renal disease: origin and development of ideas. In *The Kidney and Hypertension in Diabetes Mellitus*, 5th edn., Mogensen CE (ed.). 2000. Boston, MA: Kluwer, pp. 655–706.
64. Mogensen CE and Cooper ME. Diabetic renal disease: from recent studies to improved clinical practice. *Diabet Med* 2004; **21**: 4–17.
65. Mogensen CE, Neldam S and Tikkannen I *et al*. for the CALM Study Group. Randomised controlled trial of dual blockade of the renin–angiotensin system in hypertensive, microalbuminuric, non-insulin dependent diabetes: the Candesartan and Lisinopril Microalbuminuria (CALM) Study. *BMJ* 2000; **321**: 1440–1444.
66. Mogensen CE. Microalbuminuria and hypertension with focus on Type 1 and Type 2 diabetes. *J Intern Med* 2003; **254**: 45–66.
67. Mogensen CE. Combined high blood pressure and glucose in Type 2 diabetes: double jeopardy – British trial shows clear effects of treatment, especially blood pressure reduction. *BMJ* 1998; **317**: 693–694.
68. Mogensen CE, Viberti GC and Halimi S *et al*. Effect of low-dose perinodopril/indapamide on albuminuria in diabetes (PREterax in albuMInuria regression – PREMIER). *Hypertension* 2003; **41**: 1063–1071.
69. National Institute for Clinical Excellence (NICE). *Guideline H: Management of Type 2 Diabetes – Management of Blood Pressure and Blood Lipids*. 2002.
70. National Institute for Clinical Excellence (NICE). *Guideline G: Management of Type 2 Diabetes – Blood Glucose*. 2002.
71. National Institute for Clinical Excellence (NICE). *Guideline F: Management of Type 2 Diabetes – Renal Disease, Prevention and Early Management*. 2002.
72. National Institute for Clinical Excellence (NICE). *Guideline E: Management of Type 2 Diabetes – Retinopathy*. 2002.
73. New JP, Marshall SM and Bilous RW. Renal auto-regulation is normal in newly diagnosed normotensive NIDDM patients. *Diabetologia* 1998; **41**: 206–211.
74. Nielsen S, Schmitz A, Rehling M and Mogensen CE. The clinical course of renal function in NIDDM patients with normo- and microalbuminuria. *J Intern Med* 1997; **241**: 133–141.
75. Nielsen S, Schmitz O and Møller N *et al*. Renal function and insulin sensitivity during simvastatin treatment in Type 2 (non-insulin-dependent) diabetic patients with microalbuminuria. *Diabetologia* 1993; **36**: 1079–1086.
76. Olivarius, Andreasen AH, Keiding N and Mogensen CE. Epidemiology of renal involvement in newly-diagnosed middle-aged and elderly diabetic patients. Cross-sectional data from the population-based study 'Diabetes Care in General Practice', Denmark. *Diabetologia* 1993; **36**: 1007–1016.
77. Olsen S and Mogensen CE. How often is NIDDM complicated with non-diabetic renal disease? An analysis of renal biopsies and the literature. *Diabetologia* 1996; **39**: 1638–1645.
78. Orth SR, Ritz E and Schrier RW. The renal risks of smoking. *Kidney Int* 1997; **51**: 1669–1677.
79. Park YW *et al*. The metabolic syndrome: prevalence and associated risk factor findings in the US population from the Third National Health and Nutrition Examination Survey, 1988–1994. *Arch Intern Med* 2003; **163**: 427–436.

80. Parving HH, Lehnert H, Bröchner-Mortensen J *et al.* The effect of irbesartan on the development of diabetic nephropathy in patients with Type 2 diabetes. *N Engl J Med* 2001; **345**: 870–878.
81. Parving HH, Hovind P, Rossing K and Andersen S. Evolving strategies for renoprotection: diabetic nephropathy. *Nephrol Hypertens* 2001; **10**: 515–522.
82. Pijls LTJ, de Vries H and Donker AJ *et al.* The effect of protein restriction on albuminuria in patients with Type 2 diabetes mellitus: a randomised trial. *Nephrol Dial Transpl* 1999; **14**: 1445–1453.
83. Pijls LTJ, de Vries H, van Eijk JTM and Donker AJ. Protein restriction, glomerular filtration rate and albuminuria in patients with Type 2 diabetes mellitus: a randomized trial. *Eur J Clin Nutr* 2002; **56**: 1200–1207.
84. Pirart J. Diabetes mellitus and its degenerative complications: a prospective study of 4,400 patients observed between 1947 and 1973. *Diabetes Care* 1978; **1**: 168–188.
85. Poulsen PL and Mogensen CE. Clinical evaluation of a test for immediate and quantitative determination of urinary albumin-to-creatinine ratio. *Diabetes Care* 1998; **21**: 97–98.
86. Rachmani R, Levi Z and Lidar M *et al.* Considerations about the threshold value of microalbuminuria in patients with diabetes mellitus: lessons from an 8-year follow-up study of 599 patients. *Diabetes Res Clin Pract* 2000; **49**: 187–194.
87. Ravid M, Lang R and Rachmani R *et al.* Long-term renoprotective effect of ACE inhibition in NIDDM: a 7-year follow-up study. *Arch Intern Med* 1996; **156**: 286–289.
88. Ravid M, Brosh D, Levi Z and Bar-Dayan Y *et al.* Use of enalapril to attenuate decline in renal function in normotensive, normoalbuminuric patients with Type 2 diabetes mellitus. A randomized controlled trial. *Ann Intern Med* 1998; **128**: 982–988.
89. Rayer P. *Traité des Maladies des Reins et des Alterations de la Sécrétion Urinaire Étudiées en Elles-Mêmes et Dans Leurs Rapports avec les Maladies des Uretères de la Vessie, de la Prostate et de l'Urètre.* 1839. Paris: Librairie de l'Académie Royale de Médecine, NB.
90. Rippin J, Bain SC and Barnett AH. Rationale and design of diabetics exposed to telmisartan and enalapril (DETAIL) study. *J Diabetes Complications* 2002; **16**: 195–200.
91. Ritz E and Rychlik I (eds). *Nephropathy in Type 2 Diabetes. 1999.* Oxford: Oxford University Press.
92. Ritz E and Stefanski A. Diabetic nephropathy in Type 2 diabetes (in-depth review). *Am J Kidney Dis* 1996; **27**: 167–194.
93. Ritz E and Orth SR. Nephropathy in patients with Type 2 diabetes mellitus. *N Engl J Med* 1999; **341**: 1127–1133.
94. Ritz E. Albuminuria and vascular damage – the vicious twins. *N Engl J Med* 2003; **348**: 2349–2352.
95. Ruggenenti P and Remuzzi G. Nephropathy of Type 1 and Type 2 diabetes: diverse pathophysiology, same treatment? *Nephrol Dial Transplant* 2000; **15**: 1900–1902.
96. Sasso FC, Carbonara O and Persico M *et al.* Irbesartan reduces the albumin excretion rate in microalbuminuric Type 2 diabetic patients independently of hypertension. *Diabetes Care* 2002; **25**: 1909–1913.
97. Sato A, Hayashi K, Naruse M and Saruta T. Effectiveness of aldosterone blockade in patients with diabetic nephropathy. *Hypertension* 2003; **41**: 64–68.
98. Schmitz R. Über die prognostische Bedeutung und die Ätiologie der Albuminurie bei Diabetes. *Berlin Klin Wschr* 1891; **28**: 373–377.
99. Schrier RW, Estacio RO, Esler A and Mehler P. Effects of aggresive blood pressure control in normotensive Type 2 diabetic patients on albuminuria, retinopathy and strokes. *Kidney Int* 2002; **61**: 1086–1097.
100. Siebenhofer A, Plank J, Horvath K, Bergholdt A, Sutton AJ, Sommer R and Pieber TR. Angiotensin receptor blockers as anti-hypertensive treatment for patients with diabetes

mellitus: meta-analysis of controlled double-blind randomized trials. *Diabet Med* 2004; **21**: 18–25.
101. Sowers JR. Recommendations for Special Populations: Diabetes mellitus and the metabolic syndrome. *Am J Hypertens* 2003; **16**: S41–S45.
102. Stratton IM, Adler AI, Neil HA, Matthews DR, Manley SE, Cull CA, Hadden D, Turner RC and Holman RR. Association of glycaemia with macrovascular and microvascular complications of Type 2 diabetes (UKPDS 35): prospective observational study. *BMJ* 2000; **321**: 405–419.
103. Støvring H, Andersen M, Beck-Nielsen H, Green A and Vach W. Rising prevalence of diabetes: evidence from a Danish pharmaco-epidemiological database. *Lancet* 2003; **9383**: 537–538.
104. Tonolo G, Ciccarese M and Brizzi P *et al*. Reduction of albumin excretion rate in normotensive microalbuminuric diabetic patients during long-term simvastatin treatment. *Diabetes Care* 1997; **20**: 1891–1895.
105. UKPDS Post Study Monitoring Programme. The Oxford centre for diabetes, endocrinology and metabolism. 2003. www.dtu.ox.ac.uk/ukpds/psm.html.
106. UK Prospective Diabetes Study Group. Intensive blood-glucose control with sulfonylureas or insulin compared with conventional treatment and risk of complications in Type 2 diabetes (UKPDS33). *Lancet* 1998; **352**: 837–853.
107. UK Prospective Diabetes Study Group. Tight blood pressure control and risk of macrovascular and microvascular complications in Type 2 diabetes (UKPDS38). *BMJ* 1998; **317**: 703–712.
108. UK Prospective Diabetes Study Group. Efficacy of atenolol and captopril in reducing risk of macrovascular and microvascular complications in Type 2 diabetes (UKPDS39). *BMJ* 1998; **317**: 713–720.
109. Valmadrid CT, Klein R and Moss SE *et al*. The risk of cardiovascular disease mortality associated with microalbuminuria and gross proteinuria in persons with older-onset diabetes mellitus. *Arch Intern Med* 2000; **160**: 1093–1100.
110. van Dam RM, Rimm EB, Willett WC, Stampfer MJ and Hu FB. Dietary patterns and risk for Type 2 diabetes mellitus in US men. *Ann Intern Med.* 2002; **136**: 201–209.
111. Vedel P, Obel J and Nielsen FS *et al*. Glomerular hyperfiltration in microalbuminuric NIDDM patients. *Diabetologia* 1996; **39**: 1584–1589.
112. Vestra MD, Saller A and Bortoloso E *et al*. Structural involvement in Type 1 and Type 2 diabetic nephropathy. *Diabetes Metab* 2000; **26**: 8–14.
113. Viberti GC and Wheeldon NM. For the Microalbuminuria Reduction with Valsartan (MARVAL) Study investigators. Microalbuminuria reduction with valsartan in patients with Type 2 diabetes mellitus. A blood pressure-independent effect. *Circulation* 2002; **106**: 672–678.
114. Wang SL, Head J and Stevens L *et al*. Excess mortality and its relation to hypertension and proteinuria in diabetic patients. The WHO multinational study of vascular disease in diabetes. *Diabetes Care* 1996; **19**: 305–312.
115. Weber MA. Yet more hypertension guidelines: what do they add? *J Hypertens* 2003; **21**: 1977–1982.
116. Weir MR. Diabetes and hypertension: How low should you go and with which drugs? *Am J Hypertens* 2001; **14**: 17S–26S.
117. World Health Organization, International Society of Hypertension Writing Group. 2003 World Health Organization (WHO)/International Society of Hypertension (ISH) statement on management of hypertension. *J Hypertens* 2003; **21**: 1983–1992.
118. Williams B. Drug treatment of hypertension. *BMJ* 2003; **326**: 61–62.

119. Williams B. The unique vulnerability of diabetic subjects to hypertensive injury. *J Human Hypertens* 1999; **13** (2): S3–S8.
120. Wolf G and Ritz E. Diabetic nephropathy in Type 2 diabetes prevention and patient management. *J Am Soc Nephrol* 2003; **14**: 1396–1405.
121. Zanchetti A. Costs of implementing recommendations on hypertension management given in recent guidelines. *J Hypertens* 2003; **21**: 2207–2209.

14

Diabetic Retinopathy in the 21st Century: Screening and Visual Outcomes

Ayad Al-Bermani and **Roy Taylor**

Introduction

Around two per cent of the UK population are known to have diabetes; of these 200 000 have Type 1 diabetes, and more than a million have Type 2 diabetes.[1] At any one time up to 10 per cent of people with diabetes will have retinopathy requiring medical follow-up or treatment. It is the commonest preventable cause of registered blindness in the UK amongst working age people.[2] Screening programmes have been shown to result in marked reduction in rates of blindness due to diabetes mellitus.[3,4]

Management of diabetic retinopathy by laser photocoagulation and vitrectomy combined with glycaemic and blood pressure control is an outstanding achievement of modern times. However, successful outcomes can only be achieved by carrying out regular retinal checks to detect both any retinopathy to guide therapy of blood pressure and blood glucose and the development of the asymptomatic sight-threatening retinopathy.

Diabetic retinopathy is a progressive dysfunction of the retinal microvasculature caused by chronic hyperglycaemia. Growth of new blood vessels, known as proliferative retinopathy, may lead to blindness through haemorrhage and scarring. A deterioration of retinal blood vessel integrity causing leakage into the retina and

Prevention of Type 2 Diabetes Edited by Manfred Ganz
 ISBN: 0-470-85733-1

loss of blood vessels is known as maculopathy, and this leads to visual impairment and possibly blindness.

Epidemiology

The prevalence of retinopathy is strongly linked to the duration of diabetes.[5] Patients who have had Type 1 (insulin-dependent) diabetes mellitus for less than 5 years rarely show evidence of sight-threatening diabetic retinopathy, although some background diabetic retinopathy is already present.[6,7] About 27 per cent of those who have had diabetes for 5–10 years have diabetic retinopathy. After 20 years, the prevalence rises to 95 per cent and 30–50 per cent of these patients have proliferative diabetic retinopathy.[8] The demography of the problem is different in Type 2 (non-insulin-dependent) diabetes, patients, 37 per cent of whom will already have retinopathy at diagnosis.[9] In another study, 10 years after the diagnosis, 67 per cent of patients had retinopathy and 10 per cent had proliferative diabetic retinopathy.[8]

Good Glycaemic Control

Strict glycaemic control will reduce both the incidence and the progression of early retinopathy.[10,11] In the UKPDS study of Type 2 diabetes, one per cent lower glycated haemoglobin resulted in a 25 per cent reduction in microvascular endpoints, a 37 per cent decrease in laser treatment and a 10 per cent reduction in cataract extraction.[12] Furthermore, the EDIC study showed that there is a prolonged beneficial effect of good glycaemic control in lowering the prevalence of worsening of retinopathy and of progression to proliferative or severe nonproliferative retinopathy by 74 per cent and 78 per cent respectively despite the change in glycaemic control.[13]

Good Blood Pressure Control

In the United Kingdom prospective diabetes study, over half of the patients had high blood pressure or were receiving antihypertensive treatment. Tight control of the blood pressure, aiming at below 150/90, had a significant beneficial effect, reducing the incidence of retinopathy and its progression to photocoagulation. For every 10 mm reduction in the systolic blood pressure there was an 11 per cent reduction in the need for laser treatment. The effect was similar whether beta blocker or angiotensin-converting enzyme inhibitor was used.[14] Overall, the effect of tight blood pressure control was greater than that of tight glycaemic control (see Figures 14.1 and 14.2).

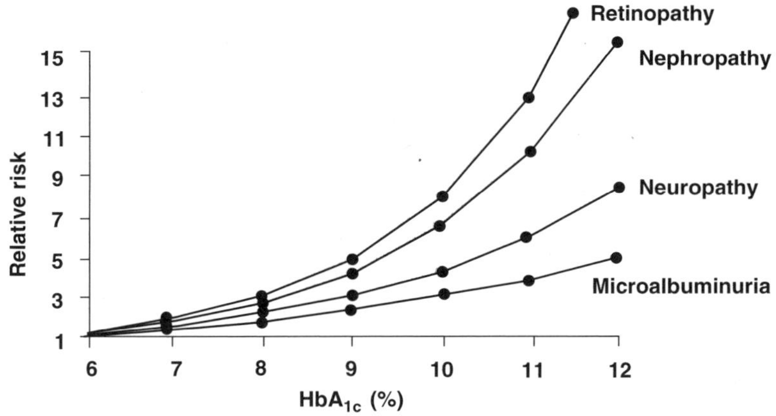

FIGURE 14.1 DCCT: relationship of HbA_{1c} to risk of microvascular complications

Other Risk Factors

Renal disease as evidenced by proteinuria, elevated blood urea nitrogen and elevated blood creatinine is a reliable predictor of the presence of retinopathy.[15] Even patients who have microalbuminuria are at high risk of developing retinopathy.[16]

In women who begin a pregnancy without retinopathy, the risk of developing nonproliferative diabetic retinopathy has been reported to be about 10 per cent. Further, those with nonproliferative diabetic retinopathy at the onset of pregnancy and those who have or who develop systemic hypertension tend to show progression.[17] About four per cent of pregnant women who have nonproliferative diabetic retinopathy progress to PDR.[17]

Aspirin has no influence on the progression of retinopathy, visual acuity or incidence of vitreous haemorrhage.[18] Ticlopidine inhibits adenosine diphosphate-induced platelet aggregation. It has been shown to decrease the risk of stroke in patients with transient ischaemic attacks. One study showed a statistical benefit in retarding the onset of diabetic retinopathy, but it was not carried out long enough to demonstrate definite clinical benefit.[19]

Screening

Regular examination of the retinae of people with diabetes is simply part of good clinical care in the same way that screening of feet helps to minimize amputation rates. Although often characterized as a free-standing screening exercise with the single aim of detecting those who require laser therapy, retinal screening informs

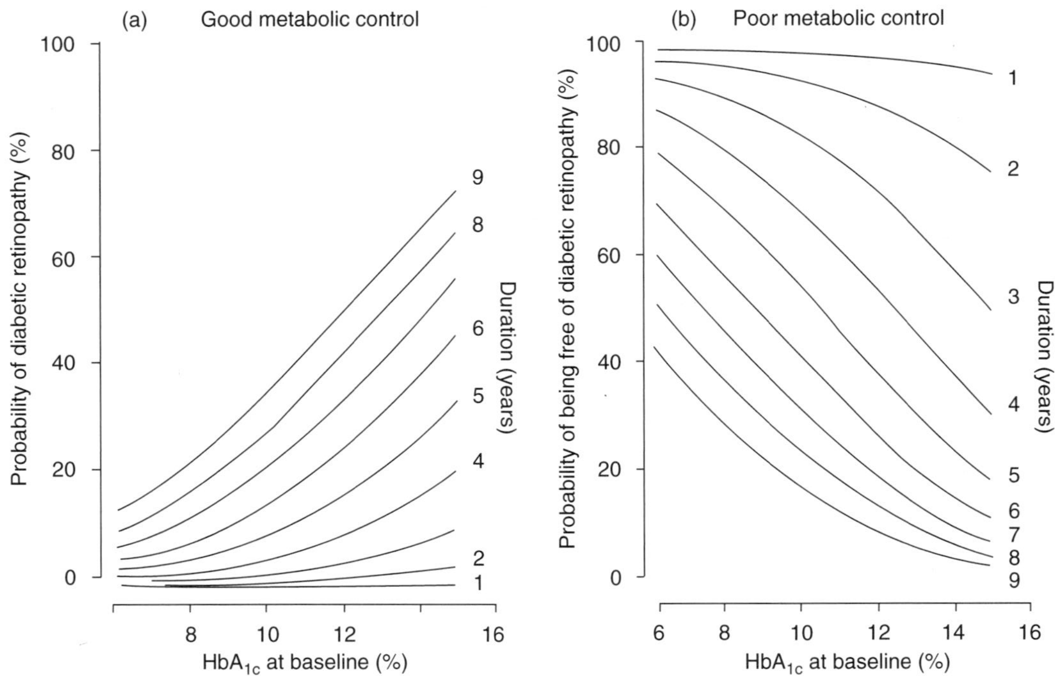

FIGURE 14.2 (a) Probability of developing retinopathy in Type 1 diabetic patients as a function of HbA_{1c} level (%) at baseline and duration (years) of good metabolic control ($HbA_{1c} < 6.87\%$). (b) Probability of not developing retinopathy in Type 1 diabetic patients as a function of HbA_{1c} level (%) at baseline and duration (years) of poor metabolic control ($HbA_{1c} > 9.49\%$). In both cases, BMI is assumed to be equal to $22\ kg/m^2$.

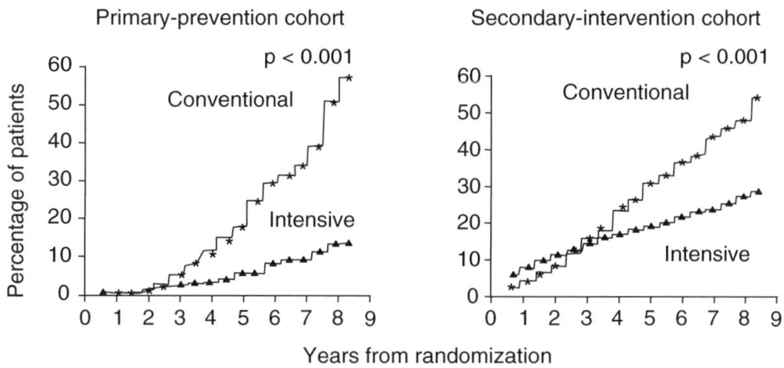

FIGURE 14.3 DCCT: effects of management on retinopathy (adapted from DCCT Research Group. Reference 10.)

the setting of clinical targets for blood pressure and blood glucose control in individual patients. From the point of view of the patient, it is important that feet, eyes, blood pressure and injection sites are examined annually. The organization of retinal screening is therefore inextricably linked with organization of the rest of clinical care in any one locality.

The single most important characteristic of a successful system is population coverage. The system must be simple to operate in order that it is robust in performing, despite changes in personnel and pressures upon health-care provision. Even the sensitivity of a screening system is less important than population coverage in determining the fall in rates of blindness in a district. Naturally, the method used must be sound, but undue concentration upon sensitivity and specificity distracts from the overall health outcomes achieved in the population by ensuring complete population coverage.

It is clear that use of the ophthalmoscope is inadequate in most circumstances, probably because of the need to spend adequate time examining each retina in the context of a busy clinic.[20] Even use of retinal photography without mydriasis is superior to ophthalmoscopy.[21] It became clear following the first large study of retinal photography as a screening modality that the occurrence of poor films was most often associated with small pupils,[21] and following this observation we have observed poor film rates of less than five per cent with routine use of 0.5 per cent tropicamide. Polaroid retinal photography was remarkably effective, and in a routine screening system dealing with approximately 9000 patients per year at the time sensitivity for detection of referable retinopathy was 85 per cent.[22] The films could easily be stored in clinical notes for comparison from year to year, and no fading has been observed over a period of almost 20 years.

The introduction of digital retinal imaging has brought further benefits. The intensity of flash required is less than for Polaroid photography, films from previous years can readily be retrieved from storage and the images can be immediately shown and explained to the patient. The latter advantage is most important in minimizing the chance of people failing to attend for the next annual review appointment. Additionally, the ease of storing and transmitting the images means that quality assurance systems are simple to organize. In routine clinical practice in Newcastle-upon-Tyne during evaluation of 13 000 patients per year a screening sensitivity of 85 per cent and specificity of 97 per cent for referral was observed.[50] Annual digital retinal screening has been recommended by the National Screening committee in the UK (http://www.diabetic-retinopathy.screening.nhs.uk/).

Operation of a successful screening system is critically dependent upon properly trained retinal screeners. In Newcastle the basic training occupies 12 weeks and consists of five domains: the clinical context of diabetes, the biology of diabetic

TABLE 14.1 Disease grading protocol in National Guidelines on Screening for Diabetic Retinopathy

	Level	Grade	Description
Retinopathy (R)	0	None	
	1	Background	Microaneurysm(s), retinal haemorrhage(s) ± any exudate
	2	Preproliferative	Venous beading, venous looping or reduplication Intraretinal microvascular abnormality (IRMA) Multiple deep, round or blot haemorrhages (CWS – careful search for above features)
	3	Proliferative	New vessels (NVD), new vessels elsewhere (NVE) Pre-retinal or vitreous haemorrhage Pre-retinal fibrosis ± tractional retinal detachment
Maculopathy (M)			Exudate within one disc diameter (DD) of the centre of the fovea Circinate or group of exudates within the macula Retinal thickening within 1 DD of the centre of the fovea (if stereo available) Any microaneurysm or haemorrhage within 1 DD of the centre of the fovea only if associated with a visual acuity of 6/12 or better (if no stereo)
Photocoagulation (P)			Focal/grid to macula or peripheral scatter
Unclassifiable (U)			

TABLE 14.2 Management of cases after completion of grading in the National Guidelines on Screening for Diabetic Retinopathy

Grade		Management
Retinopathy (R)	R 0	Annual screening
	R1	Annual screening
	R2	Refer to hospital eye service
	R3	Fast track referral to hospital eye service
Maculopathy (M)	M	Refer to hospital eye service
Photocoagulation (P)	P	New screenee – refer to hospital eye service
		Quiescent post-treatment – annual screening
Other lesions (OL)		Refer to hospital eye service or inform primary physician
Ungradable/unobtainable (U)		Poor view but gradable on biomicroscopy – refer to hospital eye service
		Unscreenable – discharge, inform GP (option to recall for photos if purely technical failure)

retinopathy, image acquisition, image interpretation and targeted ophthalmoscopy. The single most important characteristic of a retinal screener is that he or she should be good with people. Sensitive explanation of the findings of screening is essential, with the patient viewing his or her own retinal appearances. In order that this can be done, image interpretation is a necessary skill. In sharp contrast to ophthalmoscopy, image interpretation is simple to teach and the skill, based upon pattern recognition, is rapidly acquired in practice. (See Tables 14.1 and 14.2)

Effect of Screening Upon Rates of Blindness

A decrease of more than one-third in the incidence of blindness in patients with diabetes in Stockholm county has been reported over a 15 year period of regular screening. To determine the impact of systematic population screening in Newcastle-upon-Tyne since 1986, the blindness prevalence in Newcastle Health District was determined.[4] Data were collected for 1998–2000 from the Royal National Institute for the Blind Liaison Office of the Newcastle Ophthalmology department. The ophthalmology clinic notes on each individual were retrieved to verify clinical details including previous eye diagnosis, dates of previous laser photocoagulation and eye surgery. To ensure completeness of data, details of all patients registered blind attending the Newcastle diabetic centre were examined. The annual incidence of blindness and partial sight due to diabetes in the Newcastle district were 0.35 and 0.56 per 1000 respectively. Proliferative retinopathy accounted for 30 and maculopathy for 24 registrations. The times from referral to ophthalmology to registration were 6.2 ± 3.5 and 4.4 ± 3.3 years in these groups respectively. No cases resulted from false negative screening. In Newcastle district the rates of blindness and partial sight are now less than one-third of those reported in the surveys prior to 1997, confirming that objectives of the St. Vincent declarations are being achieved. However, a more dramatic observation is that in 1986 there were six people under the age of 25 years registered blind due to diabetes. By 2000, the youngest person blind due to diabetes was 35 years of age. Clearly change in blood pressure and blood glucose therapy have contributed to this change, but it is likely that systematic screening has played the largest part.

Treatment of Diabetic Retinopathy

Using timely laser photocoagulation as advocated by the Diabetic Retinopathy Study and the Early Treatment Diabetic Retinopathy Study, severe visual loss can be reduced by 95 per cent. ETDRS was a multicentre, randomized clinical trial designed to evaluate argon laser photocoagulation and aspirin treatment in the management of patients with nonproliferative or early proliferative diabetic retinopathy. A total of 3711 patients were recruited to be followed for a minimum of 4 years to provide long-term information on the risks and benefits of the treatments under study.

Panretinal Photocoagulation

When well focused, intense light is absorbed by pigmented cells (e.g. erythrocytes, retinal pigment epithelial cells), it is converted to heat, coagulating the cells and surrounding tissues. Photocoagulation burns scattered throughout the retina decreases the retina's need for oxygen and thereby prevent new vessels from developing, or might even cause regression of existent new vessels.

Eyes with high-risk characteristics have (1) NVD greater than one-half the disc area; (2) any NVD and vitreous haemorrhage or (3) NVE greater than one-half the disc area and vitreous or pre-retinal haemorrhage. The main findings of the Diabetic Retinopathy Study are summarized in Table 14.3.

After panretinal photocoagulation, retinal circulation is clearly improved. There is a better regulatory response to hypoxia and decreased blood flow.[25,26] The exact mechanism by which panretinal photocoagulation works remains unknown. Some investigators believe that it decreases production of vasoproliferative factors by (1) eliminating some of the hypoxic retina or (2) stimulating the release of antiangiogenic factors from the retinal pigment epithelium.[27] An alternative hypothesis is that vessel dilatation caused by chronic hypoxia is the direct stimulus for endothelial cell proliferation and neovascularization, and that panretinal photocoagulation works by thinning the retina. Vasodilatation is reduced by increased

TABLE 14.3 Results of the Diabetic Retinopathy Study at 3 years

Patients with final VA <5/200 = 6/240		
Without PRP	With PRP	High-risk characteristics
25.6%	4.3%	NVD < 1/2 DD with vitreous haemorrhage
26.2%	8.5%	NVD > 1/2 DD without vitreous haemorrhage
36.9%	20.1%	with vitreous haemorrhage NVD > 1/2 DD
29.7%	7.2%	with vitreous haemorrhage NVE > 1/2 DD

DD, disc diameters; NVD, neovascularization of the disc; NVE, neovascularization elsewhere; PRP, panretinal photocoagulation; VA, visual acuity.[23,24]

diffusion of oxygen from the choroids.[28–31] Another possibility is that panretinal photocoagulation decreases choroidal circulation in the midperiphery, which in turn shunts blood flow centrally (a 'reverse choroidal steal'), decreasing the stimulus for NVD.[32] Finally, others suggest that panretinal photocoagulation leads to an increase in vasoinhibitors, either by stimulating the retinal pigment epithelium to produce inhibitors of vasoproliferation[27,33] or by causing a breakdown of the blood–retinal barrier so that serum vasoinhibitors can diffuse into the vitreous.[34]

The goal of panretinal photocoagulation is to arrest or cause regression of the proliferating new vessels. The usual panretinal photocoagulation destroys approximately 14 per cent of the total retinal area.[35] Most ophthalmologists use the argon blue–green or green laser. The Early Treatment Diabetic Retinopathy Study (ETDRS) also found that panretinal photocoagulation significantly retards the development of high-risk characteristics in eyes with very severe nonproliferative diabetic retinopathy and macular oedema.[36] After 7 years of follow-up, 25 per cent of eyes that received panretinal photocoagulation developed high-risk characteristics compared with 75 per cent of eyes in which panretinal photocoagulation was deferred until high-risk characteristics developed. Nevertheless, the ETDRS concluded that treatment of nonproliferative diabetic retinopathy and proliferative diabetic retinopathy in the absence of high-risk characteristics was not indicated, based on the following findings.

1. After 7 years of follow-up, 25 per cent of eyes assigned to deferral of panretinal photocoagulation never developed high-risk characteristics.

2. When patients are closely monitored and panretinal photocoagulation is given as soon as high-risk characteristics develop, severe visual loss is prevented. After 7 years of follow-up, four per cent of eyes that did not receive panretinal photocoagulation until high-risk characteristics developed had a visual acuity of 5/200 (6/240) or less as compared with 2.5 per cent of eyes assigned to immediate panretinal photocoagulation. The difference was neither clinically

nor statistically significant. Therefore, many eyes with severe nonproliferative diabetic retinopathy that received panretinal photocoagulation would be unnecessarily treated.

3. Panretinal photocoagulation has significant complications. It often causes decreased visual acuity by increasing macular oedema[37–39] or by causing macular pucker. Fortunately, the oedema frequently regresses spontaneously over 6 months. The visual field is usually moderately decreased.[40] Colour vision and dark adaptation, which are often already impaired, are also worsened by the technique.[41] Finally, proliferative diabetic retinopathy is associated with an increased risk of myocardial infarction and increased mortality.[42] Many patients die before they develop complications from proliferative diabetic retinopathy.

Treatment of Macular Oedema

The ETDRS treatment strategy was to treat all leaking microaneurysms further than 500 mm from the centre of the macula and to place a grid of 100–200 mm burns in areas of either diffuse capillary leakage or capillary nonperfusion. After 3 years of follow-up, 15 per cent of eyes with clinically significant macular oedema had doubling of the visual angle as opposed to 32 per cent of nontreated control eyes.[43] Recent subgroup analysis showed that treatment can be deferred in eyes in which the centre of the fovea is not thickened as long as hard exudates are not threatening the centre; however, such eyes must be closely observed.[43] In people with diabetic maculopathy, one ETDRS found a significant improvement in visual acuity in eyes treated with grid photocoagulation versus untreated eyes at 12 months and at 24 months. Photocoagulation versus no photocoagulation reduced the risk of moderate visual loss by 50–70 per cent.

Vitrectomy

The major indications are nonclearing vitreous haemorrhage, traction retinal detachment and combined traction/rhegmatogenous retinal detachment. Less common indications are macular oedema with a thickened and taut posterior hyaloid,[44,45] macular heterotopia, and tight preretinal macular haemorrhage.[46]

The Diabetic Retinopathy Vitrectomy Study (DRVS) randomized 370 eyes with florid neovascularization and visual acuity of 10/200 (6/120 or counting fingers) or better to either early vitrectomy or observation.[47] After 4 years of follow-up, approximately 50 per cent of both groups had 20/60 or better, and approximately 20 per cent of each group had light perception or worse. Thus, the results indicate that such patients probably do not benefit from early vitrectomy. They should be observed closely so that vitrectomy, when indicated, can promptly be undertaken.

If a patient has a vitreous haemorrhage severe enough to cause a visual acuity of 5/200 or less, the chances of visual recovery within 1 year are only about 17 per cent.[48] The DRVS randomized patients who had a visual acuity of 5/200 or less for more than 6 months into two groups: those who received an immediate vitrectomy and those whose vitrectomy was deferred for 6 months.[49] Of those who had a deferred vitrectomy, 15 per cent had a final visual acuity of 20/40 or better as opposed to 25 per cent of those who had an immediate vitrectomy. In patients with Type 1 diabetes, 12 per cent of those who had a deferred vitrectomy had a final visual acuity of 20/40 or better as opposed to 36 per cent of those who had an immediate vitrectomy. The reason for this discrepancy was believed to be excessive growth of fibrovascular proliferation during the waiting period. For this reason, the DRVS concluded that strong consideration should be given to immediate vitrectomy, especially in Type 1 diabetic patients. (In patients with Type 2 diabetes, the final visual results were similar.)

If surgery is deferred, ultrasonography should be performed at regular intervals to make sure that traction retinal detachment is not developing behind the haemorrhage. The goals of surgery are to release all anteroposterior vitreous traction and to perform a complete panretinal photocoagulation to reduce the incidence of recurrent haemorrhage. Further, the results of vitrectomy for nonclearing vitreous haemorrhage are excellent (Table 14.4).

Before current treatments were available, the prognosis for patients with proliferative diabetic retinopathy was blindness within 5 years for more than 50 per cent of patients. Rates of blindness in ETDRS patients following the development of proliferative retinopathy are remarkably lower. Legal blindness is reduced to less than five per cent in 5 years for patients with proliferative retinopathy. Severe vision loss is reduced to one per cent.

TABLE 14.4 Overall visual results following vitrectomy

Patients (%)[49]	Visual acuity
25	20/20–20/40
29	20/50–20/100
5	20/120–20/300
7	20/400–CF
10	HM–LP
25	NLP

CF, counting fingers; HM–LP, hand movements–light perception; NLP, no light perception; DRVS, Diabetic Retinopathy Vitrectomy Study.

Summary

Good blood pressure and good blood glucose control will minimize the rate of progression of retinopathy in people with diabetes. However, it will still be necessary to screen for this, the most feared complication of the disease. There is now compelling data that rates of blindness due to diabetes can be markedly decreased by systems for retinal screening that are simple and effective and have high population coverage.

References

1. Chief Medical Officer. *The Annual Report of the Chief Medical Officer of the Department of Health for the Year 1997*. 1998. London: Stationery Office.
2. Evans J, Rooney C, Ashwood F, Dattani N and Wormald R. Blindness and partial sight in England and Wales: April 1990 to March 1991. *Health Trends* 1996; **28**: 5–12.
3. Blacklund AL, Algvere PV and Rosenqvist U. New blindness in diabetes reduced by more than one third in Stockholm County. *Diabet Med* 1997; **14**: 732–740.
4. Arun CS, Ngugi N, Lovelock L and Taylor R. Effectiveness of screening in preventing blindness due to diabetic retinopathy. *Diabet Med* 2003; **20** (3): 186–190.
5. Klein R and Klein BEK. Epidemiology of proliferative diabetic retinopathy. *Diabetes Care* 1992; **15**: 1875–1891.
6. Younis N, Broadbent DM, Harding SP and Vora JP. Incidence of sight-threatening retinopathy in Type 1 diabetes in a systematic screening programme. *Diabet Med* 2003; **20** (9): 758–765.
7. Malone JI, Morrison AD, Pavan PR and Cuthbertson DD; Diabetic control and complications trial. Prevalence and significance of retinopathy in subjects with Type 1 diabetes of less than 5 years duration screened for the Diabetes control and Complications Trial. *Diabetes Care* 2001; **24** (3): 522–526.
8. Klein R, Klein BE, Moss SE and Cruickshank KJ. The Wisconsin Epidemiologic Study of Diabetic Retinopathy. XIV. Ten-year incidence and progression of diabetic retinopathy. *Arch Ophthalmol* 1994; **112**: 1217–1228.
9. Stratton IM, Kohner EM, Adlington S, Mathews DR and Turner RC. Prevalence of diabetic retinopathy at diagnosis of NIDDM in 2964 white Caucasian subjects and association with hypertension, hyperglycaemia and impaired B cell function. *Diabetes* 1995; **44**: 117a.
10. Diabetes Control and Complications Trial Research Group. The effect of intensive treatment of diabetes on the development and progression of long term complications in insulin dependent diabetes mellitus. *N Engl J Med* 1993; **32**: 977–986.
11. United Kingdom Prospective Diabetes Study Group. Intensive blood glucose control with sulphonylureas or insulin compared with conventional treatment and risk of complications in patients with Type 2 diabetes (UKPDS 33). *Lancet* 1998; **352**: 837–853.
12. Stratton IM, Adler AI, Neil HA, Matthews DR, Manley SE and Cull CA *et al.* Association of glycaemia with macrovascular and microvascular complications of Type 2 diabetes (UKPDS 35). *BMJ* 2000; **321**: 405–412.
13. White NH, Cleary PA, Dahms W, Goldstein D, Malone J and Tamborlane WV; Diabetes Control and Complications Trial (DCCT)/Epidemiology of Diabetes Interventions and Complications (EDIC) Research Group. Beneficial effects of intensive therapy of diabetes during adolescence: outcomes after the conclusion of the Diabetes Control and Complications Trial (DCCT). *J Pediatr* 2001; **139** (6): 804–812.

14. United Kingdom Prospective Study Group. Tight blood pressure control and risk of macro and microvascular complications in Type 2 diabetes (UKPDS 38). *BMJ* 1998; **317**: 703–713.
15. Klein R and Klein BEK. Epidemiology of proliferative diabetic retinopathy. *Diabetes Care* 1992; **15**: 1875–1891.
16. Klein R, Klein BEK, Moss SE, Davis MD and DeMets DL. The Wisconsin Epidemiologic Study of Diabetic Retinopathy. II. Prevalence and risk of diabetic retinopathy when age is less than 30 years. *Arch Ophthalmol* 1984; **102**: 520–526.
17. Rosenn B, Miodovnik M and Kranias G *et al.* Progression of diabetic retinopathy in pregnancy: association with hypertension in pregnancy. *Am J Obstet Gynecol* 1992; **166**: 1214–1218.
18. Chew EY, Klein ML, Murphy RP, Remaley NA, Ferris III FL and ETDRS Study Group. Effects of aspirin on vitreous haemorrhage/preretinal haemorrhage in patients with diabetes mellitus. ETDRS Report No. 20. *Arch Ophthalmol* 1995; **113**: 52–55.
19. Ticlopidine Microangiopathy of Diabetes Study Group. Ticlopidine treatment reduces the progression of nonproliferative diabetic retinopathy. *Arch Ophthalmol* 1990; **108** (11): 1577–1583.
20. Harding SP, Broadbent DM, Neoh C, White MC and Vora J. Sensitivity and specificity of photography and direct ophthalmoscopy in screening for sight threatening eye disease: the Liverpool Diabetic Eye Study. *BMJ* 1995; **311** (7013): 1131–1135.
21. Taylor R, Lovelock L, Tunbridge WM, Alberti KG, Brackenridge RG, Stephenson P and Young E. Comparison of non-mydriatic retinal photography with ophthalmoscopy in 2159 patients: mobile retinal camera study. *BMJ* 1990; **301** (6763): 1243–1247.
22. Pandit RJ and Taylor R. Quality assurance in screening for sight-threatening diabetic retinopathy. *Diabet Med* 2002; **19** (4): 285–291.
23. Diabetic Retinopathy Study Group. Photocoagulation treatment of proliferative diabetic retinopathy: the second report of diabetic retinopathy study findings. *Ophthalmology* 1978; **85**: 82.
24. Diabetic Retinopathy Study Research Group. Four risk factors for severe visual loss in diabetic retinopathy: the third report from the diabetic retinopathy study. *Arch Ophthalmol* 1979; **97**: 654.
25. Patel V, Rassam S and Newsom R *et al.* Retinal blood flow in diabetic retinopathy. *BMJ* 1992; **305**: 678.
26. Grunwald JE, Brucker AJ and Petrig BL *et al.* Retinal blood flow regulation and the clinical response to panretinal photocoagulation in proliferative diabetic retinopathy. *Ophthalmology* 1989; **96**: 1518.
27. Glaser BM, Campochiaro PA, Davis DL Jr and Sato M. Retinal pigment epithelial cells release an inhibitor of neovascularization. *Arch Ophthalmol* 1985; **103**: 1870.
28. Stefansson E, Landers MB III and Wolbarsht ME. Oxygenation and vasodilation in relation to diabetic and other proliferative retinopathies. *Ophthalmic Surg* 1983; **17**: 209.
29. Wolbarsht ML, Landers MB III and Stefansson E. Vasodilation and the etiology of diabetic retinopathy: a new model. *Ophthalmic Surg* 198; **12**: 104.
30. Wolbarsht ML and Landers MB. The rationale of photocoagulation therapy for proliferative diabetic retinopathy: a review and a model. *Ophthalmic Surg* 1980; **11**: 235.
31. Stefansson E, Machemer R and de Juan E Jr *et al.* Retinal oxygenation and laser treatment in patients with diabetic retinopathy. *Am J Ophthalmol* 1992; **113**: 36.
32. Schiodte N. Ocular effects of panretinal photocoagulation. *Acta Ophthalmol* 1988; **66** (Suppl. 1): 9.
33. Marshall J, Clover G and Rothery S. Some new findings on retinal irradiation by krypton and argon lasers. *Doc Ophthalmol* 1984; **36**: 21.

34. Singh A, Boulton M and Lane C *et al.* Inhibition of microvascular endothelial cell proliferation by vitreous following retinal scatter photocoagulation. *Br J Ophthalmol* 1990; **74**: 328.
35. Ogden TE, Riekolf FT and Benkwith SM. Correlation of histologic and electroretinographic changes in peripheral retinal ablation in the rhesus monkey. *Am J Ophthalmol* 1976; **81**: 272.
36. Early Treatment Diabetic Retinopathy Study Research Group. Early photocoagulation for diabetic retinopathy: ETDRS Report number 9. *Ophthalmology* 1991; **98**: 766.
37. Meyers SM. Macular edema after scatter laser photocoagulation for proliferative diabetic retinopathy. *Am J Ophthalmol* 1980; **90**: 210.
38. Ferris FL, Podgor MJ and Davis MD. The Diabetic Retinopathy Research Group: macular edema in diabetic retinopathy study patients. *Ophthalmology* 1987; **94**: 754.
39. Kleiner RC, Elman MJ and Murphy RP *et al.* Transient severe visual loss after panretinal photocoagulation. *Am J Ophthalmol* 1988; **106**: 298.
40. Cambie E. Functional results following argon laser photocoagulation in eyes with diabetic retinopathy. In *Diabetic Renal–Retinal Syndrome*, Friedman EA and L'Esperance FA (eds). 1980. New York: Grune and Stratton, pp. 295–307.
41. Henson DB and North RV. Dark adaptation in diabetes mellitus. *Br J Ophthalmol* 1979; **63**: 539.
42. Miettinen H, Haffner S and Lehto S *et al.* Retinopathy predicts coronary heart disease events in NIDDM patients. *Diabetes Care* 1966; **19**: 1445.
43. Early Treatment Diabetic Retinopathy Study Research Group. Focal photocoagulation treatment of diabetic macular edema: relationship of treatment effect to fluorescein angiographic and other retinal characteristics at baseline: ETDRS Report No. 19. *Arch Ophthalmol* 1995; **113**: 1144.
44. Lewis H, Abrams GW, Blumenkranz MS and Campo RV. Vitrectomy for diabetic macular traction and edema associated with posterior hyaloidal traction. *Ophthalmology* 1992; **99**: 753.
45. Harbour JW, Smiddy WE, Flynn HW and Rubsamen PE. Vitrectomy for diabetic macular edema associated with a thickened and taut posterior hyaloid membrane. *Am J Ophthalmol* 1996; **121**: 405.
46. Ramsay RC, Knobloch WH and Cantrill HL. Timing of vitrectomy for active proliferative diabetic retinopathy. *Ophthalmology* 1986; **93**: 283.
47. Diabetic Retinopathy Vitrectomy Study Research Group. Early vitrectomy for severe proliferative diabetic retinopathy in eyes with useful vision: results of a randomized trial – Diabetic Retinopathy Vitrectomy Study Report 3. *Ophthalmology* 1988; **95**: 1307.
48. Diabetic Retinopathy Vitrectomy Study Research Group. Two year course of visual acuity in severe proliferative diabetic retinopathy with conventional management. *Ophthalmology* 1985; **92**: 492.
49. Diabetic Retinopathy Vitrectomy Study Research Group. Early vitrectomy for severe vitreous hemorrhage in diabetic retinopathy: two-year results of a randomized trial – Diabetic Retinopathy Vitrectomy Study Report 2. *Arch Ophthalmol* 1985; **103**: 1644.
50. Arun CS, Young D, Batey B, Stannard KS and Taylor R. Quality assurance in screening for diabetic retinopathy: establishing a practical and efficient system. *Diabet Med* 2004; **21**: (Suppl. 2): 77.

15

Prevention and Treatment of Diabetic Polyneuropathy (DPN)

Anders A. F. Sima

Introduction

Diabetes mellitus has reached epidemic proportions, not only in Europe and North America but also in heavily populated countries such as China, India and the Arabic World. It is estimated that the global diabetic population will reach 210 million by the year 2010. The socioeconomic implications are enormous; in the USA alone today the cost to society is approximately $150 billion annually. It therefore behooves the medical scientific community to provide the basis for the development of meaningful preventive measures and therapies.

The brunt of the costs is accounted for by the chronic complications of diabetes, which are responsible for the increased morbidity and mortality in the diabetic population. Among these, diabetic neuropathies are, as a group, the most common,[1,2] with a prevalence that varies from 10 per cent within one year of diagnosis to 50 per cent in patients with diabetes for 25 years.[2–5]

As a group, diabetic neuropathy includes several distinct syndromes of which distal sensory polyneuropathy, often associated with diabetic autonomic neuropathy (DAN), are the most common and are referred to as diabetic polyneuropathy (DPN).[5–7] DPN is a progressive disorder caused by metabolic aberrations,[8,9] which fuel the progressive degenerative process. Additional diabetic neuropathic syndromes include focal/multifocal neuropathies,[5,6] which have a vascular genesis with acute onset and partial resolution.

This review will focus on DPN, which constitutes a major clinical and therapeutic problem.[1,7] The metabolic mechanisms underlying DPN are multiple and

Prevention of Type 2 Diabetes Edited by Manfred Ganz
 ISBN: 0-470-85733-1

interrelated and are in part mutually perpetuating.[8,9] These aberrations occur consequent to hyperglycaemia and insulin/C-peptide deficiencies,[1,9] a notion that is supported by the outcome of the Diabetes Control and Complications Trial (DCCT). In this trial, five years of intense hyperglycaemic control reduced the incidence of DPN by 60 per cent in Type 1 patients.[10] However, the fact that strict hyperglycaemic control did not completely prevent DPN suggests that additional underlying mechanisms are operable, such as insulin/C-peptide deficiencies and genetic predispositions.

In recent decades, several experimental drugs have undergone clinical testing. Unfortunately the results from these clinical trials have been disappointing, in part due to the fact that the compounds have not been potent enough or they were introduced too late in the natural history of the disease. Some groups of these compounds are being reassessed and new approaches are being introduced.

In the following review, I will elaborate on the following issues:

- clinical presentation and classification of DPN
- pathogenetic mechanisms
- tested therapies
- future therapeutic opportunities
- concluding thoughts.

Clinical Presentation and Classification of DPN

Signs and symptoms

The early abnormalities indicative of DPN are asymptomatic nerve dysfunction reflected by decreased nerve conduction velocities and/or reduced heart beat variation.[7,9] These changes are followed by loss of ankle reflexes and vibratory sensation in the lower extremities. As the neuropathy progresses, there is increasing loss of sensation, starting in the feet. Clinical symptoms can be divided into negative and positive symptoms. The former include impaired tactile, thermal and pain sensation and negative autonomic symptoms such as impotence, sudomotor impairment and gastroparesis are common. Positive symptoms, due to neural hyperexcitability, include pins and needles and pain (see below), which may be of varying qualities (burning, aching or lancinating). Symptoms usually begin in the feet and progress proximally, then start in the hands with progression in the upper limbs, reflecting the dying-back nature of underlying nerve degeneration.[1,7,11,12] It is important to keep in mind that DPN may be mixed with diabetic mononeuropathies (radiculoneuropathies, femoral neuropathy, mononeuropathies of median or ulnar nerve and oculomotor neuropathy). These disorders usually occur acutely and tend to run a self-limiting course. They are more common in elderly Type 2 patients.[7]

One of the most debilitating symptoms in diabetic neuropathy is neuropathic pain. It may be the result of nociceptive stimulation of pain receptors, or more commonly the result of dysaesthetic pain due to nerve fibre damage. Dyck and coworkers found a correlation between active nerve fibre degeneration and painfulness.[13] Britland *et al.*[14] suggested that axonal atrophy may be involved in the causation of neuropathic pain. As a possible mechanism for pain we[15] have suggested that increased frequencies of spontaneous discharges from dorsal root ganglia, due to distal axonal degeneration, may activate central impulse transmission from nociceptive neurons. Increased presence of exitotoxic glutamate consequent to ischaemia may excite nociceptive interneurons in the spinal cord.[16,17] Hence, diabetic pain is a complex and poorly understood phenomenon that is probably multifactorial, affecting different anatomical levels of pain transmission, resulting in different pain qualities, which are seldom differentiated clinically.[18]

Acute painful diabetic neuropathy is an uncommon but characteristic syndrome affecting predominantly Type 1 patients. It may follow initiation of glycaemic control and is often associated with profound weight loss ('diabetic neuropathic cachexia'). Nerve conduction velocities are often normal or only slightly affected. The syndrome is self-limiting but it may take considerable time before the patient starts to gain weight, at which time the painful neuropathy usually subsides.

Staging paradigms of diabetic neuropathy

To standardize and classify DPN, several protocols have been proposed. These vary from comprehensive assessments of neurological symptom scores and neuropathy impairment scores by Dyck *et al.*[19] to simple bedside examination.[20] The former can be compared with age-matched control data and abnormalities can be expressed as percentiles of normal. From these a composite scoring system classifying DPN into four stages is obtained, providing a single score based on multiple tests. It was advantageously used in the Rochester Diabetic Neuropathy Study[19] and the DCCT study. These classifications are, however, time consuming and therefore inconvenient in daily practice.

The San Antonio Consensus Meeting on Diabetic Neuropathy[21] suggested assessment of five categories: symptom profiles, neurological examination, quantitative sensory testing, nerve conduction studies and autonomic function testing. The advantage with this scoring system is that it reflects the function of most fibre types and these measures are reasonably reproducible over time. Even this classification, however, is elaborate and best suited for research purposes.

A less time-consuming but reliable and reproducible scheme for classification of DPN was proposed by Feldman *et al.*[22] This, the Michigan Neuropathy Screening Instrument, combines quantitative evaluation of a standardized neurologic examination and nerve conduction studies. It is convenient and therefore suitable for screening, longitudinal follow-ups[23] and population-based or cross-sectional studies. It is simple, less time consuming and it has been validated *vis à vis* more comprehensive protocols.

One problem in staging and classifying DPN that is important to keep in mind is that the progression rates of objective measurements are not linear and differ from one nerve to the other.[24] The progression rate in 182 patients with established clinically overt DPN monitored over 18 months showed significant deterioration in vibratory perception threshold, the Valsalva ratio, median F-wave latencies and sensory nerve conduction velocities of the upper limb, whereas sural and peroneal nerve conduction velocities showed no significant changes.[24] Had the same patient cohort been followed for the same period at an earlier stage of their neuropathies, the distribution of significant changes would have been different. When correlating electrophysiological changes with quantitative structural changes, a similar pattern arises with respect to progression rates.[25] The phenomenon of nonlinearity and varied progression rates of DPN in various nerves is of fundamental importance for choosing efficacy end-points in future clinical neuropathy trials.[26]

Pathogenetic Mechanisms

Most data on mechanisms underlying DPN originate from experimental rodent models such as the streptozotocin- (STZ-) induced diabetic rat and the spontaneously diabetic Type 1 diabetic BB/Wor-rat. Under these experimental conditions it is increasingly clear that DPN is caused by a multitude of interacting factors and that the impact of these may vary during the course of the disease and between the two types of diabetes (Figure 15.1). The complexity of pathogenetic factors and their often direct extrapolation to the human situation may in part explain the problems associated with the design of effective therapies and the failures of earlier clinical intervention trials.[27]

Polyol pathway activation and associated abnormalities

Activation of the polyol pathway is an early and important mechanism in DPN (Figure 15.1). The polyol pathway is comprised of two steps: (1) the conversion of glucose to sorbitol by aldose reductase and (2) the conversion of sorbitol to fructose by sorbitol dehydrogenase. Shunting of excessive glucose through this pathway results in accumulation of sorbitol and fructose, which leads to compensatory depletion of other organic osmolytes such as myo-inositol and taurine.[28] Taurine not only acts as an osmolyte but also has endogenous antioxidant and neurotrophic functions.[28] Polyol pathway activation promotes oxidative stress via depletion of NADPH, a cofactor of both aldose reductase and glutathione reductase, resulting in a decrease in reduced glutathione and an increase in

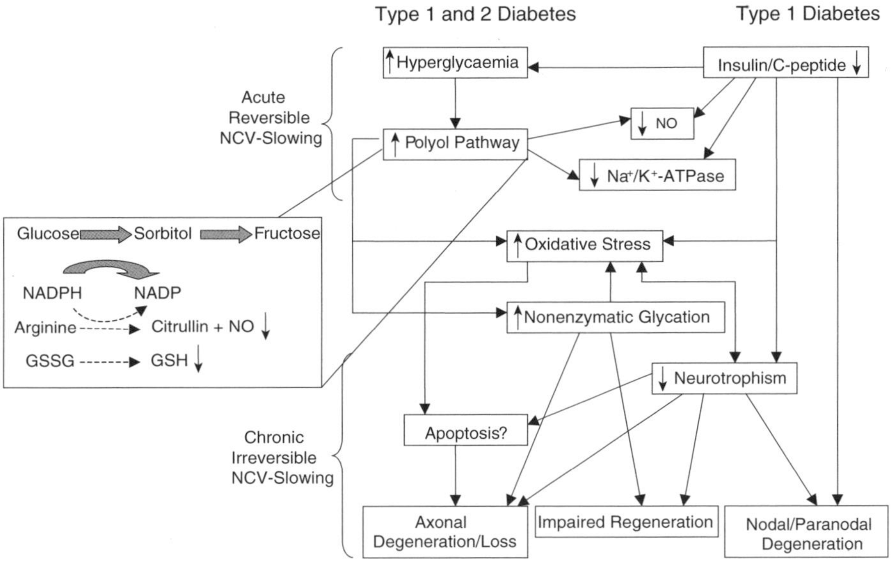

Figure 15.1 Simplified scheme of pathogenetic mechanisms operable in Type 1 and Type 2 DPN. Major underlying factors occur sequentially and often become mutually perpetuating. For further explanation see the text

oxidized glutathione[29] (Figure 15.1). Depletion of NADPH impairs nitric oxide synthase, resulting in compromised NO activity.[9,30] Furthermore, increased accumulation of fructose as a result of polyol pathway activity enhances oxidative stress via nonenzymatic glycation (see below). *Myo*-inositol depletion perturbs phosphoinositide turnover with decreased diacylglycerol synthesis and impaired activation of protein kinase C (PKC), particularly the beta isoform, believed to contribute to impaired neural Na^+/K^+-ATPase activity.[12] Decreased Na^+/K^+-ATPase activity results in decreased nodal Na^+ membrane potentials, increased intra-axonal Na^+, and reduced nerve conduction.[31] Other metabolic derangements such as carnitine deficiency[32,33] and impaired prostanoid metabolism[33,34] as well as C-peptide deficiency[35,36] contribute to impaired Na^+/K^+-ATPase activity in experimental (Figure 15.1) and possibly human Type 1 DPN without affecting the polyol pathway, suggesting multiple mechanisms underlying the Na^+/K^+-ATPase defect. In experimental Type 1 DPN, the initial activity of the polyol pathway subsides with progression of DPN, whereas in Type 2 DPN its activity is significantly more protracted.

Non-enzymatic glycation

In non-enzymatic glycation, reducing sugars such as glucose and fructose react initially with free amino groups of proteins, lipids or nucleic acids to form early reversible Schiff bases and Amadori products. These undergo chemical rearrangements to form advanced glycation end products (AGEs) (Figure 15.1). *In vivo*, AGEs accumulate during normal aging and at an accelerated rate in diabetes in various tissues including peripheral nerve.[37] The receptor for AGE (RAGE) has been cloned and identified as a member of the immunoglobulin superfamily of cell-surface molecules.[38] Accumulation of AGEs may play a crucial role in the pathogenesis of DPN through generation of oxidative stress and altered endoneurial haemodynamics (Figure 15.1) (see below).

In peripheral nerve, the glycation process is enhanced in diabetes[39,40] via an increased production of fructose through activation of the polyol pathway (Figure 15.1), since cross-linking of proteins by fructose occurs with a 10-fold higher affinity compared with glucose.[41]

Oxidative stress

There are several potential sources of oxidative stress in diabetes including altered redox status,[42] dysregulation of glutathione synthesis[43] and hypoxia and ischaemic reperfusion injury (Figure 15.1). Glucose autoxidation and glycoxidation, which are catalysed by trace amounts of transition metal ions, generate reactive oxygen species.[44] Low-dose transition metal chelators such as deferoxamine and trientine improve nerve blood flow and nerve conduction velocity. Furthermore, superoxide generated not only via nonenzymatic glycation but also by inactivation of Cu–Zn superoxide dismutase attenuates nitric oxide activity, leading to reduced blood flow[45] (Figure 15.1). Interaction of AGEs with RAGE depletes intracellular reduced glutathione and vitamin C, thereby further enhancing oxidative stress[46] (Figure 15.1). This process gives rise to breakdown of endothelial barrier functions and NF-κB-mediated gene inductions of tissue necrosis factor and endothelin-1, both of which contribute to reduced vascular blood flow.[46,47]

Short-term treatment with aminoguanidin, which inhibits AGE formation, ameliorates the nerve conduction velocity and the Na^+/K^+-ATPase defects, but not endothelial damage as reflected by systemic thrombomodulin concentrations. On the other hand, long-term aminoguanidin treatment has beneficial effects on the structural alterations of endoneurial microvessels.[48]

Lipid metabolism

Impaired microvascular function, in part due to abnormal lipid metabolism, plays an essential role in the pathogenesis of diabetic neuropathy[49] (Figure 15.1). The synthesis of vasoactive prostanoids is compromised in diabetes.[30,50] Reduced tissue and plasma concentrations of gamma-linoleic acid and arachidonic acid result in impaired synthesis of vasodilatory and antiplatelet prostaglandins. Prostaglandins PGI_2 and PGE_2 are reduced in sciatic nerve of the diabetic BB/Wor and STZ rats.[33,51,52] These deficits are overcome by treating diabetic rats with evening primrose oil, or with acetyl-L-carnitine, thereby preventing decreased nerve blood flow, nerve hypoxia and impaired NCV.[32,33,51]

Plasma and tissue L-carnitine concentrations are reduced in diabetes.[32] In diabetic neuropathy replacement with acetyl-L-carnitine prevents the nerve conduction deficits and structural and morphometric abnormalities and improves nerve regeneration.[33] Acetyl-L-carnitine improves cellular energy metabolism by promoting mitochondrial transport of long-chain fatty acids for beta oxidation and restores Na^+/K^+-ATPase activity, NO synthesis and prostaglandins[32,33] (Figure 15.1). Therefore, abnormal essential fatty acid metabolism perturbs vasoactive prostanoids and plays an important pathogenetic role in DPN. These defects often act in concert with other elements such as increased polyol pathway activity and nonenzymatic glycation with additive affects on vascular dysfunction.

Neutrophism

There is now overwhelming evidence indicating that impaired neurotrophic support is involved in diabetes-related neuronal dysfunctions.[53,54] Recent studies, though, suggest that neurotrophism is more severely affected in Type 1[55,56] than in Type 2 diabetes (Figure 15.1). NGF administration prevents the reduction of neuropeptides such as substance P and calcitonin gene-related peptide in dorsal root ganglion neurons and sciatic nerve of the diabetic rat.[57,58] These neuropeptides are confined to small-fibre sensory neurons, mediating nociceptive or thermoreceptive sensation.

The expression of neurotrophin-3 (NT-3), which is trophic for sympathetic neurons and sensory neurons of large-diameter fibres,[59] is also reduced in the diabetic muscle. Administration of NT-3 ameliorates only sensory nerve conduction deficits, not those of motor nerves. Recent clinical trials have been inconclusive with respect to the effect of recombinant human NGF.[60]

Insulin-like growth factors (IGFs) have neurotrophic actions on sensory, sympathetic and motor neurons.[61] Reduction in systemic IGF-I levels and increased IGF-I binding protein levels contribute to impaired IGF-I activity in Type 1 diabetic patients and the diabetic rat.[61–64] Subcutaneous infusion of IGF-I or IGF-II prevents the progression of hyperalgesia in the STZ diabetic rat, and local administration of IGFs protects against impairment of sensory nerve regeneration.[65] It is worth noting that IGFs exert their ameliorating effects on diabetic neuropathy without improving hyperglycaemia. The abnormalities of NGF, IGF-1 and their receptors are normalized by C-peptide replacement in the spontaneously diabetic type 1 BB/W-rat.[66,67]

Insulin/C-peptide action

Physiological concentrations of insulin stimulate neurite outgrowth and are required for survival of sensory and sympathetic neurons. Insulin up-regulates and stabilizes neurofilament and tubulin in a dose-dependent manner.[68] In the STZ rat, local unilateral administration of insulin to sciatic nerve results in an increased number of small myelinated fibres and prevention of nerve conduction slowing in the treated nerve, suggesting that insulin is involved in peripheral nerve fibre regeneration and repair.[69]

The insulin signalling comprises two major pathways: the phosphatidylinositol 3-kinase (PI 3-kinase) pathway and the mitogen-activated protein (MAP) kinase pathway. The PI 3-kinase pathway is linked to metabolic effects such as glucose transport, glycolysis, glycogen synthesis and protein synthesis. The MAP kinase pathway is associated with cell proliferation and differentiation. It appears that the MAP kinase pathway predominates in the insulin signalling transduction in peripheral nerve.

Recently, we demonstrated that peripheral nerve expresses mainly the high-affinity isoform of the insulin receptor, which is concentrated to the nodal and paranodal apparatus.[70] Nodal plasma membranes of myelinated fibres possess a highly organized molecular structure with a nonuniform clustering of several molecules (ion channels, Na^+/K^+-ATPase, glucose transporter, aldose reductase and cell adhesion molecules, casprs and ankyrin$_G$),which are involved in the integrity of normal nodal function and structure as well as fibre maturation, regeneration and repair. Hence they co-localize with the insulin receptor, suggesting that insulin may regulate some of their biological activities.

It is known that proinsulin C-peptide enhances the effects of insulin[71–74] and phosphorylates the insulin receptor.[75] C-peptide also normalizes the expression of IGF-1 and its receptor both in peripheral and central nervous tissue. In peripheral nerve it dose-dependently prevents the Na^+/K^+-ATPase defect and corrects endothelial NO and blood-flow.[76,77] These effects occur in the absence of any effects on the polyol pathway by C-peptide.[36] C-peptide substitution in the Type 1 diabetic BB/Wor rat prevents and ameliorates paranodal pathology and related nerve conduction deficits and promotes nerve fibre regeneration.[36,67,78] Preliminary data[77] indicate that C-peptide has no effect on oxidative stress. These findings indicate that insulin and/or C-peptide deficiencies play pathogenic roles in the functional and structural abnormalities characterizing Type 1 human and murine DPN, changes that are not present in hyper- or normoinsulinaemic Type 2 DPN.[79]

Tested Therapies

Over the last two decades, several classes of compounds have been developed targeting specific pathogenetic mechanisms. Most compounds showed promising results in short-term animal studies, but failed to deliver convincing data in human trials. This may in part be due to the fact that animal studies were almost exclusively prevention studies as contrasted to human intervention trials.

Inhibition of the polyol pathway

Initially aldose reductase inhibitors held promise for the treatment of the chronic diabetic complications. It was reasoned that blockage of the activated polyol pathway, one of the earliest metabolic abnormalities, would prevent or ameliorate subsequent consequences of polyol pathway activation (Figure 15.1). Numerous pre-clinical, often short-term, prevention studies seemed to confirm this concept.

However, the optimism caused by the data from animal studies turned into disappointments when several clinical trials failed to demonstrate any clinically meaningful improvements (Table 15.1). Although some studies showed effects on sorbitol levels, minimal improvements of NCVs and increased fibre regeneration, these effects did not translate into significant clinical improvements. So what went so drastically wrong? Several confounding factors have been identified, some of which include pharmacokinetic aspects, such as penetration of the drug into human nerve and retina and probably more importantly the potency of the compounds, factors that may have had limiting effects. It has recently been shown that the inhibitory effect of aldose reductase inhibitors (ARIs) on sorbitol concentrations is nonlinear and that almost 100 per cent inhibition of aldose reductase is required for efficacy.[106] Other factors include the length of the trials, which in general were too short, and probably most importantly the timepoint in the natural history of DPN when treatment was initiated was too late. As mentioned above, the progression of commonly used end-points such as NCVs, QSTs and even morphometry[24,107,108] is not linear over time and is different in different nerves. It is therefore important to choose end-points when they have their most rapid decline during the natural history of the disease, in order to optimize the potential therapeutic effects. Furthermore, any intervention by pharmacological means is more likely to be efficacious during the early metabolic stage of DPN, rather than during the chronic stage, when advanced structural changes bear the brunt of the neurologic deficits. This may indeed pertain to the polyol pathway, whose activity in experimental DPN is significantly greater in acute DPN as compared with chronic DPN.[79] One of the most significant effects of clinical ARI trials has been increased regeneration of fibres[88,92,102,105] (Table 15.1). The same response has been noted in experimental ARI trials in diabetic rats.[109,110] Unfortunately, it was shown in the latter that, despite a multifold increase in nerve fibre regeneration following ARI treatment, regenerating fibres did not mature either functionally or structurally.[108,110]

Recent studies have identified dinucleotide repeat polymorphism of the osmotic response region of the aldose reductase gene (ARZ), in which the 'Z-2' polymorphism is associated with high risk for the development of microvascular

Table 15.1 Double-blind placebo controlled neuropathy trials with ARIs

Type of ARI	Duration (weeks)	No. of patients	Result	Authors
Alrestatin	12	30	Improved ulnar NCV and QST; improved subjective symptoms.	Fagius and Jameson[80]
Sorbinil	9	39	NCV improved.	Judzewitsch *et al.*[81]
Sorbinil	16	15	Improved sensory amplitude; pain improved.	Young *et al.*[82]
Sorbinil	6	36	Improved somato-sensory evoked potentials.	Jaspan *et al.*[83]
Sorbinil	24	55	Electrophysiologic measures improved.	Fagius *et al*[84]
Sorbinil	4	31	No improvement.	Lehtinen *et al.*[85]
Sorbinil	24	22	No improvement.	Martyn *et al.*[86]
Sorbinil	52	39	No improvement.	Guy *et al.*[87]
Sorbinil	52	16	Increased number of regenerating fibres.	Sima *et al.*[88]
Sorbinil	52	31	No improvement.	O'Hare *et al.*[89]
Sorbinil	4	23	No improvement.	Gieron *et al.*[90]
Sorbinil	52	30	No effect on endoneurial vascular pathology.	Sima *et al.*[91]
Sorbinil	52	16	Improved axoglial dysjunction; sural NCV and decreased axonal atrophy.	Sima *et al.*[92]
Ponalrestat	4	30	No improvement.	Sundkvist *et al.*[93]
Ponalrestat	24	54	No improvement.	Florkowski *et al.*[94]
Ponalrestat	52	50	No improvement.	Krenz *et al.*[95]
Ponalrestat	78	259	No improvement.	Sundkvist *et al.*[96]
Ponalrestat	52	60	No improvement.	Ziegler *et al.*[97]
Tolrestat	52	219	Improvement of pain and NCV.	Boulton *et al.*[98]
Tolrestat	24	190	Improved NCV; improved vibration sense.	Macleod *et al.*[99]
Tolrestat	24	35	Improved motor NCV.	Van Gerven *et al.*[100]
Tolrestat	52	45	Vibration improved.	Guigliano *et al.*[101]
Tolrestat	52	27	Increased fibre regeneration; decreased nerve sorbitol and fructose.	Sima *et al.*[102]
Tolrestat	52	372	Motor NCV decreased in placebo patients.	Santiago *et al.*[103]
Epalrestat	12	196	Improved NCVs and vibration; improvement in pain.	Goto *et al.*[104]
Zenarestat	52	113	Improved NCVs; increased regeneration.	Greene *et al.*[105]

complications.[106] The data from clinical diabetic neuropathy ARI trials are summarized in Table 15.1.

In summary, based on previous experience, it can be stated that ARIs will probably be efficacious (provided they are safe and at the same time potent enough to prevent sorbitol accumulation) during the early metabolic phase of diabetic neuropathy, when their effects will probably be due to prevention of further deterioration rather than reversal of already established deficits. Therefore, with respect to the design of clinical trials, early intervention is preferred to late; efficacy end-points have to be carefully selected as to reflect the natural history of the disease. Trials have to extend over two years at a minimum, with strict standardization and monitoring of efficacy end-points, and to have sufficient power (at least 300 patients in each arm of the study).[26,111] Finally, potential responders may be identified genetically based on the individual polymorphism profile of the ARZ gene.[106]

Aminoguanidine

Aminoguanidine inhibits the producton of AGEs and secondarily free radical formation. This compound has in experimental DPN beneficial effects on nerve blood flow, vascular permeability, NCVs and structural parameters.[112–114] No clinical trials targeting DPN have been performed to date. The results from the ACTION II trial comparing two doses of aminoguanidine and placebo on the progression of neuropathy and retinopathy[115] in Type 2 patients have not been published.

Gamma-linoleic acid (GLA) and prostaglandins

Essential fatty acids are needed for normal membrane structure and prostanoid metabolism. Several prostacyclins are perturbed in diabetic nerve, where they impair endoneurial blood flow. Placebo-controlled clinical trials employing GLA (360–480 mg/d) have reported improvement in sensory or motor NCV, thermal threshold and symptoms.[116–118]

Some prostaglandin trials have reported positive treatment effects following short-term intravenous administration of lipo-PGE. Clinical improvement as well as improvement in motor NCV and vibratory threshold were reported.[119,120] No serious adverse effects were noted following lipo-PGE administration.

Nerve growth factor

Although the early phase II trial on the effect of recombinant human NGF appeared to show beneficial effects on specific sensory modalities,[60,172] phase III studies showed no significant effects. Administration of neurotrophic factors is a difficult problem and is associated with hyperalgesia and pressure allodynia at the site of NGF-injection.[57,121]

Alpha-lipoic acid (ALA) trials (thioctic acid)

Experimental data have shown that alpha-lipoic acid is a potent lipophilic free radical scavenger[122] and enhances glucose uptake in muscle[123] and stimulates pyruvate dehydrogenase activity, thereby reducing serum lactate and pyruvate concentrations.[124] In humans it increases insulin sensitivity in Type 2 patients.[125] Several short-term studies with intravenous infusion of ALA over 3 weeks have demonstrated significant improvement in total symptoms score, pain score and neuropathy symptom score.[126–128] Long-term studies over 7 months did not improve further total symptom score or neuropathy impairment score.[129] A 2 year multi-centre double-blind placebo-controlled trial with alpha-lipoic acid showed small but significant improvements in sural and tibial NCVs, whereas no differences were found in neuropathy disability scores.[130] Less convincing data have been obtained with respect to cardiac autonomic neuropathy.[131]

In summary, therefore, several extensive clinical trials have been undertaken to test potential ethiology-targeted treatments. With few exceptions, these have been disappointing, indicating that the therapeutic approach to DPN has to be reconsidered. It appears that this multifactorial disease has to be attacked by multi-drug algorithms preventing and/or blocking several pathogenetic pathways simultaneously. Furthermore, it seems logical that the sooner the course of this chronic disorder can be influenced therapeutically, the greater the expected benefits. Such approaches however require in-depth knowledge of the natural history of the disease, which is only starting to emerge. Equally important, potentially efficacious drugs to be tested and eventually used in clinical practice have to be safe, since they will provide lifelong therapy for the individual patient.

Future Therapeutic Opportunities

Re-evaluation of the polyol pathway

Since activation of the polyol pathway is one of the earliest metabolic abnormalities and fuels many of the more downstream abnormalities (Figure 15.1), it appears that this should be a prime therapeutic target. However, it is well known that some patients develop diabetic complications early in their course of diabetes, regardless of glycaemic control, while others do not develop significant complications regardless of glycaemic control or duration of diabetes. This suggests the existance of genotypic determinants of diabetic complications, as mentioned above. Increased flux through the polyol pathway is either caused by increased availability of glucose or by exposure to hypertonicity.[132] It has been demonstrated repeatedly that increased aldose reductase activity and sorbitol levels are higher in patients with severe diabetic complications as compared with patients without complications with the same duration of diabetes and HbA_{1c} levels,[133–135] strongly suggesting a genetic link and predisposition. This predisposition has recently been linked to dinucleotide CA repeat polymorphism of the osmotic response element, the ORE enhancer of the aldose reductase gene promotor.[136,137] In this polymorphism repeats exceeding the average 24 repeats appears to have a protective effect on complications such as neuropathy,[138] whereas lesser repeats predispose to the development of complications. The induction of aldose reductase by hypertonicity is promoter driven.[139] To this should be added a third potential regulator and that is insulin itself. A number of years ago we showed in the Type 1 insulin-deficient BB-rat increased aldose reductase activity, protein and mRNA in lens, sciatic nerve, kidney and retina. Aldose reductase inhibitor treatment suppressed aldose reductase activity only, whereas intensive insulin treatment also normalized protein and mRNA levels. Hence only insulin controlled intracellular enzyme levels.[140] It is therefore plausible that insulin signalling intermediaries may regulate the gene-enhancing effects of the osmotic response element.

This area of active research is likely to provide new insights into the polyol pathway and how it is regulated. Results to date suggest that genotyping of the response element would predict who would be responsive to enzyme inhibition and that Type 1 patients (insulin deficient) would be more responsive than Type 2 patients. In a general sense, susceptible subgroups are likely to benefit from early intervention (or prevention) rather than late.

Antioxidants and vasodilators

The activated polyol pathway consumes the cofactor NADPH, which is also an obligate cofactor for both glutathione and NO, linking the ability to scavenge radical oxygen species. Increased oxidative stress and reduced levels of systemic antioxidants such as ascorbic acid, vitamin E and taurin in human diabetes have also been implicated in increased DAG and altered PKC in the vasculature. However, in diabetic peripheral nerve PKC activity is decreased rather than increased. Furthermore glucose auto-oxidation is catalysed by transition metals such as iron and copper and leads to oxidative stress. The transition metal handling is impaired in diabetes. Hence, there are several metabolic events that lead to a vicious circle of oxidative stress, resulting in mitochondrial dysfunction, nerve ischaemia and perhaps neuronal apoptosis.[141,169]

Lipoic acid, one of the most powerful antioxidants, functions as a coenzyme of hydrogen transfer. It has been suggested that lipoic acid may not be sufficient to eliminate severe oxidative stress occurring in diabetic neuropathy.[142] A review of several clinical trials employing alpha-lipoic acid showed reduction in neuropathic symptoms and small improvements of autonomic function.[143]

The likelihood for antioxidant therapy to be successful will probably require multiple antioxidant compounds targeting the different mechanisms and would include alpha-lipoic acid, vitamins E and C and probably therapies targeting the related perturbed lipid metabolism using compounds such as gamma-linoleic acid, evening primrose oil, acetyl-L-carnitine and/or fish liver oils.[144] There is experimental evidence demonstrating a synergistic effect in this type of combination therapy.[30,145] Finally, since oxidative stress is in part the consequence of endoneurial hypoxia, additional therapies that have proven successful under experimental conditions include ACE inhibition, endothelin-1 ET_A antagonists and PKC inhibitors.[30]

In summary therefore, to therapeutically correct oxidative stress in diabetic neuropathy, a multi-targeted approach holds the greatest promise and this should, like any other therapy, be initiated as early as possible in the natural history of the disease.

C-peptide

In recent years it has become clear that hyperglycaemia, although an important aetiological factor, is not the sole culprit in the development of diabetic complications. Increasing attention is being paid to insulin and/or C-peptide deficiencies or even hyperinsulinaemia in the case of accelerated atherosclerosis for instance. Both insulin and C-peptide exert neuroprotective and antiapoptotic effects.[36]

Therefore, the physiological role of the proinsulin C-peptide has received increasing attention, focusing on the potential therapeutic value of C-peptide replacement in preventing and ameliorating Type 1 diabetic complications.[146]

In Type 1 diabetic patients, autonomic nerve function as measured by heart rate variability during deep breathing improves after intravenous C-peptide infusion for 3 h.[147] and in patients who received C-peptide for 3 months. A subgroup of the latter patients with signs of sensory neuropathy exhibited improved temperature threshold discrimination after C-peptide replacement for 3 months.[148] In a recent study, the Karolinska group[149] demonstrated progressive improvements in sensory nerve conduction velocities at 6 and 12 weeks of C-peptide treatment of Type 1 diabetic patients. None of these effects were seen in patients who received insulin therapy alone. C-peptide stimulates nerve Na^+,K^+-ATPase activity, resulting in improved electrolyte balance and enzyme state. Additionally, C-peptide normalizes endothelial NO with consequent improvement in neural blood flow.[77,150] Several studies have demonstrated an effect of C-peptide on NO release. It stimulates eNOS with release of NO from bovine aortic endothelial cells in a concentration-dependent manner, an effect that is abolished by NO synthase inhibitors.[151] This is in keeping with the finding that C-peptide induces increased forearm blood flow in Type 1 diabetic patients, which is blocked by an NO synthase blocker.[152] It is also consistent with the demonstration of a C-peptide concentration-dependent dilatation of rat skeletal muscle arterioles in the presence of insulin.[72]

C-peptide elicits concentration-dependent stimulation of Na^+/K^+-ATPase activity in a variety of tissues including renal tubular cells, rat sciatic nerve, pancreatic islets, granulation tissue and red blood cells.[76,147,153] Further support for the effect of C-peptide on Na^+/K^+-ATPase is provided by its effect on rat sciatic nerve Na^+/K^+-ATPase in Type 1 diabetic BB/Wor-rats treated with C-peptide for 8 months.[36] This is substantiated by partial correction of the associated defect in nerve conduction velocity and paranodal swelling, secondary to axonal Na^+ accumulation. Furthermore, in the C-peptide-deficient diabetic BB/Wor-rat model the expression of both the insulin receptor and the IGF-I receptor mRNA and protein in peripheral nerve and brain tissue are normalized by C-peptide replacement, probably via a nuclear factor κB-mechanism.[75] These effects translate into a normalization of the expression of neurocytoskeletal proteins such as tubulins and neurofilaments and eventually a normalization of nerve regeneration[67] and the diabetes-induced hippocampal apoptosis was prevented by C-peptide replacement.[154]

Recent studies show that C-peptide has an insulinomimetic effect and modulates insulin signalling activity.[73,74] These data strongly suggest a role for C-peptide in the treatment of the more severe neuropathy accompanying Type 1 diabetes. Its beneficial effects should be tested in large-scale clinical trials.

Glutamate inhibition

Hyperglutamatergic activity induced by ischaemia is believed to underlie neuronal damage in a variety of neurological disorders, such as stroke, ALS and neuropathic pain.[155,156] Glutamate carboxypeptidase II (GCPII): EC#3.4.17.21, also known as N-acetylated-alpha-linked acidic dipeptidase (NAALADase), is a neuropetidase that hydrolyses the neuropeptide N-acetyl-aspartyl-glutamate (NAAG) to liberate free glutamate and N-acetyl aspartate. GCPII is found in the brainstem, spinal cord, dorsal root ganglion cells and Schwann cells.[157]

Recent potent and selective GCPII inhibitors have been reported to provide neuroprotection against ischaemic injury in a neuronal culture model of stroke and in rats following middle cerebral artery occlusion.[158] Consistent with inhibition of GCPII, these compounds increase NAAG and attenuate the ischaemia-induced rise in extracellular glutamate.[159] They protect motor neurons against glutamate toxicity, and enhance nerve regeneration in mice.[160]

Glutamate has been implicated in the generation and maintenance of neuropathic pain. Several drugs that attenuate glutamate neurotransmission have been shown to be effective in relieving neuropathic pain in various animal models.[161,162] The mechanism is believed to be their ability to attenuate glutamate spinal 'wind-up' or sensitization. Pain is a common and poorly understood symptom of DPN. In the BB/Wor-rat we have previously suggested that chronic diabetic pain may be mediated by increased spontaneous firing of afferent neurons,[15] which is associated with increased voltage-dependent calcium currents in dorsal root ganglion cell with increase in neuronal calcium load,[163,164] which may be related to opening of glutamate-regulated calcium channels.[161,165]

We recently demonstrated a partial preventive effect of GCPII inhibition on hyperalgesia, nerve conduction velocity and myelinated fibre morphology in the spontaneously diabetic BB/Wor-rat,[17] indicating that inhibition of GCPII has a beneficial effect on both large myelinated fibres and unmyelinated and small myelinated nociceptive fibres. The latter effect may be related to inhibition of ischaemia-induced glutamate release and opening of glutamate-regulated calcium channels,[163,164] thereby decreasing the hyperexcitability of nociceptive neurons. Decreased nerve conduction velocity and length-dependent axonal degeneration and atrophy are characteristic of DPN and are believed to be due to impaired synthesis, transport and content of neuroskeletal proteins such as tubulins and neurofilaments.[9,144] Since neural ischaemia is a central component in the pathogenesis of experimental DPN,[144,166] and is associated with loss of high-energy phosphate compounds,[167] increases in cytosolic Ca^{2+} are likely to result in a series of events. One is activation of calpains with subsequent inhibition of neurocytoskeletal protein synthesis.[166,168] Another is phospholipase activation and lipid peroxidation with free radical generation, mitochondrial dysfunction and apoptosis.[169,170] These constructs are consistent with the effects of GCPII inhibition on glucotoxic DRG/Schwann cell co-cultures, in which it prevents apoptosis and promotes axonal growth.[171] These findings suggest that, as in other ischaemic conditions, production of glutamate produces hyperalgesia and is likely to contribute to progressive nerve dysfunction and degeneration in diabetes. GCPII inhibition may therefore be a valuable adjunct to other therapies counteracting peripheral nerve hypoxia and free radical production.

Concluding Thoughts

The prevention and treatment of DPN have eluded us for decades. However, recent advances of our understanding of this common disease should allow us an optimistic outlook. It is clear that hyperglycaemia plays a major role in the genesis of DPN in both Type 1 and Type 2 diabetes. Therefore, strict glycaemic control remains a prime goal in the prevention and treatment of any diabetic complication. As an adjuvant to glycaemic control, ARIs are likely to be most effective, *provided* that safe and at the same time potent compounds can be developed. These drugs will and should probably be used as preventive drugs in genetically susceptible patients. It is now increasingly clear that the complications differ in Type 1 and Type 2 diabetes and by extension insulin and C-peptide deficiencies play not unimportant pathogenetic roles. Both clinical and experimental studies have demonstrated the beneficial effects of the combined replenishment of insulin and C-peptide on Type 1 complications. However, this regimen may be equally applicable to insulin-deficient Type 2 patients. Hence, it would be feasible to imitate 'nature's own way' by using a combination of these two hormones from onset of Type 1 diabetes to prevent the complications from occurring rather than treating already existing abnormalities.

Finally, it is obvious that it will be more meaningful and beneficial to prevent DPN rather than to treat already existing DPN with sometimes advanced structural degenerative changes. Interventions should be the same as the preventive measures mentioned above. However, to this should be added a multi-drug therapy targeting the different facets of oxidative stress as well as those of relative neural ischaemia. This may include antioxidants, vitamin C, essential fatty acids, supplements, glutamate inhibitors, acetyl-L-carnitine and other vasodilators. These latter tailor-made approaches, however, will require full attention by the treating diabetologist or neurologist familiar with the natural history of the disease.

Correction of neurotrophic factors by systemic administration of specific factor is not likely to be successful, due to their extremely diverse effects on a multitude of tissues. A potentially more rational approach would be to influence specific growth factor gene expressions further upstream. In this respect, C-peptide has shown promising experimental results.

I therefore believe that the future approach to DPN should be more focused on prevention. When faced with intervention the expectations must be realistic, even following the most sophisticated multi-therapy.

In view of the complexity and heterogeneity of the pathogenetic mechanism of DPN, it is unlikely that one single drug will provide the magic bullet. Instead, this disease most likely requires a multi-therapy approach, which is likely to differ between the neuropathies accompanying the two major types of diabetes and should be tailored to underlying adverse metabolic events.

References

1. Greene DA, Sima AAF, Feldman EL and Stevens MJ. Ellenberg and Rifkin diabetic neuropathy. In *Diabetes Mellitus*, Rifkin H, Porte D and Sherwin R (eds). 1997. Stanford, CT: Appleton and Lange, pp. 1009–1076.
2. Melton LJ III and Dyck PJ. Diabetic polyneuropathy. Epidemiology. In *Diabetic Neuropathy*, Dyck PJ and Thomas PK (eds). 1999. Philadelphia, PA: Saunders, pp. 239–254.
3. Pirart J. Diabetes mellitus and its degenerative complications: a prospective study of 4,400 patients observed between 1947 and 1973. *Diabetes Metab* 1977; **3**: 97–107.
4. Vinik AI, Liuzze FJ, Holland MT, Stansberry KB, LeBean JM and Colen LB. Diabetic neuropathies. *Diabetes Care* 1992; **15**: 1926–1975.
5. Sima AAF, Thomas PK, Ishii D and Vinik A. Diabetic neuropathies. *Diabetologia* 1997; **40** (Suppl. 3): B74–B77.

6. Thomas PK. Classification, differential diagnosis, and staging of diabetic peripheral neuropathy. *Diabetes* 1997; **46** (Suppl. 2), S54–S57.
7. Dyck PJB and Dyck PJ. Diabetic polyneuropathy. In *Diabetic Neuropathy*, Dyck PJ and Thomas PK (eds). 1999. Philadelphia, PA: Saunders, pp. 255–278.
8. Feldman EL, Russell JW, Sullivan KA and Golovoy D. New insight into the pathogenesis of diabetic neuropathy. *Curr Opin Neurol* 1999; **12**: 553–563.
9. Sugimoto K, Murakawa Y and Sima AAF. Diabetic neuropathy – a continuing enigma. *Diab Metab Res Rev* 2000; **16**: 408–433.
10. The DCCT Research Group. The effect of intensive treatment of diabetes on the development and progression of long-term complications in insulin-dependent diabetes mellitus. The Diabetes Control and Complications Trial Research Group. *N Engl J Med* 1993; **329**: 977–986.
11. Said G, Slama G and Selva J. Progressive centripetal degeneration of axons in small fibre diabetic polyneuropathy. *Brain* 1983; **106**: 791–807.
12. Greene DA, Sima AAF, Stevens MJ, Feldman EL and Lattimer SA. Complications: neuropathy, pathogenetic considerations. *Diabetes Care* 1992; **15**: 1902–1925.
13. Dyck PJ, Lambert EH and O'Brien PC. Pain in peripheral neuropathy is related to rate and kind of fibre degeneration. *Neurology* 1976; **26**: 466–471.
14. Britland ST, Young RJ, Sharma AK and Clarke BF. Association of painful and painless diabetic polyneuropathy with different patterns of nerve fibre degeneration and regeneration. *Diabetes* 1990; **39**: 898–908.
15. Burchiel KJ, Russel LC, Lee RP and Sima AAF. Spontaneous activity of primary afferent neurons in diabetic BB-Wistar rats: a possible mechanism of chronic diabetic pain. *Diabetes* 1985; **34**: 1210–1213.
16. Chiechio S, Caricasole A, Barletta E, Storto M, Catania MV, Copani A, Vertechy M, Nicolai R, Calvani M, Melchiorri D and Nicoletti F. L-acetylcarnitine induces analgesia by selectively up-regulating mGlu2 metabotropic glutamate receptors. *Mol Pharmacol* 2002; **61**: 989–996.
17. Zhang W, Slusher B, Murakawa Y, Wozniak KM and Sima AAF. GCPII (NAALADase) inhibition prevents long-term diabetic neuropathy in Type I BB/Wor-rats. *J Neurol Sci* 2002; **194**: 21–28.
18. Thomas PK. Mechanisms and treatment of pain. In *Diabetic Neuropathy*, Dyck PJ and Thomas PK (eds). 1999. Philadelphia, PA: Saunders, pp. 387–397.
19. Dyck PJ, Davies JL, Litchy WJ and O'Brien PC. Longitudinal assessment of diabetic polyneuropathy using a composite score in the Rochester Diabetic Neuropathy Study cohort. *Neurology* 1997; **49**: 229–239.
20. Valk GD, de Sonnaville JJ, van Houtum WH, Heine RJ, van Eijk JT, Bouter LM and Bertelsmann FW. The assessment of diabetic polyneuropathy in daily clinical practice: reproducibility and validity of Semmes Weinstein monofilaments examination and clinical neurological examination. *Muscle Nerve* 1997; **20**: 116–118.
21. American Diabetes Association. Consensus statement. Report and recommendations of the San Antonio conference on diabetic neuropathy. American Diabetes Association American Academy of Neurology. *Diabetes Care* 1988; **11**: 592–597.
22. Feldman EL, Stevens MJ, Thomas PK, Brown MB, Canal N and Greene DA. A practical two-step quantitative clinical and electrophysiological assessment for the diagnosis and staging of diabetic neuropathy. *Diabetes Care* 1994; **17**: 1281–1289.
23. Fedele D, Comi G, Coscelli C, Cucinotta D, Feldman EL, Ghirlanda G, Greene DA, Negrin P and Santeusanio F. A multicenter study on the prevalence of diabetic neuropathy in Italy. Italian diabetic neuropathy committee. *Diabetes Care* 1997; **20**: 836–843.

24. Laudadio C and Sima AAF. The Ponalrestat Study Group. Progression rates of diabetic neuropathy in placebo patients in an 18-month clinical trial. *J Diab Compl* 1998; **12**: 121–127.
25. Sima AAF and Cherian PV. Neuropathology of diabetic neuropathy and its correlations with neurophysiology. *Clin Neurosci* 1997; **4**: 359–364.
26. Laudadio C and Sima AAF. Design of controlled clinical trials for diabetic polyneuropathy. *Semin Neurol* 1996; **16**: 187–192.
27. Sima AAF. Diabetic neuropathy; pathogenetic backgrounds, current and future therapies. *Exp Rev Neurotherapeut* 2001; **1**: 225–238.
28. Stevens MJ, Lattimer SA, Kamijo M, Van Huysen C, Sima AAF and Greene DA. Osmotically-induced nerve taurine depletion and the compatible osmolyte hypothesis in experimental diabetic neuropathy in the rat. *Diabetologia* 1993; **36**: 608–614.
29. El Idrissi A and Trenkner E. Growth factors and taurine protect against excitotoxicity by stabilizing calcium homeostasis and energy metabolism. *J Neurosci* 1999; **19**: 9459–9468.
30. Cameron NE and Cotter MA. Oxidative stress and abnormal lipid metabolism in diabetic complications. In *Chronic Complications in Diabetes. Animal Models and Chronic Complications*, Sima AAF (ed.) 1999. Amsterdam: Harwood, pp. 97–130.
31. Sima AAF and Brismar T. Reversible diabetic nerve dysfunction: structural correlates to electrophysiological abnormalities. *Ann Neurol* 1985; **18**: 21–29.
32. Stevens MJ, Lattimer SA, Feldman EL, Helton ED, Millington DS, Sima AAF and Greene DA. Acetyl-L-carnitine deficiency as a cause of altered nerve myo-inositol content, Na, K-ATPase activity, and motor conduction velocity in the streptozotocin-diabetic rat. *Metabolism* 1996; **45**: 865–872.
33. Sima AAF, Ristic H, Merry A, Kamijo M, Lattimer SA, Stevens MJ and Greene DA. Primary preventive and secondary interventionary effects of acetyl-L-carnitine on diabetic neuropathy in the bio-breeding Worcester rat. *J Clin Invest* 1996; **97**: 1900–1907.
34. Sonobe M, Yasuda H, Hisanaga T, Maeda K, Yamashita M, Kawabata T, Kikkawa R, Taniguchi Y and Shigeta Y. Amelioration of nerve Na(+)–K(+)-ATPase activity independently of myo-inositol level by PGE1 analogue OP-1206.alpha-CD in streptozocin-induced diabetic rats. *Diabetes* 1991, **40**. 726–730.
35. Ido Y, Vindigni A, Chang K, Stramm L, Chance R, Heath WF, DiMarchi RD, Di Cera E and Williamson JR. Prevention of vascular and neural dysfunction in diabetic rats by C-peptide. *Science* 1997; **277**: 563–566.
36. Sima AAF, Zhang W, Sugimoto K, Henry D, Li Z-G, Wahren J and Grunberger G. C-peptide prevents and improves chronic Type I diabetic poly neuropathy in the BB/Wor rat. *Diabetologia* 2001; **44**: 889–897.
37. Vogt BW, Schleicher ED and Wieland OH. e-amino-lysine-bound glucose in human tissues obtained at autopsy. Increase in diabetes mellitus. *Diabetes* 1982; **31**: 1123–1127.
38. Schmidt AM, Vianna M, Gerlach M, Brett J, Ryan J, Kao J, Esposito C, Hegarty H, Hurley W and Clauss M. Isolation and characterization of two binding proteins for advanced glycosylation end products from bovine lung which are present on the endothelial cell surface. *J Biol Chem* 1992; **267**: 14 987–14 997.
39. Vlassara H, Brownlee M and Cerami A. Nonenzymatic glycosylation of peripheral nerve protein in diabetes mellitus. *Proc Natl Acad Sci, USA* 1981; **78**: 5190–5192.
40. Ryle C, Leow CK and Donaghy M. Nonenzymatic glycation of peripheral and central nervous system proteins in experimental diabetes mellitus. *Muscle Nerve* 1997; **20**: 577–584.
41. McPherson JD, Shilton BH and Walton DJ. Role of fructose in glycation and cross-linking of proteins. *Biochemistry* 1988; **27**: 1901–1907.

42. Williamson JR, Chang K and Frangos M. Hyperglycemic pseudohypoxia and diabetic complications. *Diabetes* 1993; **42**: 801–813.
43. Yoshida K, Hirokawa J, Tagami S, Kawakami Y, Urata Y and Kondo T. Weakened cellular scavenging activity against oxidative stress in diabetes mellitus: regulation of glutathione synthesis and efflux. *Diabetologia* 1995; **38**: 201–210.
44. Hunt JV and Wolff SP. Oxidative glycation and free radical production: a causal mechanism of diabetic complications. *Free Rad Res Communs* 1991; **12**, **13**: 115–123.
45. Gryglewski RJ, Palmer RM and Moncada S. Superoxide anion is involved in the breakdown of endothelium-derived vascular relaxing factor. *Nature* 1986; **320**: 454–456.
46. Wautier JL, Zoukourian C and Chappey O. Receptor-mediated endothelial cell dysfunction in diabetic vasculopathy. Soluble receptor for advanced glycation end products blocks hyperpermeability in diabetic rats. *J Clin Invest* 1996; **97**: 238–243.
47. Bierhaus A, Chevion S and Chevion M. Advanced glycation end product-induced activation of NF-kB is suppressed by a-lipoic acid in cultured endothelial cells. *Diabetes* 1997; **46**: 1481–1490.
48. Sugimoto K and Yagihashi S. Effects of aminoguanidine on structural alterations of microvessels in peripheral nerve of streptozotocin diabetic rats. *Microvasc Res* 1997; **53**: 105–112.
49. Cameron NE and Cotter MA. Metabolic and vascular factors in the pathogenesis of diabetic neuropathy. *Diabetes* 1997; **46** (Suppl.2): S31–S37.
50. Horrobin DF. Essential fatty acids in the management of impaired nerve function in diabetes. *Diabetes* 1997; **46** (Suppl. 2): S90–S93.
51. Ward KK, Low PA, Schmelzer JD and Zochodne DW. Prostacyclin and noradrenaline in peripheral nerve of chronic experimental diabetes in rats. *Brain* 1989; **112**: 197–208.
52. Cameron NE, Cotter MA and Robertson S. Essential fatty acid diet supplementation. Effects on peripheral nerve and skeletal muscle function and capillarization in streptozocin-induced diabetic rats. *Diabetes* 1991; **40**: 529–532.
53. Tomlinson DR and Fernyhough P. Neurotrophism in diabetic neuropathy. In *Chronic Complications in Diabetes. Animal Models and Chronic Complications*, Sima AAF (ed.). 1999. Amsterdam: Harwood, pp. 167–182.
54. Sima AAF (ed.). Trophic factors and inflammatory mediators in diabetic complications. *Exp Diab Res* 2003; **4**: 201–312.
55. Pierson CR, Zhang W, Murakawa Y and Sima AAF. Early gene responses of trophic factors differ in nerve regeneration in Type 1 and Type 2 diabetic neuropathy. *J Neuropath Exp Neurol* 2002; **61**: 857–871.
56. Pierson CR, Zhang W, Murakawa Y and Sima AAF. Tubulin and neurofilament expression and axonal growth differ in Type 2 and Type 2 diabetic polyneuropathy. *J Neuropath Exp Neurol* 2003; **62**: 260–271.
57. Apfel SC, Arezzo JC, Brownlee M, Federoff H and Kessler JA. Nerve growth factor administration protects against experimental diabetic sensory neuropathy. *Brain Res* 1994; **634**: 7–12.
58. Diemel LT, Brewster WJ, Fernyhough P and Tomlinson DR. Expression of neuropeptides in experimental diabetes; effects of treatment with nerve growth factor or brain-derived neurotrophic factor. *Brain Res Mol Brain Res* 1994; **21**: 171–175.
59. Ernfors P, Lee KF, Kucera J and Jaenisch R. Lack of neurotrophin-3 leads to deficiencies in the peripheral nervous system and loss of limb proprioceptive afferents. *Cell* 1994; **77**: 503–512.
60. Apfel SC, Kessler JA, Adornato BT, Litchy WJ, Sanders C and Rask CA. Recombinant human nerve growth factor in the treatment of diabetic polyneuropathy. *Neurology* 1998; **3**: 695–702.

61. Ishii DN, Guertin DM and Whalen LR. Reduced insulin-like growth factor-I mRNA content in liver, adrenal glands and spinal cord of diabetic rats. *Diabetologia* 1994; **37**: 1073–1081.
62. Crosby SR, Tsigos C and Anderton CD. Elevated plasma insulin-like growth factor binding protein-1 levels in Type 1 (insulin-dependent) diabetic patients with peripheral neuropathy. *Diabetologia* 1992; **35**: 868–872.
63. Xu G and Sima AAF. Altered immediate gene expression is impaired in diabetic nerve; implications in regeneration. *J Neuropath Exp Neurol* 2001; **60**: 972–983.
64. Sima AAF, Li Z-G and Zhang W. The insulin-like growth factor system and neurological complications in diabetes. *Exp Diab Res* 2003; **4**: 235–256.
65. Zhuang HX, Snyder CK, Pu SF and Ishii DN. Insulin-like growth factors reverse or arrest diabetic neuropathy: effects on hyperalgesia and impaired nerve regeneration in rats. *Exp Neurol* 1996; **140**: 198–205.
66. Sima AAF, Zhang W, Murakawa Y, Wahren J and Pierson CR. C-peptide corrects aberrations in immediate early gene responses and cytoskeletal protein expression in regenerating nerve in Type 1 neuropathy. *Proc 12th Neurodiab* 2002; Vol. 12 [abstract].
67. Pierson CR, Zhang W and Sima AAF. Proinsulin C-peptide replacement in Type 1 diabetic BB/Wor-rats prevents deficits in nerve fibre regeneration. *J Neuropath Exp Neurol* 2003; **62**: 765–779.
68. Wang C, Li Y, Wible B, Angelides KJ and Ishii DN. Effects of insulin and insulin-like growth factors on neurofilament mRNA and tubulin mRNA content in human neuroblastoma SH-SY5Y cells. *Mol Brain Res* 1992; **13**: 289–300.
69. Singhal A, Cheng C, Sun H and Zochodne DW. Near nerve local insulin prevents conduction slowing in experimental diabetes. *Brain Res* 1997; **763**: 209–214.
70. Sugimoto K, Murakawa Y, Zhang W, Xu G and Sima AAF. Insulin receptor in rat peripheral nerve: its localization and alternatively spliced isoforms. *Diab Metab Res Rev* 2000; **16**: 354–363.
71. Johansson BL, Kernell A, Sjoberg S and Wahren J. Influence of combined C-peptide and insulin administration on renal function and metabolic control in diabetes Type 1. *J Clin Endocrinol Metab* 1993; **77**: 976–981.
72. Jensen ME and Messina EJ. C-peptide induces a concentration-dependent dilation of skeletal muscle arterioles only in presence of insulin. *Am J Physiol* 1999; **276**: H1223–H1228.
73. Grunberger G, Qiang X, Li Z, Mathews ST, Sbriessa D, Shisheva A and Sima AAF. The molecular basis for the insulinomimetic effects of C-peptide. *Diabetologia* 2001; **44**: 1247–1257.
74. Grunberger G and Sima AAF. The C-peptide signaling. *Exp Diab Res* 2004; **5**: 25–36.
75. Li Z-G, Zhang W and Sima AAF. C-peptide enhances insulin-mediated cell growth and protection against high glucose-induced apoptosis in SH-5YSY cells. *Diab Metab Res Rev* 2003; **19**: 375–385.
76. Zhang W, Yorek M, Pierson CR, Murakawa Y, Breidenbach A and Sima AAF. Human C-peptide dose dependently prevents early neuropathy in the BB/Wor-rat. *Int J Exp Diab Res* 2001; **7**: 187–194.
77. Stevens MJ, Zhang W and Sima AAF. C-peptide prevents impaired endoneurial blood flow but does not effect oxidative stress in Type 1 BB/Wor-rats. *J Periph Nerv Syst* 2003; **8**: 196.
78. Sima AAF, Pierson CR and Zhang W. C-peptide prevents the molecular abnormalities of the paranode in Type 1 diabetic polyneuropathy. *Diabetologia* 2003; **46**: (Suppl. 2): A314.
79. Sima AAF, Zhang W, Xu G, Sugimoto K, Guberski DL and Yorek MA. A comparison of diabetic polyneuropathy in Type 1 diabetic BBBZDR/Wor rats and Type 1 diabetic BB/Wor rats. *Diabetologia* 2000; **43**: 786–793.

80. Fagius J and Jameson S. Effects of aldose reductase inhibitor treatment in diabetic polyneuropathy. *J. Neurol Neurosurg Psychiatry* 1981; **44**: 991–1001.
81. Judzewitsch RG, Jaspan JB, Polansky KS, Weinberg CR, Halter JB, Halar E, Pfeifer MA, Vukadinovic C, Bernstein L, Schneider M, Liang KY, Gabbay KH, Rubenstein AH and Porte D Jr. Aldose reductase inhibition improves nerve conduction velocity in diabetic patients. *N Engl J Med* 1983; **308**: 119–125.
82. Young RJ, Ewing DJ and Clarke BF. A controlled trial of sorbinil, an aldose reductase inhibitor, in chronic painful diabetic neuropathy. *Diabetes* 1983; **32**: 938–942.
83. Jaspan JB, Herold K and Bartkus C. Effects of sorbinil therapy in diabetic patients with painful peripheral neuropathy and autonomic neuropathy. *Am J Med* 1985; **79** (Suppl. 5A): 24–37.
84. Fagius J, Brattberg A, Jameson S and Berne C. Limited benefits of treatment of diabetic polyneuropathy with an aldose reductase inhibitor: a 24-week controlled trial. *Diabetologia* 1985; **28**: 323–329.
85. Lehtinen JM, Hyvonen SK, Unsitupa M, Puhakainen E, Halonen T and Kilpelainen H. The effect of sorbinil treatment on red cell sorbitol levels and clinical and electrophysiological parameters of diabetic neuropathy. *J Neurol* 1986; **233**: 174–177.
86. Martyn CN, Reid W, Young RJ, Ewing DJ and Clarke BF. Six-month treatment with sorbinil in asymptomatic diabetic neuropathy. *Diabetes* 1987; **36**: 987–990.
87. Guy RJC, Gilbey SG, Sheehy M, Asselman P and Watkins PJ. Diabetic neuropathy in the upper limb and the effects of twelve months sorbinil treatment. *Diabetologia* 1988; **31**: 214–220.
88. Sima AAF, Bril V, Nathaniel V, McEwen TAJ, Brown M, Lattimer SA and Greene DA. Regeneration and repair of myelinated fibres in sural nerve biopsies from patients with diabetic neuropathy treated with an aldose reductase inhibitor. *N Engl J Med* 1988; **319**: 548–555.
89. O'Hare JP, Morgan MH, Alden P, Chissel S, O'Brien IAD and Cosrall RJM. Aldose reductase inhibition in diabetic neuropathy: clinical and neurophysiological studies of one year's treatment with sorbinil. *Diabet Med* 1988; **5**: 537–542.
90. Gieron MA, Malone JI, Lowitt S and Korthals JK. Improvement in peripheral nerve function after one year of sorbinil. *Neuroreport* 1991; **2**: 348–350.
91. Sima AAF, Nathaniel V, Prashar A, Bril V and Greene DA. Endoneurial microvessels in human diabetic neuropathy: endothelial cell dysfunction and lack of treatment effect by aldose reductase inhibitor. *Diabetes* 1991; **40**: 1090–1099.
92. Sima AAF, Prashar A, Nathaniel V, Bril V, Werb MR and Greene DA. Overt diabetic neuropathy: repair of axo-glial dysjunction and axonal atrophy by aldose reductase inhibition and its correlation to improvement in nerve conduction velocity. *Diabet Med* 1993; **10**: 115–121.
93. Sundkvist G, Lilia B, Rosen I and Agardh CD. Autonomic and peripheral nerve function in early diabetic neuropathy. *Acta Med Scand* 1987; **221**: 445–453.
94. Florkowski CM, Rowe BR, Nightingale S, Harvey TC and Barnett AH. Clinical and neurophysiological studies of aldose reductase inhibitor ponalrestat in chronic symptomatic diabetic peripheral neuropathy. *Diabetes* 1991; **40**: 129–133.
95. Krenz AJ, Honigsberger L, Ellis SH, Hardman M and Nattrass M. A 12 month randomized controlled study of the aldose reductase inhibitor ponalrestat in patients with chronic symptomatic diabetic neuropathy. *Diabet Med* 1992; **9**: 463–468.
96. Sundkvist G, Arenstrong FM, Bradbury JE, Chaplin C, Ellis SH, Owens DR, Rosen I and Sonksen P. Peripheral and autonomic nerve function in 259 diabetic patients with peripheral neuropathy treated with ponalrestat (an aldose reductase inhibitor) or placebo for 18 months. *J Diab Compl* 1992; **6**: 123–130.

97. Ziegler D, Mayer P, Rothmann W and Gries FA. One-year treatment with aldose reductase inhibitor, ponalrestat, in diabetic neuropathy. *Diab Res Clin Pract* 1991; **14**: 63–74.
98. Boulton AJM, Levin S and Comstock J. A multicenter trial of the aldose reductase inhibitor tolrestat, in patients with symptomatic diabetic neuropathy. *Diabetologia* 1990; **33**: 431–437.
99. Macleod AF, Boulton AJM, Owens DR, Van Rooy P, Wan Gerven JM, Macrury S, Scarpello JH, Segers O, Heller SR and Van Der Veen EA. A multicenter trial of the aldose reductase inhibitor tolrestat, in patients with symptomatic diabetic peripheral neuropathy. *Diabetes Metab* 1992; **18**: 14–20.
100. Van Gerven JMA, Lemkes HHPJ and Van Dijk JG. Long-term effects of tolrestat on symptomatic diabetic sensory polyneuropathy. *J Diab Compl* 1992; **6**: 45–48.
101. Guigliano D, Marfella R and Quatraro A *et al*. Tolrestat for mild diabetic neuropathy. *Ann Intern Med* 1993; **118**: 7–11.
102. Sima AAF, Greene DA, Brown MB, Hohman TC, Hicks D, Graepel GJ, Bochenek WJ, Beg M, Gonen B and the Tolrestat Study Group. Effect of hyperglycemia and the aldose reductase inhibitor tolrestat on sural nerve biochemistry and morphometry in advanced diabetic peripheral polyneuropathy. *J Diab Compl* 1993; **7**: 157–169.
103. Santiago JV, Sönksen PH, Boulton AJ, Macleod A, Beg M, Bochenek W, Graepel GJ and Gonen B. Withdrawal of the aldose reductase inhibitor tolrestat in patients with diabetic neuropathy: effect on nerve function. *J Diab Compl* 1993; **7**: 170–178.
104. Goto Y, Hotta N, Shigeta Y, Sakamoto N, Kito S, Matsuoka K, Takahashi A, Kikkawa R and Sakuma A. A placebo-controlled double-blind study of epalrestat (Ono-2235) in patients with diabetic neuropathy. *Diabet Med* 1993; **10**: S39–S43.
105. Greene DA, Arezzo JC, Brown MB and the Zenarestat Study Group. Effect of aldose reductase inhibition on nerve conduction and morphometry in diabetic neuropathy. *Neurology* 1999; **53**: 580–591.
106. Oates PJ and Mylari BL. Aldose reductase inhibitors: therapeutic implications for diabetic complications. *Expert Opin Investig Drugs* 1999; **8**: 2095–2119.
107. Sima AAF. Pathological definition and evaluation of diabetic neuropathy and clinical correlations. *Can J Neurol Sci* 1994; **21** (Suppl. 4): 513–517.
108. Sima AAF. Diabetic neuropathy – the utility of nerve biopsy. In *Clinical Neurophysiology: From Receptors to Perception*, Comi G, Lücking CH, Kimura J and Rossini PM (eds). 1999. Amsterdam: Elsevier, Chapter 64, pp. 525–533.
109. Sima AAF, Prashar A, Zhang W-X, Chakrabarti S and Greene DA. Preventive effect of long term aldose reductase inhibition (Ponalrestat) on nerve conduction and sural nerve structure in the spontaneously diabetic BB-rat. *J Clin Invest* 1990; **85**: 1410–1420.
110. Sima AAF, Merry AC and Levitan I. Increased regeneration in ARI-treated diabetic nerve is associated with upregulation of IGF-1 and NGF receptors. *Exp Clin Endocrin Diab* 1997; **105**: 60–62.
111. Pfeifer MA, Schumer MP and Gelber DA. Aldose reductase inhibitors: the end of an era or the need for different trial designs? *Diabetes* 1997; **46** (Suppl. 2): 582–589.
112. Yagihashi S, Kamijo M, Baba M, Yagahashi N and Nagai K. Effect of aminoguanidine on functional and structural abnormalities in peripheral nerve of STZ-induced diabetic rats. *Diabetes* 1990; **41**: 47–52.
113. Kihara M, Schmelzer JD, Podulso JF, Curran FF, Nickander KK and Low PA. Aminoguanidine effect on nerve blood flow, vascular permeability, electrophysiology and oxygen free radicals. *Proc Natl Acad Sci, USA* 1991; **88**: 6107–6111.
114. Cameron NE, Cotter MA, Dines K and Low PA. Effects of aminoguanidine on peripheral nerve function and polyol pathway metabolites in streptozotocin-diabetic rats. *Diabetologia* 1992; **35**: 46.

115. Freedman BI, Wuerth JP, Cartwright K, Bain RP, Dippe S, Hershon K, Mooradian AD and Spinowitz BS. Design and baseline characteristics for the aminoguanidine clinical trial in overt Type 2 diabetic nephropathy (ACTION II). *Contr Clin Trials* 1999; **20**: 493–510.
116. Jamal GA and Carmichael H. The effects of gamma-linoleic acid on human diabetic peripheral neuropathy: a double-blind, placebo controlled trial. *Diabet Med* 1990; **7**: 319–323.
117. Keen H, Payan J, Allaiw J, Walker J, Jamal GA, Weir AI, Henderson LM, Bissessar EA, Watkins PJ and Sampson M. Treatment of diabetic neuropathy with γ-linoleic acid. *Diabetes Care* 1993; **16**: 8–15.
118. Boulton AJM, Ziegler D, Scarpello J, Jamal G, Keen H, Almer LO and Gamstedt A. A multicentre double-blind trial of gamolenic acid in diabetic peripheral sensorimotor neuropathy. *Diabetologia* 1997; **40** (Suppl. 1), A32: 117.
119. Toyota T, Hirata Y, Ikeda Y, Matsuoka K, Sakuma A and Mizushima Y. Lipo-PGE, a new lipid encapsulated preparation of prostaglandin E_1: placebo and prostaglandin E_1-controlled multicenter trials in patients with diabetic neuropathy and leg ulcers. *Prostaglandins* 1993; **46**: 453–468.
120. Shindo H, Tawata M, Inoue M, Yokomori N, Hosaka Y, Ohtaka M and Onaya T. The effect of prostaglandin E_1 alpha CD on vibratory threshold determined with the SMV-5 vibrometer in patients with diabetic neuropathy. *Diab Res Clin Prac* 1994; **24**: 173–180.
121. Dyck PJ, Peroutka S, Rask C, Burton E, Baker MK, Lehman KA, Gillen DA, Hokanson JL and O'Brien PC. Intracameral recombinant human nerve growth factor induces pressure allodynia and lowered heat-pain threshold in humans. *Neurology* 1997; **48**: 501–505.
122. Nagamatsu M, Nickander KK, Schmelzer JD, Raya A, Wittrock DA, Tritschler H and Low PA. Lipoic acid improves nerve blood flow, reduces oxidative stress and improves distal nerve conduction in experimental diabetic neuropathy. *Diabetes Care* 1995; **18**: 1160–1167.
123. Jacob S, Streeper RS, Fogt DL, Hokama JY, Tritschler HJ, Dietze GJ and Henriksen EJ. The antioxidant α-lipoic acid enhances insulin-stimulated glucose metabolism in insulin resistant rat skeletal muscle. *Diabetes* 1996; **45**: 1024–1029.
124. Wagh SS, Natraj CV and Merion KKL. Mode of action of lipoic acid in diabetes. *J Biochem* 1987; **11**: 59–74.
125. Konrad T, Vicini P, Kusterer K, Hoflich A, Assadkhani A, Bohles HJ, Sewell A, Tritschler HJ, Cobelli C and Usadel KH. α-lipoic acid treatment decreases serum lactate and pyruvate concentrations and improves glucose effectiveness in lean and obese patients with Type 2 diabetes. *Diabetes Care* 1999; **22**: 280–287.
126. Ziegler D, Hanefeld M, Ruhnua KJ, Meissner HP, Lobisch M, Schutte K and Gries FA. Treatment of symptomatic diabetic peripheral neuropathy with the anti-oxidant alpha-lipoic acid. A 3-week multi-center randomized controlled trial (ALADIN Study). *Diabetologia* 1995; **38**: 1425–1433.
127. Ruhnau KJ, Meissner HP, Finn JR, Reljanovic M, Lobisch M, Schutte K, Nehrdich D, Tritschler HJ, Mehnert H and Ziegler D. Effects of 3-week oral treatment with the antioxidant thioctic acid (α-lipoic acid) in symptomatic diabetic polyneuropathy. *Diabet Med* 1999; **16**: 1040–1043.
128. Haak ES, Vsadel KH, Kohleisen M, Yilmaz A, Kusterer K and Haak T. The effect of alpha-lipoic acid on the neurovascular reflex are in patients with diabetic neuropathy assessed by capillary microscopy. *Microvasc. Res* 1999; **58**: 28–34.
129. Ziegler D, Hanefeld M, Ruhnau K-J, Hasche H, Lobisch M, Schutte K, Kerum G and Malessa R. Treatment of symptomatic diabetic polyneuropathy with the anti-oxidant α-lipoic acid. *Diabetes Care* 1999; **22**: 1296–1301.

130. Reljanovic M, Reichel G, Rett K, Lobisch M, Schuette K, Moller W, Tritschler HJ and Mehnert H. Treatment of diabetic polyneuropathy with the anti-oxidant thioctic acid (α-lipoic acid): a two year multi-center randomized double-blind placebo-controlled trial (ALADIN II). *Free Rad Res* 1999; **31**: 171–179.
131. Ziegler D, Schalz H, Conrad F, Gries FA, Ulrich H and Reichel G. Effects of treatment with the anti-oxidant alpha-lipoic acid on cardiac autonomic neuropathy in NIDDM patients. A 4-month randomized controlled multi-center trial (DEKAN-study). Deutsche Kardiale Autonome Neuropathie. *Diabetes Care* 1997; **20**: 369–373.
132. Burg MB, Kwon ED and Kultz D. Regulation of gene expression by hypertonicity. *Annu Rev Physiol* 1997; **59**: 437–455.
133. Hamada Y, Hammon K and Raskin P. No correlation between glycemic control and an increase in erythrocyte aldose reductase activity in Type I and Type II diabetic patients. *J Diabetes Compl* 1992; **6**: 111–115.
134. Hamada Y, Kitoh R and Raskin P. Association of erythrocyte aldose reductase activity with diabetic complications in Type 1 diabetes mellitus. *Diab Med* 1993; **10**: 33–38.
135. Nishimura C, Saito T, Ito T, Omori Y and Tanimoto T. High levels of erythrocyte aldose reductase and diabetic retinopathy in NIDDM patients. *Diabetologia* 1993; **73**: 328–330.
136. Ko BC, Lam KS, Wat NM and Chung SS. An $(A–C)_n$ dinucleotide repeat polymorphic marker at the 5′ end of the aldose reductase gene is associated with early-onset diabetic retinopathy in NIDDM patients. *Diabetes* 1995; **44**: 727–732.
137. Ruepp B, Bohren KM and Gabbay KH. Characterization of the osmotic response element of the human aldose reductase gene promoter. *Proc Natl Acad Sci, USA* 1996; **93**: 8624–8629.
138. Heesom AE, Millward A and Demaine AG. Susceptibility to diabetic neuropathy in patients with insulin dependent diabetes mellitus is associated with a polymorphism at the 5′ end of the aldose reductase gene. *J Neurol Neurosurg Psychiatry* 1998; **64**: 213–216.
139. Ko BB, Ruepp B, Bohren KM, Gabbay KH and Chung SS. Identification and characterization of multiple osmotic response sequences in the human aldose reductase gene. *J Biol Chem* 1997; **272**: 16 431–16 437.
140. Ghahary A, Chakrabarti S, Murphy LJ and Sima AAF. Effect of insulin and statil on aldose reductase expression in diabetic rats. *Diabetes* 1991; **40**: 1391–1396.
141. Low PA, Nickander KK and Tritschler HJ. The roles of oxidative stress and antioxidant treatment in diabetic neuropathy. *Neurosci Res Commun* 1997; **21**: 41–48.
142. Lipinski B. Pathophysiology of oxidative stress in diabetes mellitus. *J Diab Compl* 2001; **15**: 203–210.
143. Ziegler D, Reljanovic M, Meknert H and Gries FA. Alpha lipoic acid in the treatment of diabetic polyneuropathy in Germany: current evidence from clinical trials. *Exp Clin Endocrin-Diab* 2000; **107**: 421–430.
144. Sima AAF and Sugimoto K. Experimental diabetic neuropathy: an update. *Diabetologia* 1999; **42**: 773–788.
145. Cameron NE and Cotter MA. Metabolic and vascular factors in the pathogenesis of diabetic neuropathy. *Diabetes* 1997; **46** (Suppl. 2): S31–S37.
146. Sima AAF (ed). Physiology and pathophysiology of C-peptide. *Exp Diab Res* 2004; **5** (special issue): 1–96.
147. Johansson B-L, Borg K, Fernquist-Forbes E, Odergren T, Remahl S and Wahren J. C-peptide improves autonomic nerve function in patients with Type 1 diabetes. *Diabetologia* 1996; **39**: 687–695.
148. Johansson B-L, Borg K, Fernquist-Forbes E, Kernell A, Odergren T and Wahren J. 2000 Beneficial effects of C-peptide on incipient nephropathy and neuropathy in patients with Type 1 diabetes – a three-month study. *Diabet Med* 2000; **17**: 181–188.

149. Ekberg K, Brismar T, Johansson B-L, Jonsson B, Lindström P and Wahren J. Amelioration of sensory nerve dysfunction by C-peptide in patients with Type 1 diabetes. *Diabetes* 2003; **52**: 536–541.
150. Cotter MA, Ekberg K, Wahren J and Cameron NE. Effects of proinsulin C-peptide in experimental diabetic neuropathy: vascular actions and modulation by nitric oxide synthase inhibition. *Diabetes* 2003; **53**: 1812–1817.
151. Forst T, De La Tour DD, Kunt T, Pfutzner A, Goitom K, Pohlmann T, Schneider S, Johansson BL, Wahren J, Lobig M, Engelbach M, Beyer J and Vague P. Effects of proinsulin C-peptide on nitric oxide, microvascular blood flow and erythrocyte Na^+, K^+-ATPase activity in diabetes mellitus Type 1. *Clin Sci (Lond)* 2000; **98**: 283–290.
152. Johansson B-L, Pernow J and Wahren J. Muscle vasodilatation by C-peptide is NO-mediated. *Diabetologia* 1999; **42**: A324.
153. Wahren J, Ekberg K, Johansson J, Henriksson M, Pramanik A, Johansson BL, Riegler R and Jörnvall H. Role of C-peptide in human physiology. *Am J Physiol Endocrinol Metab* 2000; **278**: E759–E768.
154. Li Z-G, Zhang W and Sima AAF. C-peptide prevents hippocampal apoptosis in Type 1 diabetes. *Int J Exp Diab Res* 2002; **3**: 241–246.
155. Fagg GE and Foster AC. Excitatory amino acid synaptic mechanisms and neurological function. *Trends Pharmacol Sci* 1986; **7**: 357–363.
156. Butcher SP, Bullock R, Graham DI and McCulloch J. Correlation between amino acid release and neuropathologic outcome in rat brain following middle cerebral artery occlusion. *Stroke* 1990; **21**: 1727–1733.
157. Berger UV and Schwab ME. N-acetylated alpha-linked acidic dipeptidase may be involved in axon–Schwann cell signaling. *J Neurocytol* 1996; **25**: 499–512.
158. Jackson PF, Cole DC, Slusher BS, Stetz SL, Ross LE, Donzanti BA and Trainor DA. Design, synthesis and biological activity of a potent inhibitor of the neuropeptidase N-acetylated-α-linked acidic dipeptidase. *J Med Chem* 1996; **39**: 619–622.
159. Slusher BS, Vornov JJ, Thomas AG, Hurn PD, Harukuni I, Bhardwaj A, Traystman RJ, Robinson MB, Britton P, Lu XC, Tortella FC, Wozniak KM, Yudkoff M, Potter BM and Jackson PF. Selective inhibition of NAALADase, which converts NAAG to glutamate, reduces ischemic brain injury. *Nature Med* 1999; **5**: 1396–1402.
160. Wozniak KM, Callizot N, Poindron P and Slusher BS. NAALADase inhibition enhances behavioral and morphological recovery following sciatic nerve crush in mice. [abstract] *Soc Neurosci* **43** 11.
161. Kawamata M and Omote K. Involvement of increased excitatory amino acids and intracellular Ca^{2+} concentration in the spinal dorsal horn in an animal model of neuropathic pain. *Pain* 1996; **68**: 85–96.
162. Malcangio M and Tomlinson DR. A pharmacological analysis of mechanical hyperalgesia in streptozotocin diabetic rats. *Pain* 1998; **76**: 151–157.
163. Hall KE, Sima AAF and Wiley JW. Voltage-dependent calcium currents are enhanced in dorsal root ganglion neurons from the BB/W diabetic rat. *J Physiol (Lond)* 1995; 486: 313–322.
164. White BC, Sullivan JM, DeGarcia DJ, O'Neil BJ, Neumar RW, Grossman LI, Rafols JA and Krause GS. Brain ischemia and reperfusion: molecular mechanisms of neuronal injury. *J Neurol Sci* 2000; **179**: 1–33.
165. Thayer SA and Wang GJ. Glutamate-induced calcium loads: effects on energy metabolism and neuronal viability. *Clin Exp Pharmacol Physiol* 1995; **22**: 303–304.
166. Stevens EJ, Carrington AL and Tomlinson DR. Nerve ischemia in diabetic rats: time-course of development, effect of insulin treatment plus comparison of streptozotocin and BB models. *Diabetologia* 1994; **37**: 43–48.

167. Krause GS, White BC, Aust SD, Nayini NR and Kumar K. Brain cell death following ischemia and reperfusion: a proposed biochemical sequence. *Crit Care Med* 1998; **16**: 714–726.
168. Cooper HK, Zalewska T, Kawakani S and Hossman KA. The effect of ischemia and recirculation on protein synthesis in the rat brain. *J Neurochem* 1977; **28**: 929–934.
169. Greene DA, Stevens MJ, Obrosova I and Feldman EL. Glucose-induced oxidative stress and programmed cell death in diabetic neuropathy. *Eur J Pharm* 1999; **375**: 217–223.
170. Stevens MJ, Obrosova I, Cao X, Van Huysen C and Greene DA. Effects of DL-α-lipoic acid on peripheral nerve conduction, blood flow, energy metabolism and oxidative stress in experimental diabetic neuropathy. *Diabetes* 2000; **49**: 1006–1015.
171. Gong C, Berent A, Golovoy D, Slusher B and Russell JW. Inhibition of NAALADase protects neurons against glucose-induced programmed cell death models of diabetic neuropathy. *Soc Neurosci* 2000; **227**, **20**; **26**: 605.
172. Apfel SC. Neurotrophic factors in the therapy of diabetic neuropathy. *Am J Med* 1999; **107**: S34–S42.

16

The Cardiologist's View: Prevention of Macrovascular Complications

Michael Faust, Sabine Wiedenmann and **Reinhard Griebenow**

Prevalence of Cardiovascular Complications in Patients with Diabetes Mellitus

Cardiovascular disease continues to be the leading cause of death among patients with diabetes mellitus, being responsible for about 80 per cent of all cases of death in diabetic patients and accounting for a shortened life expectancy. Three-quarters of these cardiovascular deaths are due to coronary heart disease (CHD).[1]

The *Framingham Heart Study* showed a two- to fourfold higher risk for CHD for patients with diabetes mellitus than without diabetes mellitus. Since then diabetes – beside elevated cholesterol, arterial hypertension and smoking – has been considered as one of the four major well established risk factors for the development of CHD. The increase of risk is particularly dramatic in female patients. The occurrence of diabetes can even eliminate the statistic benefit that premenopausal women show compared to men. Unfortunately, diabetes particularly leads to an increase in severe cardiac events, such as myocardial infarction or sudden cardiac death, compared with less threatening manifestations such as stable angina.[2,3]

A prospective observational study in a large Finnish cohort recently revealed a similar cardiovascular mortality risk over 7 years for Type 2 diabetic patients without known myocardial infarction compared with a group of patients without diabetes but with post-myocardial infarction.[4]

Prevention of Type 2 Diabetes Edited by Manfred Ganz
 ISBN: 0-470-85733-1

Although these results could not be confirmed by a Scottish cohort trial,[5] the risk of cardiovascular complications in patients with Type 2 diabetes mellitus is dramatically increased compared with non-diabetic individuals.

It has yet to be proven whether Type 1 diabetic patients also have to be considered as high-risk patients. In the DCCT trial, one of the most revealing endpoint studies in Type 1 diabetes, barely any cardiovascular events were registered due to young age.[6] A large prospective analysis of a Finnish cohort of more than 5000 Type 1 diabetic patients from 1965 to 1979 revealed that the cardiovascular risk in Type 1 diabetic patients does show a 10-fold increase if a diabetic nephropathy exists.[7] Therefore, Type 2 diabetic patients and Type 1 diabetic patients with nephropathy are considered as high-risk patients for the development of cardiovascular diseases.

Various epidemiological observations suggest that even preliminary stages of diabetes mellitus, such as impaired fasting glucose (IFG) and impaired glucose tolerance (IGT), carry an increased risk for cardiovascular complications, considering a different risk profile for patients with increased fasting glucose (IFG) versus patients with pathological glucose tolerance (IGT). The DECODE trial, a meta-analysis of 13 European prospective cohort trials with a total of more than 18 000 male and 7000 female participants, revealed at a mean observation time of 7.3 years that mortality risk in impaired glucose tolerance (IGT) is explicitly higher than in impaired fasting glucose (IFG) (Figure 16.1).

This however has not been unequivocally proven in all trials. As an example, the *National Health and Nutrition Examination Survey* (NHANES III) showed no statistically significant increase of nonfatal myocardial infarction and strokes in patients with impaired glucose tolerance (IGT).[9]

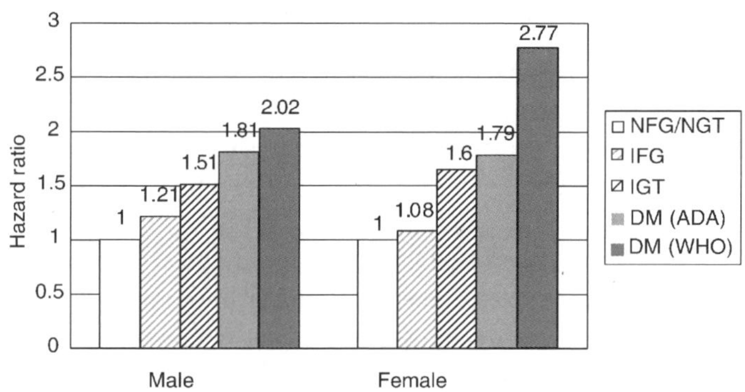

NFG = normal fasting glucose; NGT = normal glucose tolerance; IFG = impaired fasting glucose; DM (ADA) = diabetes mellitus (American Diabetes Association); DM (WHO) = diabetes mellitus (World Health Organization)[8].

FIGURE 16.1 Risk of mortality depending on metabolic disorders (DECODE trial)

Occurrence of Diabetes in Patients with Cardiovascular Disease

The percentage of diabetic patients among cardiological patients is high and steadily growing due to the increasing prevalence of metabolic disorders in the population as well as high susceptibility of these patients to cardiovascular diseases. A dramatic increase in the number of patients with diabetes mellitus being admitted to the hospital because of acute myocardial infarction in 1970–1985 was recorded in the *Minnesota Heart Survey*, a cardiological register kept since the 1970s. The number has more than doubled from 8.2 per cent in 1970 to 16.8 per cent in 1985. This has even been more staggering in female patients: whereas in 1970 16 per cent of female patients with acute myocardial infarction had diabetes, there were 25.8 per cent in 1985.[10] Furthermore, long-term outcome of diabetic patients among all who survived the first infarct was worse. Mortality rate was 40 per cent higher in diabetic versus nondiabetic patients.

Furthermore, a European trial showed 21 per cent of patients admitted because of myocardial infarction having diagnosed diabetes mellitus. In another four per cent, diagnosis was primarily found during the in-patient stay, so that altogether one-quarter of all patients with acute infarction had diabetes.[11]

In the course of the MONICA project of the WHO, 244 patients have been reassessed with an oral glucose tolerance test 4–9 years (mean 6.5 years) after having suffered from myocardial infarction. So far no metabolic disorder had been found in these patients. As a result, diabetes mellitus was diagnosed in every eighth individual and a pathologic glucose tolerance in 27 per cent.[12] More interestingly, only 17 per cent of these patients were diagnosed with an impaired fasting glucose according to the diagnostic criteria of the American Diabetes Society. This again strongly points out that the oral glucose tolerance test is a highly sensitive test for the detection of patients with metabolic disorders, in particular in individuals with cardiovascular diseases.

Prognosis and Course of Coronary Heart Disease in Diabetic Patients

Mortality after acute myocardial infarction in diabetic versus non-diabetic patients is already greatly increased during hospital stay. As an example, a retrospective study by Yudkin and colleagues demonstrated a hospital mortality of 24.7 per cent in 380 non-diabetic (patients defined by normal HbA_{1c} values) after infarction versus 42.2 per cent in diabetic patients, which is almost doubled.[13]

Medium- and long-term survival is also decreased in diabetic patients with coronary heart disease. In the aforementioned Finnish observation trial by Haffner *et al.* only a little more than half of the patients with Type 2 diabetes survived the 7 year observation time after myocardial infarction.[4] Similar results were seen in the diabetes subgroup analysis of the placebo arms of the statin intervention trials, such as the 4S-trial.[14]

In the OASIS trial, which was conducted in six different countries, male patients with diabetes mellitus admitted due to unstable angina or non-Q-wave infarction showed a 1.5-fold increased mortality in the following 2 years compared with nondiabetic patients. In female diabetic patients the 2 year mortality rate was even twice as high.[15]

Coronary heart disease in diabetic patients shows significantly more frequently a multi-vessel disease pattern with diffuse coronary sclerosis than in nondiabetic patients. Acute coronary syndrome in diabetic patients leads more often to impaired left ventricular function. The occurrence of cardiac dysrhythmias also seems to be higher. The primary size of infarction, however, does not differ significantly.[16]

Explanatory Models for the Particular Fatal Course of Coronary Heart Disease in Diabetic Patients (Risk Factors)

The most obvious biochemical change in diabetes mellitus is the elevated fasting and/or postprandial blood glucose. Therefore the question has been raised of to what extent hyperglycaemia is responsible for the increased susceptibility for cardiovascular complications and the worse prognosis of diabetic patients.

As a matter of fact, elevated blood sugar values as defined by elevated HbA_{1c} values seem to be correlated with a higher probability for the development of a cardiovascular event. In the UKPD trial, which includes more than 5000 newly diagnosed Type 2 diabetic patients in different treatment arms being observed for several years, a positive correlation between elevated HbA_{1c} values and cardiovascular events was detected. 574 participants of this trial suffered from a total of 597 myocardial infarctions, of which 351 had a lethal course. Furthermore, 199 participants suffered from a total of 234 strokes, including 48 lethal courses. Expressed in figures, a one per cent reduction in the HbA_{1c} leads to a decrease in the risk of diabetes-related fatal events of 21 per cent. The risk of myocardial infarction is decreased by 14 per cent.[17]

Another multivariate analysis showed that the risk for fatal cardiovascular events depends on glycated haemoglobin (HbA_{1c}), age, blood pressure and urinary albumin excretion. The odds ratio for a one per cent HbA_{1c} increase is 1.17 for fatal myocardial infarctions and 1.37 for fatal strokes.[18] The DCCT trial also demonstrated a trend in Type 1 diabetic patients towards more frequent cardiovascular complications in patients with higher blood sugar and HbA_{1c} values, respectively. Due to low absolute figures a statistical significance level was not reached.[19]

Cardiovascular Complications – Preventive and Therapeutic Options

Blood sugar control

No proof exists that any existing glycaemic control treatment option is able to prevent macrovascular complications. Merely for acute myocardial infarction,[20] a strict reduction in blood glucose level was linked to an improved prognosis. Furthermore, strong glycaemic control may lead to a distinct reduction of microvascular, particularly ocular, complications.[19,21,22]

Frequently discussed is the question of whether the use of sulfonylurea may increase the probability of cardiac events and unfavourably influence their course, respectively. The discussion is among other things based on the proof of sulfonylurea receptors in the myocardium. A retrospective trial by Klamann *et al.* examined this question in a German cohort by determing size of infarction and mortality rate of nondiabetic individuals, diabetic patients treated with sulfonylurea and differently treated diabetic patients. As in other trials the mortality rate of 30 per cent in patients with known diabetes mellitus was significantly higher than in nondiabetic individuals (20.2 per cent). The difference in mortality between diabetic patients with sulfonylurea treatment (32.9 per cent) and diabetic patients without this therapy (29 per cent), however, was not statistically significant. Moreover, no significant difference in size of infarction was found.[23]

Antihypertensive therapy

ACE inhibitors/angiotensin II receptor blockers

The strict reduction of an elevated blood pressure in diabetic patients has an even greater prognostic importance than strict glycaemic control[49] as expressed in a significant reduction of cardiovascular complications. Unfortunately, only limited data are available concerning a specific organ-protective effect as most data for patients with diabetes mellitus result from (not always prospective) subgroup analyses.

In this sense, ACE inhibitors significantly lower the occurrence of cardiac complications,[24] even independently from a simultaneous blood pressure control. Similar trials for angiotensin II receptor blockers are ongoing.[25]

Furthermore, the risk of stroke is decreased.[26,27] According to the LIFE trial, the angiotensin II receptor blocker losartan has led to a 21.8 per cent stroke reduction in diabetic patients, which is, however, not significant ($p = 0.19$).[28]

As principles for treatment of cardiac insufficiency do not differ in patients with and without diabetes, ACE inhibitors are the treatment of first choice. Similar effectiveness holds true for angiotensin II receptor blockers.[29–32]

In addition, a particular nephroprotective effect for both substance groups has also been proven.[33–35] As a consequence, several scientific societies[36,37] recommend inhibition of the renin–angiotensin system as the therapy of first choice for antihypertensive combination therapy. Therefore, treatment with the goal of reaching normotensive values is of particularly special importance in diabetic patients.[38]

Unfortunately, no further investigations exist of to what extent ACE inhibitors/angiotensin II receptor blockers may positively influence the clinical course of peripheral arterial disease.

Beta-adrenergic antagonists

In diabetic patients beta-adrenergic antagonists have proven their value as part of an antihypertensive regimen, as well as other substance groups.[39,40] Furthermore, the application of beta-adrenergic antagonists may lead to a profound improvement of symptoms and prognosis of stable and unstable angina in diabetic patients. A positive effect in secondary prevention post-myocardial infarction is also known.[41,42]

Concerning treatment of cardiac failure, the addition of beta-adrenergic antagonists to an existing regimen with ACE inhibitors leads to a further improvement of prognosis. Particular organprotective effects regarding stroke or peripheral arterial disease, however, have not been shown for beta-adrenergic antagonists. On the contrary, beta-adrenergic antagonists are rather cautiously applied in patients with peripheral arterial disease due to possible worsening of symptoms.[43]

Other antihypertensive substances

Diuretics are one of the main substances for antihypertensive therapy (ALLHAT). Regarding diabetes mellitus, loop diuretics are preferred due to a less negative influence on glucose metabolism. Calcium antagonists have also been successfully applied in antihypertensive treatment regimens[38,39] and are even allowed to be applied in stable angina without any negative effects on prognosis.[44,45]

Inhibition of platelet aggregation

In diabetic patients acetylsalicylic acid (aspirin) represents an important tool for primary and secondary prevention of coronary heart disease and is therefore to be administered in all diabetic patients.[46] The same holds true for all diabetic patients with peripheral arterial disease,[43] whereas the effect is less obvious in stroke patients. For these patients favourable results for stroke prevention have been demonstrated for ticlopidin (due to severe adverse events no longer recommended) and lately also clopidogrel.[47] The use of acetylsalicylic acid does not increase the risk of ocular bleeding.[48]

Hypolipidaemic drugs

The most substantial data for the importance of lipid reduction in coronary heart disease were derived from the Pravastatin Pooling Project,[49] which, however, could not prove any clear preventive effect of the application of statins in diabetic patients.[50] In contrast, the HPS trial recently revealed a primary and secondary preventive effect for lipid-reducing therapy with statins for cardiac complications as well as for stroke patients with diabetes mellitus. As data for peripheral arterial disease are limited, indication for lipid-reducing therapy complies with concomitant cardiac or cerebral complications.[43]

Interventional Revascularization

Data for different methods of interventional revascularization in patients with diabetes mellitus are merely to be obtained by subgroup analysis partially, lacking any comparison of techniques.

Regarding coronary heart disease subgroup analysis reveals a higher cumulative risk for complications after interventional procedures for diabetic patients resulting from an increased risk profile, greater age, more severe cardiac disease and higher-grade reduction in left ventricular function in comparison with nondiabetic patients.[51]

Balloon dilatation of coronary arteries in diabetic patients shows a similar high initial success rate[52] with a higher restenosis rate[53] and worse long-term outcome.[54] The use of GP II/IIIa antagonists has proven to be favourable particularly in diabetic patients.[55–57] The BARI trial showed a randomized comparison of revascularization by balloon dilatation or bypass surgery for a subgroup of diabetic patients. Superior results have been retrieved for bypass surgery, whereas in nondiabetic patients balloon dilatation and bypass surgery performed comparatively with regard to long-term mortality.[58,59]

Indication for operative therapy of carotid artery stenosis depends on a combined assessment of grade of stenosis and clinical symptoms. Alternatively, percutaneous stent implantation has been established as a valid method, for which results with concomitant administration of GP IIb/IIIa antagonists turned out to be favourable. A direct comparison of endarterectomy with percutaneous stent implantation has so far not been performed. Primary success rates are comparably high for both techniques as well as data concerning periprocedural mortality, which is slightly lower after stent implantation. Data particularly for diabetes patients are not available so far.[60] Postinterventionally, a combination therapy of acetylsalicylic acid and clopidogrel is suggested for several weeks after stent implantation.

Interventional therapy of peripheral artery disease is pursued depending on clinical stage and technical accessibility of stenosis. Comparative methodological examinations (balloon dilatation versus bypass surgery) do not exist. Specific data for patients with diabetes mellitus are also lacking.

Procedure in Critical Ischaemia

In acute myocardial infarction thrombolysis is as well indicated in diabetic as in nondiabetic patients, leads to comparable results and is even supposed to be applied in patients with diabetic retinopathy.[61,62]

Thrombolytic therapy in ischaemic stroke has also been increasingly investigated during the recent years and has shown positive results, whereas detailed data for patients with diabetes mellitus do not exist.[26]

For management of critical limb ischaemia a multidisciplinary teaching and treatment approach seems to be as neccessary as well as revascularization and drug therapy.[43]

References

1. Aronson D, Rayfield EJ and Chesebro JH. Mechanisms determining course and outcome of diabetic patients who have had acute myocardial infarction. *Ann Intern Med* 1997; **126** (4): 296–306.
2. Kannel WB and McGee DL. Diabetes and cardiovascular disease. The Framingham Study. *JAMA* 1979; **241** (19): 2035–2038.
3. Haffner SM. Coronary heart disease in patients with diabetes. *N Engl J Med* 2000; **342** (14): 1040–1042.
4. Haffner SM *et al.* Mortality from coronary heart disease in subjects with Type 2 diabetes and in nondiabetic subjects with and without prior myocardial infarction. *N Engl J Med* 1998; **339** (4): 229–234.
5. Evans JM, Wang J and Morris AD. Comparison of cardiovascular risk between patients with Type 2 diabetes and those who had a myocardial infarction: cross sectional and cohort studies. *BMJ* 2002; **324** (7343): 939–942.
6. The Diabetes Control and Complications Trial Research Group. The effect of intensive treatment of diabetes on the development and progression of long-term complications in insulin-dependent diabetes mellitus. *N Engl J Med* 1993; **329** (14): 977–986.
7. Tuomilehto J *et al.* Incidence of cardiovascular disease in Type 1 (insulin-dependent) diabetic subjects with and without diabetic nephropathy in Finland. *Diabetologia* 1998; **41** (7): 784–790.
8. The DECODE Study Group. European diabetes epidemiology group. Diabetes epidemiology: Collaborative Analysis of Diagnostic Criteria in Europe. Glucose tolerance and

mortality: comparison of WHO and American Diabetes Association diagnostic criteria. *Lancet* 1999; **354** (9179): 617–621.

9. Qureshi AI, Giles WH and Croft JB. Impaired glucose tolerance and the likelihood of nonfatal stroke and myocardial infarction: the Third National Health and Nutrition Examination Survey. *Stroke* 1998; **29** (7): 1329–1332.
10. Sprafka JM *et al.* Trends in prevalence of diabetes mellitus in patients with myocardial infarction and effect of diabetes on survival. The Minnesota Heart Survey. *Diabetes Care* 1991; **14** (7): 537–543.
11. Tenerz A *et al.* Myocardial infarction and prevalence of diabetes mellitus. Is increased casual blood glucose at admission a reliable criterion for the diagnosis of diabetes? *Eur Heart J* 2001; **22** (13): 1102–1110.
12. Rathmann W *et al.* Undiagnosed diabetes mellitus among patients with prior myocardial infarction. *Z Kardiol* 2002; **91** (8): 620–625.
13. Yudkin JS and Oswald GA. Determinants of hospital admission and case fatality in diabetic patients with myocardial infarction. *Diabetes Care* 1988; **11** (4): 351–358.
14. Pyorala K *et al.* Cholesterol lowering with simvastatin improves prognosis of diabetic patients with coronary heart disease. A subgroup analysis of the scandinavian simvastatin survival study (4S). *Diabetes Care* 1997; **20** (4): 614–620.
15. Malmberg K *et al.* Impact of diabetes on long-term prognosis in patients with unstable angina and non-Q-wave myocardial infarction: results of the OASIS (Organization to assess strategies for ischemic syndromes) registry. *Circulation* 2000; **102** (9): 1014–1019.
16. Hasdai D *et al.* Diabetes mellitus and outcome after primary coronary angioplasty for acute myocardial infarction: lessons from the GUSTO-IIb angioplasty substudy. Global use of strategies to open occluded arteries in acute coronary syndromes. *J Am Coll Cardiol* 2000; **35** (6): 1502–1512.
17. Stratton IM *et al.* Association of glycaemia with macrovascular and microvascular complications of Type 2 diabetes (UKPDS 35): prospective observational study. *BMJ* 2000; **321** (7258): 405–412.
18. Stevens RJ *et al.* Risk factors for myocardial infarction case fatality and stroke case fatality in Type 2 diabetes: UKPDS 66. *Diabetes Care* 2004; **27** (1): 201–207.
19. Effect of intensive diabetes management on macrovascular events and risk factors in the diabetes control and complications trial. *Am J Cardiol* 1995; **75** (14): 894–903.
20. Malmberg K *et al.* Randomized trial of insulin-glucose infusion followed by subcutaneous insulin treatment in diabetic patients with acute myocardial infarction (DIGAMI study): effects on mortality at 1 year. *J Am Coll Cardiol* 1995; **26** (1): 57–65.
21. Abraira C *et al.* Cardiovascular events and correlates in the veterans affairs diabetes feasibility trial. Veterans affairs cooperative study on glycemic control and complications in Type 2 Diabetes. *Arch Intern Med* 1997; **157** (2): 181–188.
22. UK Prospective Diabetes Study (UKPDS) Group. Intensive blood-glucose control with sulphonylureas or insulin compared with conventional treatment and risk of complications in patients with Type 2 diabetes (UKPDS 33). *Lancet* 1998; **352** (9131): 837–853.
23. Klamann A *et al.* Myocardial infarction in diabetic vs non-diabetic subjects. Survival and infarct size following therapy with sulfonylureas (glibenclamide). *Eur Heart J* 2000; **21** (3). 220–229.
24. Yusuf S *et al.* Effects of an angiotensin-converting-enzyme inhibitor, ramipril, on cardiovascular events in high-risk patients. The heart outcomes prevention evaluation study investigators. *N Engl J Med* 2000; **342** (3): 145–153.
25. Unger T. The ongoing telmisartan alone and in combination with ramipril global endpoint trial program. *Am J Cardiol* 2003; **91** (10A): 28G–34G.

26. Hoogwerf BJ. Diabetes and cardiovascular disease. In *Diabetes and Cardiovascular Risk*, Ritz E (ed.). 2002. Cologne: Academy pp. 192–221.
27. PROGRESS Collaborative Group Randomised trial of a perindopril-based blood-pressure-lowering regimen among 6105 individuals with previous stroke or transient ischaemic attack. *The Lancet* 2001; **358** (9287): 1033–1041.
28. Dahlof B *et al.* Cardiovascular morbidity and mortality in the losartan intervention for endpoint reduction in hypertension study (LIFE): a randomized trial against atenolol. *Lancet* 2002; **359** (9311): 995–1003.
29. The SOLVD Investigators. Effect of enalapril on survival in patients with reduced left ventricular ejection fractions and congestive heart failure. *N Engl J Med* 1991; **325** (5): 293–302.
30. Pfeffer MA *et al.* Effect of captopril on mortality and morbidity in patients with left ventricular dysfunction after myocardial infarction. Results of the survival and ventricular enlargement trial. The SAVE investigators. *N Engl J Med* 1992; **327** (10): 669–677.
31. Pitt B *et al.* Effect of losartan compared with captopril on mortality in patients with symptomatic heart failure: randomised trial – the losartan heart failure survival study ELITE II. *Lancet* 2000; **355** (9215): 1582–1587.
32. Yusuf S *et al.* Effects of candesartan in patients with chronic heart failure and preserved left-ventricular ejection fraction: the CHARM-preserved trial. *Lancet* 2003; **362** (9386): 777–781.
33. Heart Outcomes Prevention Evaluation Study Investigators. Effects of ramipril on cardiovascular and microvascular outcomes in people with diabetes mellitus: results of the HOPE study and MICRO-HOPE substudy. *Lancet* 2000; **355** (9200): 253–259.
34. Parving HH *et al.* The effect of irbesartan on the development of diabetic nephropathy in patients with Type 2 diabetes. *N Engl J Med* 2001; **345** (12): 870–878.
35. Lewis EJ *et al.* Renoprotective effect of the angiotensin-receptor antagonist irbesartan in patients with nephropathy due to Type 2 diabetes. *N Engl J Med* 2001; **345** (12): 851–860.
36. European society of hypertension–European society of cardiology guidelines for the management of arterial hypertension. *J Hypertens* 2003; **21** (6): 1011–1053.
37. Chobanian AV *et al.* Seventh report of the joint national committee on prevention, detection, evaluation, and treatment of high blood pressure. *Hypertension* 2003; **42** (6): 1206–1252.
38. Hansson L *et al.* Effects of intensive blood-pressure lowering and low-dose aspirin in patients with hypertension: principal results of the hypertension optimal treatment (HOT) randomised trial. HOT study group. *Lancet* 1998; **351** (9118): 1755–1762.
39. Hansson L *et al.* Randomised trial of old and new antihypertensive drugs in elderly patients: cardiovascular mortality and morbidity. The swedish trial in old patients with hypertension-2 study. *Lancet* 1999; **354** (9192): 1751–1756.
40. Efficacy of atenolol and captopril in reducing risk of macrovascular and microvascular complications in Type 2 diabetes: UKPDS 39. UK prospective diabetes study group. *BMJ* 1998; **317** (7160): 713–720.
41. Kjekshus J *et al.* Diabetic patients and beta-blockers after acute myocardial infarction. *Eur Heart J* 1990; **11** (1): 43–50.
42. Chen J *et al.* Beta-blocker therapy for secondary prevention of myocardial infarction in elderly diabetic patients. Results from the National Cooperative Cardiovascular Project. *J Am Coll Cardiol* 1999; **34** (5): 1388–1394.
43. Kröger K. Prevention of peripheral artery atherosclerosis. In *Panvascular Medicine*, Lanzer P and Topol EJ (eds). 2002. Berlin: Springer, pp. 1347–1350.
44. Fox KM *et al.* The Total Ischaemic Burden European Trial (TIBET). Effects of atenolol, nifedipine SR and their combination on the exercise test and the total ischaemic burden in 608 patients with stable angina. The TIBET Study Group. *Eur Heart J* 1996; **17** (1): 96–103.

45. Rehnqvist N *et al.* Effects of metoprolol vs verapamil in patients with stable angina pectoris. The Angina Prognosis Study in Stockholm (APSIS). *Eur Heart J* 1996; **17** (1): 76–81.
46. American Diabetes Association. Aspirin therapy in diabetes. *Diabetes Care* 1997; **20** (11): 1772–1773.
47. CAPRIE Steering Committee. A randomized, blinded, trial of clopidogrel versus aspirin in patients at risk of ischaemic events (CAPRIE). *Lancet* 1996; **348** (9038): 1329–1339.
48. ETDRS Investigators. Aspirin effects on mortality and morbidity in patients with diabetes mellitus. Early Treatment Diabetic Retinopathy Study report 14. *JAMA* 1992; **268** (10): 1292–1300.
49. Simes J *et al.* Effects of pravastatin on mortality in patients with and without coronary heart disease across a broad range of cholesterol levels. The prospective pravastatin pooling project. *Eur Heart J* 2002; **23** (3): 207–215.
50. Sacks FM *et al.* Effect of pravastatin on coronary disease events in subgroups defined by coronary risk factors: the prospective pravastatin pooling project. *Circulation* 2000; **102** (16): 1893–1900.
51. Cohen Y *et al.* Comparison of factors associated with 30-day mortality after coronary artery bypass grafting in patients with versus without diabetes mellitus. Israeli Coronary Artery Bypass (ISCAB) Study Consortium. *Am J Cardiol* 1998; **81** (1): 7–11.
52. Baim DS *et al.* Coronary angioplasty performed within the Thrombolysis in Myocardial Infarction II study. *Circulation* 1992; **85** (1): 93–105.
53. Van Belle E *et al.* Restenosis rates in diabetic patients: a comparison of coronary stenting and balloon angioplasty in native coronary vessels. *Circulation* 1997; **96** (5): 1454–1460.
54. Kip KE *et al.* Coronary angioplasty in diabetic patients. The National Heart, Lung, and Blood Institute Percutaneous Transluminal Coronary Angioplasty Registry. *Circulation* 1996; **94** (8): 1818–1825.
55. Platelet Receptor Inhibition in Ischemic Syndrome Management in Patients Limited by Unstable Signs and Symptoms (PRISM-PLUS) Study Investigators. Inhibition of the platelet glycoprotein IIb/IIIa receptor with tirofiban in unstable angina and non-Q-wave myocardial infarction. *N Engl J Med* 1998; **338** (21): 1488–1497.
56. The EPILOG Investigators. Platelet glycoprotein IIb/IIIa receptor blockade and low dose heparin during percutaneous coronary revascularization. *N Engl J Med* 1997; **336** (24): 1689–1696.
57. Lincoff AM *et al.* Complementary clinical benefits of coronary-artery stenting and blockade of platelet glycoprotein IIb/IIIa receptors. Evaluation of Platelet IIb/IIIa Inhibition in Stenting Investigators. *N Engl J Med* 1999; **341** (5): 319–327.
58. The Bypass Angioplasty Revascularization Investigation (BARI) Investigators. Comparison of coronary bypass surgery with angioplasty in patients with multivessel disease. *N Engl J Med* 1996; **335** (4): 217–225.
59. Detre KM *et al.* The effect of previous coronary-artery bypass surgery on the prognosis of patients with diabetes who have acute myocardial infarction. Bypass Angioplasty Revascularization Investigation Investigators. *N Engl J Med* 2000; **342** (14): 989–997.
60. Mathias K and Gissler HM. Carotid artery disease: percutaneous approach. In *Panvascular Medicine*, Lanzer P and Topol EJ (eds). 2002. Berlin: Springer, pp. 1302–1315.
61. Woodfield SL *et al.* Angiographic findings and outcome in diabetic patients treated with thrombolytic therapy for acute myocardial infarction: the GUSTO-I experience. *J Am Coll Cardiol* 1996; **28** (7): 1661–1669.
62. Mahaffey KW *et al.* Diabetic retinopathy should not be a contraindication to thrombolytic therapy for acute myocardial infarction: review of ocular hemorrhage incidence and location in the GUSTO-I trial. Global Utilization of Streptokinase and t-PA for Occluded Coronary Arteries. *J Am Coll Cardiol* 1997; **30** (7): 1606–1610.

17

Milestones and New Perspectives in Prevention of Type 2 Diabetes and its Complications

Carl Erik Mogensen

During the last 80 years or more, we have witnessed an extraordinary development within practically all areas of medicine and this is certainly also the case regarding diabetes treatment and care; an area where especially in the last 25 years we have seen many decisive steps of progress. Obviously, the seminal progress was the isolation of insulin and the first treatment of a patient with severe Type 1 diabetes and, probably, imminent ketosis with otherwise deadly outcome.[7,8]

Compared with this major milestone, other progress may seem less important, but still involves even many more patients profoundly.

It should be mentioned that the major issue of solving key questions such as a more radical treatment of Type 1 and Type 2 diabetes is still pending on the horizon. In this short chapter a number of important steps forward are reviewed more or less from the author's personal experience and evaluation, especially in Type 2 diabetes.

Classification of Diabetes

As indicated in Table 17.1, the classification of diabetes has always been and still is somewhat problematic. A completely correct classification is probably not possible, mainly because there are changes over time in the status of our patients, in particular patients with Type 2 diabetes, and, indeed, transition forms between

Prevention of Type 2 Diabetes Edited by Manfred Ganz
 ISBN: 0-470-85733-1

TABLE 17.1 The designation of diabetes (main types)

Obese diabetes	Lean diabetes
Maturity-onset diabetes	Juvenile diabetes
Non-insulin-dependent diabetes	Insulin-dependent diabetes
Type 2 diabetes	Type 1 diabetes

All the above designations have their weaknesses and the classification is not relevant for treatment where the focus is more and more on best possible glycaemic control with all measures as well as a pharmacological intervention, especially with focus on end-points.

Type 1 and Type 2 diabetes; the present classification is also prevalent. The well-known popular expression is Type 1.5 diabetes, an interesting concept of a clinical subgroup.

Usually, I do not measure plasma C-peptide to assess the capacity of insulin secretion; I rather rely on clinical judgements. With regard to treatment strategy, it is generally similar regardless of aetiologies (the goal is optimal glycaemic control and control of other risk factors). A patient with typical Type 1 diabetes needs immediate insulin treatment, but such treatment is often neglected in many patients with Type 2 or Type 1.5 diabetes, where insulin secretion deteriorates over the years.

TABLE 17.2 Problematic ideas within diabetology (often with weak theoretical background/foundation)

1. Pancreas or cell transplantation is a realistic possibility.
2. HLA genotyping is important.
3. Delivery of 'prophylactic' nicotinamide or insulin to individual at risk for Type 1 diabetes.
4. Routine measurements of C-peptide in the classification of diabetes.
5. Complications are genetically controlled.
6. Renal biopsy is necessary in evaluation of albuminuria in diabetes.
7. Kidney disease in diabetics is often caused by glomerulonefritis.
8. Diabetes diet needs to be low in carbohydrates, but rich in fat and proteins (later the opposite).
9. Glycaemic control is not essential for preventing complications.
10. High blood pressure ensures renal perfusion (BP lowering potentially harmful).
11. Hypofysectomy useful for diabetic retinopathy.
12. Growth hormone treatment relevant in Type 2 diabetes.
13. Diabetic vascular disease very specific ('only' diabetic, not ordinary arteriosclerosis).
14. Careful investigation for renal stenosis is important, especially before inhibiting the renin–angiotensin system.
15. Insulin pump treatment should be used in most patients with Type 1 diabetes.
16. SU preparations may be cardiotoxic and increase mortality.
17. Insulin preparations may be aterogenic or may promote arteriosclerosis in certain situations.
18. Cyclosporin or/immune-suppressive treatment relevant for newly diagnosed Type 1 diabetes.
19. Low doses ACE-i relevant.
20. Diabetes treatment only antihyperglycaemic.

Thus, the emerging concept is that many patients with Type 2 diabetes need insulin treatment when control becomes poorer over time. This is the pattern in many patients after some years with diabetes. In countries where insulin is expensive and not readily available, this is a serious problem.

It is well known from the UKPDS Project that the capacity of insulin secretion becomes reduced with time due to deterioration of the function of the beta cells where insulin sensitivity is relatively stable.[29] Genetic analysis is not clinically useful, also not in the classification of diabetes (see also Table 17.2 for controversial issues).

Insulin Treatment with Focus on Euglycaemia in Type 2 Diabetic Patients

Insulin treatment is now increasingly used in patients with Type 2 diabetes in order to obtain the best possible control, but the first patient treated in Toronto was indisputably a Type 1 diabetic patient, Leonard Thomson.[8] The picture of this patient before and after treatment still goes around the world. This was the major revolution in the treatment of Type 1 diabetes and soon insulin production became possible on a larger scale in the US and Canada. Also in Denmark, the Nobel laureate August Krogh very quickly obtained permission to establish insulin production. It may be known to some that August Krogh's wife, Marie Krogh, had diabetes, and this may have been a very personal incentive for Professor Krogh.[57]

In a way, Denmark seemed an ideal country for insulin production because of the very large 'population' of pigs that could be used for porcine insulin production. The pancreases of these millions of pigs were otherwise to be largely wasted. Obviously, it was a question of a refining cleaning procedure, going from the raw glands to purified insulin.

The insulin production started at Nordisk Insulin, and very quickly a new manufacturer, Novo, also introduced insulin. It has been reported many times that one day a very prominent co-worker at Nordisk did not turn up in the laboratory. Later, it became clear that he had created his own new company, Novo. However, about 1980, it was also an important step forward that the two competitors merged into one company known as Novo Nordisk, one of the major insulin producers today.

It is increasingly clear that patients with Type 2 diabetes often develop poor glycaemic control and high glycated Hb values and need insulin treatment. Indeed, there was no alternative to insulin and diet until the mid-1950s, when sulfonylureas (SU) was introduced on the market.[20]

Obviously, the long-term diabetic complications have been known for a long time, but this was only observed in Type 2 diabetes, often in elderly persons, and it was difficult to recognize the specificity of the complications. However, a breakthrough came with the classical observation of the specific renal lesions described by Kimmelstiel and Wilson observed in patients with Type 2 diabetes. Autopsy examinations revealed the typical lesions, published in a classical paper, a clear milestone.[37]

Insulin treatment had a new breakthrough with the production of long-acting insulin, protaphane or NPH insulin, based upon a principle that is still widely used.[7,8] However, in the opinion of many people, this led, in fact, to poorer glycaemic control because the main target was to relieve the patients from the typical acute symptoms of diabetes, which was quite easy by one or two injections per day. However, this probably meant that the glycaemic control may have become poorer, at least in some patients.

There was not much progress in insulin production until the early 1980s, when insulin pens and pumps were introduced. This was an important step forward since many patients had much easier means to obtain better glycaemic control with these instruments. Treatment was simply much easier with insulin pens, and the pens we now have at our disposal are really small technical wonders and clearly superior to traditional injections. Indeed, injection needles have also improved considerably in quality so the injection is only minimally disturbing to the patients, increasing compliance.

On the other hand, the total production costs for insulin delivered in advanced insulin pens are higher than insulin furnished in old-fashioned 10 ml ampoules. Porcine insulin may also be cheaper than new 'human' insulin preparations, a major concern in many developing countries.[10]

Insulin pumps have also been used widely, but it may be argued that it is possible to obtain as good long-term glycaemic control with pens compared with pumps,[39,52] as indicated by the DCCT study (HbA_{1c} 6.8 with pumps, 7.0 with pens, David Nathan, personal communication). Insulin pens are now widely used for Type 2 diabetes.

Further progress made by the industry was the so-called 'human' insulin at the beginning of the 1980s. Whether this was real progress can still be discussed; indeed, it was hardly proven that glycaemic control was any better with insulin of this type. However, the slogan was quite appealing: 'human insulin for human beings'.

Interestingly, major attempts over recent years and currently are being made to either make insulin molecules more long acting or more short acting according to patients' potential needs. This means that we are coming back to insulins that are not strictly human, just like insulin used earlier, which could be porcine or bovine, chemically somewhat different from 'human insulin'.

Newly developed and modified insulins may have more rapid and longer action. This could in theory constitute an advantage, although not a major one. It is certainly difficult to prove superior long-term glycaemic control in the clinical trials,[17,33,50,55] also with inhaled insulin.[13] However, there is some evidence that many patients with Type 2 diabetes with advantage can use long-acting insulin analogues in order to obtain better glycaemic control with few injections. Often patients with Type 2 diabetes need very large insulin doses, which may be given once or twice a day. Many studies document that 'once a day' is a very good concept for compliance, but often in these patients injections twice a day are needed.

I believe that Type 2 diabetes is now the major market for the insulin producers. We simply see many more patients that need larger doses to near-normalize their blood glucose values, often more than 100 units per day in many people. This is certainly likely to increase in the future considering the increasing number of patients with Type 2 diabetes and the increasing demand for better glycaemic control.

However, in principle, there is no radical progress in insulin treatment; it is still a question of giving insulin in the correct doses in the right time at the right place. This is now practically much easier, but the principles are not different from what we have seen earlier. Whether modulation of the entero-insular axis is a durable treatment strategy is still under evaluation. As shown at the 2004 EASD congress in Munich there is no specific advantage of using insulin in Type 2 diabetics with myocardial infarction. It is glycaemic control that counts.[2,19,45]

Sulphonylurea (SU) Preparations

The discovery and identification of insulin for clinical use were a result of systematic research, but there were many elements of pure luck in the story.

On the other hand, it can be argued that as regards the SU preparations this was a matter of typical serendipity.[20] During the Second World War in Montpellier, France, smart clinicians observed that sulfa preparations commonly used for typhus in some patients resulted in symptoms typical for low blood glucose during the treatment.[20] Thus it was possible, at least in theory, to use these agents designed for treatment of infections to reduce blood glucose. It became clear that SU preparations stimulated insulin production (although not in Type 1 diabetes), but it lasted many years before these clinical observations were implemented into the general patient treatment, first in Germany.

SU preparations are widely used because of their low price and clear cut efficiency.[1,5,12,32,35,51] We realize that doctors should be aware of change to insulin treatment in due time with poor control, possibly combined with metformin. Still good glycaemic control is a major issue, and as time passes in patients with Type 2 diabetes insulin production is reduced and a shift to insulin is commonly needed. The indication in elderly patients is still debated and new trials are still being conducted.[1]

Several generations of SU preparations have been marketed, and these agents are probably the most widely used in diabetic care throughout the world. The new generations of SU preparations have a more and more specific effect on beta cells, which is probably important. Another may be more important element in the treatment strategy is that new SU preparations can be given once a day, which certainly improves compliance. The new preparations simply have longer duration of action, very useful in clinical action.

It has been suggested that SU preparations may be cardiotoxic with cardiovascular side-effects, and early studies on SU supported this phenomenon.[51,60] More careful investigations, in fact, negated this possibility, especially the UKPDS study.[59] In this way, treatment with SU preparations is very common in the treatment of Type 2 diabetes. A major problem is, however, that these patients have more than one element in their diabetes genesis, not only insulin secretory defects, but the patients are also insulin resistant. The Steno-II study included the use of a sulfonylurea with clear benefits also on cardiovascular–renal end-points.

New agents that stimulate insulin secretion have also been marketed, but are not widely used apart from specific trials.[51]

Metformin

Treatment with metformin is important because the mode of action is different from that of SU preparations. Metformin was discovered years ago and has been used in diabetes care for many years in France and Europe.[61,62,70,72] Now it has a renaissance in the US. Indeed, in the UKPDS study it was also shown to be very advantageous to use, resulting in less weight gain and also importantly and somewhat surprisingly in ameliorating cardiovascular complications.

Metformin is a very commonly used preparation in the treatment of Type 2 diabetes, often in combination with insulin or an SU preparation. A mechanism of action is not clearly defined and it has also been suggested that metformin reduces appetite.

Metformin was originally identified from French lilac[70] (Latin *Galega officinalis*), used for symptoms in the urinary tract. The active ingredient seems to be a guanidine preparation that was also explored in infusion treatment, but it appeared to be toxic, although it reduced blood glucose. This was the start of trying to develop new guanidine preparations for diabetes care. Guanidine was too toxic, but biguanide seemed to be less toxic, and was introduced in the 1950s. Initially, phenformin was used, but this resulted in some cases in lactic acid doses. In the present situation, metformin is the only agent that has been used in Europe for the last 40 years, and in the US for the last 7–8 years.[44]

In prevention of Type 2 diabetes, metformin has shown its therapeutic strength in the American Diabetes Prevention Project, although lifestyle modifications may be more effective, at least in the short-term situation.[22]

Glitazones

Glitazones were introduced a few years ago as new oral anti-diabetic agents[30] and are already widely used in the US, but much less in Europe. The mechanism of action of these molecules is related to an effect on insulin resistance, although the exact mode of action is not really known. It seems to work on nuclear receptor level and has reasonable effects by reducing the blood glucose values in patients with Type 2 diabetes, but probably not more than any other anti-diabetic agent. However, combinations with all agents could be useful.

The important point is that we do not yet have long-term clinical trials with end-point analyses, in contrast to insulin, sulfonylurea and metformin.

In many European countries, diabetologists have been a little reluctant to use these agents on a large scale and further analyses are awaited.

The Metabolic Syndrome

It has been known for many years that patients often suffer from a constellation of overweight, Type 2 diabetes, increased blood pressure and dyslipaedimia, sometimes associated with high uric acid in the blood.[9,38,56] However, this syndrome became much better defined after Reaven's efforts, followed by de Franzo, Ferranini etc. It was realized that this syndrome was really increasing in frequency and that an important element in the genesis was overweight, too little physical activity and lifestyle-related diseases. This was a very clinically relevant observation since it became clear that if one abnormality is observed it is important to screen for the other abnormalities in the syndrome, since each abnormality needs a specific treatment. So far the 'super-pill' or the 'poly-pill' for the insulin resistance syndrome has not been identified.[59,66,67]

Microalbuminuria is not usually related to this syndrome, but quite often also seen in these patients. This is important in relation to the Steno2 study,[26–28] where it was shown that pharmacological treatment of the syndrome's elements such as high blood glucose, high blood pressure and dyslipidaemia was quite relevant. On the other hand, lifestyle intervention was not easy.[28] However, important results were obtained in this study, as discussed later. Whether postprandial glucose level is a risk factor important for treatment is still debated.[43] Growth hormone administration is very controversial in Type 2 diabetes.[6,25]

Home Monitoring of Blood Glucose

Home monitoring of blood glucose appeared in the late 1970s and is now extremely common, indeed also in patients with Type 2 diabetes.[21,42] To obtain better glycaemic control, this is a critical requisite. Many patients, including elderly patients, can easily measure their blood glucose with a refined apparatus, often connected to their home computers. A quick and reliable answer can be obtained with respect to blood glucose. It is difficult to imagine modern diabetes care without home monitoring of blood glucose in both Type 1 and Type 2 diabetes.

Automatic subcutaneous continuous monitors are still being developed. However, one has to be careful because potential defects in the measurements can be catastrophic; on the other hand, measurement with stix is easy and reliable, and in elderly people this may not need to be done so often as in Type 1 diabetes.

Glycated Haemoglobin

By chance, haematologists identified a strange fraction of haemoglobin in some patients who appeared to be diabetic.[4,33,41] This was the creation of the A1c measurement that is now a key parameter in the treatment of patients diagnosed with Type 1 and Type 2 diabetes. It is hardly possible to conduct and interpret studies such as the DCCT and the UKPDS without HbA_{1c} values or as now termed A1c values.

This is really a breakthrough in the treatment strategy, and before this event it was very difficult to obtain reliable measurements of glycaemic control because many patients were keen to pretend good control by a visit to the doctors, making reliable observations very difficult, although this was possible in Pirart's milestone study about 25 years ago.[53]

At last we now have guidelines for good glycaemic control, which indicate that A1c should be below 6.5 or 7.0 per cent (but higher in elderly patients), but at most diabetic clinics the mean value is probably around 8.5, so there is still much work to do to improve glycaemic control. Most patients are very much aware of the A1c values and try hard to have the best possible control with continued measurements; still, patients seem to end up on a level they are able to achieve; it may be 7.5 or 9.5 or even higher, especially in non-compliant patients. This means that have we have to go for other measures to reduce the severity of the complications. Also individual goals for A1c are highly important.

Diabetes Nurses, 'Diabetes School' and Dietary Help

Obviously a major benefit in diabetes care is the introduction of the diabetes nurse, who maintains education and information to many patients;[64] in the last few years in particular, patients with Type 2 diabetes have been a great task for the nurses since we have an increasing number of patients that need instruction. Most elderly patients, indeed, can easily be taught the importance of diet, exercise and glycaemic control, as well as blood pressure control and lipid control. Most patients with Type 2 diabetes are quite aware that it is not only the blood glucose that needs to be controlled, but also blood pressure and cholesterol, which tend to increase with age. Clearly dieticians also play a great role in these programmes, which are usually highly valued by the patients.

Thus, the so-called 'diabetes schools' have emerged in practically all diabetes units as a major contribution to better diabetes care.

Laser Treatment of Retinopathy, including Maculopathy, in Type 2 Diabetes

This is without doubt an area with extremely important progress. In most diabetes centres, eye status is now evaluated by regular retinal photographs taken routinely at certain intervals according to the status of the patient. Thus, it is possible to follow the development of diabetic retinopathy and to introduce laser treatment quite early.[16,24,71] Further major progress is laser treatment for maculopathy in Type 2 diabetes. Such patients usually also have background, typically diabetic, retinopathy.

Clearly, the incidence of prevalence of blindness due to vascular proliferations and bleedings has been remarkably reduced, and the method is also highly effective in treating diabetic maculopathy. The exact mechanism is still not known, but the number of younger patients that are becoming blind due to diabetes is decreasing. Obviously, these patients may lose some visual function, but still they are able to manage much better than earlier.

It has been suggested that laser treatment was also discovered by serendipity, and it was proposed by Meyer-Schwickerath that a patient realized amelioration of diabetic retinopathy by looking directly at the sun. This is probably the way that laser treatment was invented.[46–48]

Diabetic Foot Care and Related Neuropathy

This is also an area with great progress regarding better practical foot-care observation and treatment of foot ulcers and neuropathy.[36] So far, there is no very good specific treatment for neuropathy. It is rather a matter of prevention with better glycaemic control and optimizing observation of early lesions in the feet and rapid treatment of foot ulcers as well as relief of the consequences of improper footwear. Many patients with Type 2 diabetes have great benefits from frequent visits to the foot therapist, and it was observed that the number of observations has been reduced in the last few decades, although we now see a stabilization or a slight increase, probably because the patients become older and older.

The major progress in this area, besides prophylactic measures, is effective treatment of infections as related to ischaemia and neuropathy.

High Blood Pressure: Blood Pressure Lowering and Microalbuminuria

Clinical investigations in Denmark at the beginning of the 1970s and early 1980s clearly showed that high blood pressure was an important risk factor for diabetic renal disease.[49] Previously, it was believed that high blood pressure was important to maintain renal perfusion, but this was clearly a wrong and problematic idea.[69]

Very soon, small intervention studies showed that the rate of fall in renal function could be reduced dramatically by ordinary antihypertensive treatment.[3,11,40]

This was remarkable progress in the practical implementation of diabetes care, in Type 1 and now many in Type 2, where we have recently seen results from major trials in Type 2 diabetes. In these trials, agents blocking renin–angiotensin systems have been used, which is an advantage, especially as the side effects are much smaller than with earlier agents, such as beta blockers and other agents. It is argued that these new preparations reduce more specifically the intra-glomerular pressure, and this is probably correct. The fall rate of the GFR can be reduced by anti-hypertensive treatment, but certainly not stopped or reduced to the normal rate of fall with age. Therefore, a major issue is to identify the patients before proteinuria, which means introducing the concept of microalbuminuria.

It is well known that microalbuminuria is common in Type 2 diabetic patients, which is below the proteinuric level, as observed by the usual stix tests. Many studies have been performed, and it is now clinical practise that patients with microalbuminuria, even with 'normotension', should be treated with blood-pressure-lowering agents, especially agents that block the renin–angiotensin system, often combined with diuretics. Now, it is therefore quite common to start treatment with a combination strategy with these agents plus diuretics (Figure 17.1). The use of ACEi or ARBs results in similar outcome.[2,5]

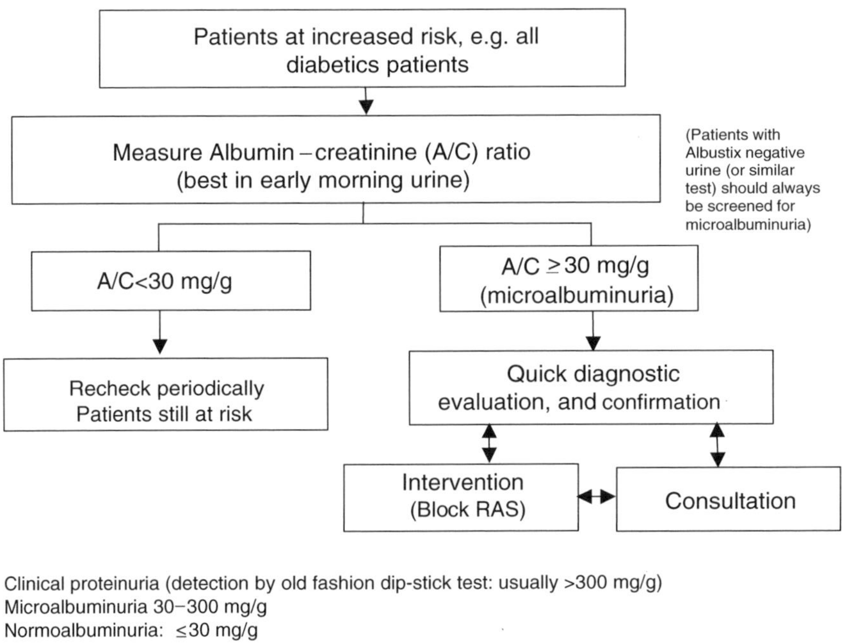

FIGURE 17.1 Search for patients with early renal disease, especially early diabetic nephropathy

This means an amelioration of the course of renal disease that can be followed very efficiently by the fall or stabilization of microalbuminuria. This strategy of early screening and treatment has led to considerably fewer patients with diabetic renal disease in the case of patients with Type 1 diabetes. However, the number of patients with Type 2 diabetes is increasing, which is probably due to the fact that more patients are being diagnosed earlier and also due to the fact that patients live longer because of better cardiac care; this means that many patients reach the state of renal insufficiency also in Type 2 diabetes. Clearly, cardiological treatment using bypass and stents is fantastic progress probably also for the diabetic patients with cardiovascular diseases. In many patients, ACE inhibitors or receptor blockers are used, and it has been shown that mortality and progression of renal disease and cardiovascular diseases can be ameliorated.[14] Dual blockade using both ACE inhibitors and receptor blockers has also been introduced as an efficient treatment strategy for reducing blood pressure and albuminuria, but we still need long-term follow-up studies.[2]

More strategies need to be developed to accomplish a further reduction of blood pressure without side-effects for the patient. It is quite clear that blood pressure is an important risk factor for developing cardiovascular lesions in Type 2 diabetes, both microvascular and macrovascular. Blood pressure lowering by beta blockers is also important, and, indeed, treatment with modern diabetes diet is important too. Studies suggest that it is important to increase the volume of vegetables and fruits as regards reduction of blood pressure along with a reduction of salt intake.

Lipid-Lowering Agents; Focus on Type 2 Diabetes

It has long been known that there seems to be a correlation between high cholesterol (especially high LDL cholesterol), low HDL cholesterol and cardiovascular complications, but it is only recently that clinical trials have been performed in order to document a positive effect using statin preparations reducing serum cholesterol, especially LDL cholesterol and, to some extent, an increasing HDL cholesterol. This has led to the concept that almost all patients with Type 2 diabetes need treatment with statins according to the results of the Heart Protection Study from the UK (with many Type 2 diabetic patients) and also according to other studies.[31] Interestingly, in the Heart Protection Study patients were treated even with a so-called normal cholesterol down to a level of 3.5 mmol/l. Anyway, there seems to be a positive effect which is not related to the actual cholesterol level, and it is clearly important also to reduce cholesterol level by introducing an efficient diabetes diet. In the Steno2 study[27] preliminary analysis suggests that especially lipid-lowering therapy is important for cardiovascular outcome (Oluf Pedersen, personal communication). Aspirin is also recommended in prevention of cardiovascular disease.[18]

The Diet of Diabetic Patients

The diet of diabetic patients is a topic that has been discussed for centuries, and for many years diabetic patients, for instance in the 1960s and 1970s, used a diet that was rich in fat and proteins; carbohydrates were not really allowed because it was thought that they resulted in an increase of the blood glucose. Therefore, many patients were put on a high-fat or high-protein diet, still with many vegetables.[23] This concept has clearly changed and now in 2003 we have seen the development of the new food pyramid, which is relevant for diabetic patients.[34,65,68] There is focus on mono- and poly-unsaturated fatty acids in plant oil and obviously non-starch, carbohydrates; carbohydrates with so-called fibre are useful for ameliorating high glucose levels and also for slower absorption from the intestinal system. Potatoes, rice, white bread etc. should be eaten sparingly.

This is the so-called Mediterranean diet that may also be useful with diabetic patients (as well as non-diabetic individuals). It is necessary to reduce the amount of animal fat, with the exception of fish. New studies also suggest that moderate alcohol intake is useful and, indeed, multivitamin tablets seem to be of importance, especially for Type 2 diabetes. Clearly, reduction in salt intake is important for reducing blood pressure. The major basic element in the new food pyramid is weight control and exercise. Although some patients may have benefits from eating according to relevant dietary rules, it is really disadvantageous if there is a weight gain, so the basis for the new food pyramid is exercise and weight control.

Multi-Factorial Intervention with Treatment Goals

This is the main concept introduced by the Steno2 study with goals for the treatment strategy.[27] Not only should glycaemic control be optimal, with HbA_{1c} values below 6.5 or 7, but also blood pressure is extremely important to control, aiming a blood pressure below 130/80 or even lower if the patient can tolerate this pressure level. According to this study, most patients also need treatment with statins, and clearly the result of this eight-year follow-up study comparing multi-factorial intervention with standard treatment with GPs had a beneficial effect on micro- and macrovascular complications.

Neuropathy

As regards neuropathy, there is only limited radical progress,[15] both in the diagnosis and treatment complication, related to neuropathy. Readers are referred to the relevant chapter. However erectile dysfunction can be efficiently treated according to several studies by using Viagra and similar agents.[58] This is an important step forward, but we still need more efficient and especially cheaper agents.

Conclusion

Many other steps of progress have been made for the last 40 years, for instance treatment of ketoacidosis; better glycaemic control is important, but, ketoacidosis may still develop; the programmes developed about 20 years ago were an important step forward, and all clinics now have an important outline for treatment with ketoacidosis using administration of insulin in a pre-planned manner.

The treatment of pregnant diabetic patients obviously has been greatly optimized in the last 30–40 years. It is a surprising observation that many patients (but certainly not all), otherwise difficult to control, are usually better controlled during pregnancy, which is maybe due to better motivation of these patients.

It is quite clear that much formidable progress has been made in the management of diabetes, in both Type 1 and Type 2 diabetes. Still, unfortunately, we are not able definitely to cure diabetes, either Type 1 or Type 2. Many trials have been performed in both Type 1 and Type 2 diabetes, but so far to little avail. Lately, we have seen the results of preventative trials in Type 1 diabetes with nicotinamide or prophylactic insulin treatment in all risk patients; unfortunately, there has been no progress in this area.

Genetic analyses are of no or limited clinical value although the optimism has been great.[54] This is also the case regarding genetic analyses and diabetic complications.

Especially for Type 2 diabetes, a real cure is still beyond the horizon, although billions of dollars, Euros or pounds are invested in many pharmaceutical companies. On the contrary, we see an increasing number of patients with Type 2 diabetes all over the world, and unless we develop more radical preventative measures by better diet and exercise programmes we have to realize that there will be more and more patients with Type 2 diabetes in the years to come. Some hope for the future is any way shown in the final Table 17.3.

TABLE 17.3 Some hope for future progress

1) Better defined insulin preparations with more predictable absorption profile.
2) All oral anti-diabetic agents will have positive effects on strong end-points (according to A1c level).
3) Prevention of diabetes would be possible in high-risk patients.
4) The ideal anti-hypertension combination pill will be created.
5) The poly-pill will be a reality.
6) Closed-loop systems for blood-glucose monitoring and insulin administration will prove safe.
7) Controlled clinical trials with the 'Mediterranean diet' will show positive results in the US and Northern Europe.
8) More patient-friendly dialysis systems will be developed.
9) Neuropathy can be treated pharaceutically.
10) Cheap insulin in poor countries.

References

1. Abraira C, Duckworth W, McCarren M, Emanuele N, Arca D, Reda D and Henderson W. Design of the cooperative study on glycemic control and complications in diabetes mellitus Type 2. Veterans Affairs Diabetes Trial. *J Diabetes Complications* 2003; **17**: 314–322.
2. Andersen NA, Poulsen PL, Knudsen ST, Poulson SH, Eiskjcer H, Hansen KW, Helleberg K and Mogensen CE. Long-term dual blockade with candesartan and lisinopril in hypertensive patients with diabetes mellitus. The CALM II Study. *Diabetes Care* 2005; in press.
3. Bakris G. Hypertension and nephropathy. *Am J Med* 2003; **115** (8A): S49–S54.
4. Balkau B, Forhan A, Simon D and Eschwège E. HbA_{1c} as a diagnostic tool for diabetes. In *The Metabolic Syndrome: Diabetes, Obesity, Hyperlipidemia and Hypertension*, Crepaldi G, Tiengo A and Avogaro A (eds). 2003. Amsterdam: Elsevier, pp. 19–26.
5. Barnett AH, Bain SC, Bouter P, Karlberg B, Madsbad S, Jervell J and Ustonen JM. Comparison of Angiotensin II receptor blockade and angiotensin-converting enzyme inhibition in subjects with Type 2 diabetes and nephropathy. *New Engl J Med* 2004; in press.
6. Blackman MR, Sorkin JD, Münzer T, Bellantoni MF, Busby-Whitehead J, Stevens TE, Jayme J, O'Connor KG, Christmas C, Tobin JD, Stewart KJ, Cottrell E, St. Clair C, Pabst KM and Harman SM. Growth hormone and sex steroid administration in healthy aged women and men. A randomized controlled trial. *JAMA* 2002; **288**: 2282–2292.
7. Bliss M. Research methods and the discovery of insulin. In *Research Methodologies in Human Diabetes* Part 1, Mogensen CE and Standl E (eds). 1994. Berlin: de Gruyter, pp. 1–10.
8. Bliss M. The Discovery of Insulin. 1982. Chicago, IL: University of Chicago Press.
9. Bonora E, Kiechl S, Willeit J, Oberhollenzer F, Egger G, Bonadonna RC and Muggeo M. Prevalence, ancillary clinical features and cardiovascular disease in the metabolic syndrome: the Bruneck study. In *The Metabolic Syndrome: Diabetes, Obesity, Hyperlipidemia and Hypertension*, Crepaldi G, Tiengo A and Avogaro A (eds). 2003. Amsterdam: Elsevier, pp. 13–18.
10. Bouter PK (ed.). Diabetes: a Global Perspective. 20 Interviews with Leading Experts. 2003. AK Leusden, The Netherlands: Mark Two Communications.
11. Brenner BM. AMGEN International Prize. The history and future of renoprotection. *Kidney Int* 2003; **64**: 1163–1168.
12. Caulfield M and O'Brien KD. Cardiovascular Safety of Oral Antidiabetic Agents: The Insulin Secretagogues. *Clin Diabetes* 2002; **20**: 81–84.
13. Cefalu WT, Skyler JS, Kourides IA, Landschulz WH, Balagtas CC, Cheng SL and Gelfand RA. Inhaled human insulin treatment in patients with Type 2 diabetes mellitus. *Ann Intern Med* 2001; **134**: 203–207.
14. Chalmers JP and Arnolda LF. Clinical update. Lowering blood pressure in 2003. *MJA* 2003; **179**: 306–312.
15. Charcot JM. Sur un case de paraplegie diabetique. *Arch Neurol* 1890; 305–335.
16. Chew EY, Ferris FL, Csaky KG, Murphy RP, Agrón E, Thompson DJ, Reed GF and Schachat AP. The long-term effects of laser photocoagulation treatment in patients with diabetic retinopathy. The early treatment diabetic retinopathy follow-up study. *Ophthalmology* 2003; **110**: 1683–1689.
17. Christiansen JS, Vaz JA, Metelko Z, Bogoev M and Dedov I. Twice daily biphasic insulin aspart improves postprandial glycaemic control more effectively than twice daily NPH insulin, with low risk of hypoglycaemia, in patients with Type 2 diabetes. *Diabetes Obesity Metab* 2003; **5**: 446–454.
18. Colwell JA. Aspirin for primary prevention of cardiovascular events in diabetes. *Diabetes Care* 2003; **26**: 3349–3350.

19. Creutzfeldt W. The entero-insular axis in Type 2 diabetes – incretins as therapeutic agents. *Exp Clin Endocrinol Diabetes* 2001; **109** (Suppl. 2): S288–S303.
20. Creutzfeldt W. The discovery of the oral treatment of diabetes mellitus with sulphonylureas. In *Research Methodologies in Human Diabetes* Part 1, Mogensen CE and Standl E (eds). 1994. Berlin: de Gruyter, pp. 11–20.
21. Day J. Patient self-empowerment: the route to improved clinical outcome and patient satisfaction. In Betteridge DJ (ed.). Diabetes Current Perspectives. 2000. London: Dunitz, pp. 341–353.
22. Diabetes Prevention Program Research Group. Reduction in the incidence of Type 2 diabetes with lifestyle intervention or metformin. *N Engl J Med* 2002; **346**: 393–403.
23. Eckel RH. Editorial. A new look at dietary protein in diabetes. *Am J Clin Nutr* 2003; **78**: 671–672.
24. Frank RN. Medical progress. Diabetic retinopathy. *N Engl J Med* 2004; **350**: 48–58.
25. Frohman LA. Controversy about treatment of growth hormone-deficient adults: a commentary. *Ann Intern Med* 2002; **137**: 202–204.
26. Gaede P, Vedel P, Parving HH and Pedersen O. Intersified multifactorial intervention in patients with Type 2 diabetes mellitus and microalbuminuria: the Steno 2 randomized study. *Lancet* 1999; **353**: 617–622.
27. Gaede P, Vedel P, Larsen N, Jensen GV, Parving HH and Pedersen O. Multifactorial intervention and cardiovascular disease in patients with Type 2 diabetes. *N Engl J Med* 2003; **348**: 383–393.
28. Gaede P, Beck M, Vedel P and Pedersen O. Limited impact of lifestyle education in patients with Type 2 diabetes mellitus and microalbuminuria: results from a randomized intervention study. *Diabet Med* 2001; **18**: 104–108.
29. Genuth S, Eastman R, Kahn R, Klein R, Lachin J, Lebovitz H, Nathan D and Vinicor F. Position statement. Implications of the United Kingdom Prospective Diabetes Study. *Diabetes Care* 2003; **26** (Suppl. 1): S28–S32.
30. Hardy E and Jabbour SA. Thiazolidinediones. In *Textbook of Type 2 Diabetes*, Goldstein BJ and Müller-Wieland D (eds). 2003. London: Dunitz, pp. 117–130.
31. Heart Protection Study Collaborative Group. The Heart Protection Study of cholesterol lowering with simvastatin in 28 536 high-risk individuals: a randomized placebo-controlled trial. *Lancet* 2002; **360**: 7–22.
32. Heine RJ, de Sonnaville JJ and Bakker SJ. Optimal control of Type 2 diabetes: current and future prospects. In *Diabetes Current Perspectives*, Betteridge DJ (ed.). 2000. London: Dunitz, pp. 295–315.
33. Hermansen K, Fontaine P, Kukolja KK, Peterkova V, Leth C and Gall MA. Insulin analogues (insulin detemin and insulin aspart) versus traditional human insulins (NPH insulin and regular human insulin) in a basal-bolus therapy for patients with Type 1 diabetes. *Diabetologia* 2004; **47**: 622–629.
34. Hu FB. The Mediterranean diet and mortality – olive oil and beyond. *N Engl J Med.* 2003; **348**: 2595–2596.
35. Inzucchi SE. Oral antihyperglycemic therapy for Type 2 diabetes. Scientific review. *JAMA* 2002; **287**: 360–372.
36. Jude EB and Boulton AJ. The diabetic foot. In *Diabetes Current Perspectives*, Betteridge DJ (ed.). 2000. London: Dunitz, pp. 179–196.
37. Kimmelstiel P and Wilson C. Intercapillary lesions in the glomeruli of the kidney. *Am J Pathol* 1936; **12**: 83–95.
38. Lefèbvre PJ. The metabolic syndrome revisited. In *The Metabolic Syndrome: Diabetes, Obesity, Hyperlipidemia and Hypertension*, Crepaldi G, Tiengo A and Avogaro A (eds). 2003. Amsterdam: Elsevier, pp. 3–10.

39. Lenhard MJ and Reeves GD. Continuous subcutaneous insulin infusion. A comprehensive review of insulin pump therapy. *Arch Intern Med.* 2001; **161**: 2293–2300.
40. Levey AS, Coresh J, Balk E, Kausz AT, Levin A, Steffes MW, Hogg RJ, Perrone RD, Lau J and Eknoyan G. National Kidney Foundation practice guidelines for chronic kidney disease: evaluation, classification, and stratification. *Ann Intern Med* 2003; **139**: 137–147.
41. Little RR and Goldstein DE. Measurements of glycated haemoglobin and other circulating glycated proteins. In *Research Methodologies in Human Diabetes* Part 1, Mogensen CE and Standl E (eds). 1994. Berlin: de Gruyter, pp. 299–317.
42. Lotz N. Self-monitoring of blood glucose: how to organize education. In *Concepts for the Ideal Diabetes Clinic*, Mogensen CE and Standl E (eds). 1992. Berlin: de Gruyter, pp. 119–130.
43. Madsbad S, Brock B and Schmitz O. Postprandial hyperglykæmi. *Ugeskr Læger* 2003; **165**: 3149–3153.
44. McCall AL and Riddle MC. Combination therapy for treatment of Type 2 diabetes. In *Textbook of Type 2 Diabetes*, Goldstein BJ and Müller-Wieland D (eds). 2003. London: Dunitz, pp. 155–170.
45. Meneilly GS, Greig N, Tildesley H, Habener JF, Egan JM and Elahi D. Effects of 3 months of continuous subcutaneous administration of glucagon-like peptide 1 in elderly patients with Type 2 diabetes. *Diabetes Care* 2003; **26**: 2835–2841.
46. Meyer-Schwickerath G. Indications and limitations of light coagulation of the retina. *Trans Am Acad Ophthalmol Otolaryngol* 1959; **63**: 725.
47. Meyer-Schwickerath G. Light Coagulation, Drance SM (transl.) 1960. St. Louis: Mosby.
48. Meyer-Schwickerath G and Schott K. Diabetic retinopathy and photocoagulation. *Am J Ophthalmol* 1968; **66**: 597.
49. Mogensen CE. Microalbuminuria and hypertension with focus on Type 1 and Type 2 diabetes. *J Intern Med* 2003; **254**: 45–66.
50. Owens D and Barnett A. Designer insulins: have they revolutionized insulin therapy? In *Diabetes Current Perspectives*, Betteridge DJ (ed.). 2000. London: Dunitz, pp. 223–265.
51. Pfeiffer AF. Oral hypoglycaemic agents: sulfonylureas and meglitinides. In *Textbook of Type 2 Diabetes*, Goldstein BJ and Müller-Wieland D (eds). 2003. London: Dunitz, pp. 77–85.
52. Pickup J and Keen H. Continuous subcutaneous insulin infusion at 25 years. *Diabetes Care* 2002; **25**: 593–598.
53. Pirart J. Diabetes mellitus and its degenerative complications; a prospective study of 4,400 patients observed between 1947 and 1973. *Diabetes Care* 1978; **1**: 168–188.
54. Poulsen P, Vaag A, Kyvik K and Beck-Nielsen H. Genetic versus environmental aetiology of the metabolic syndrome among male and female twins. *Diabetologia* 2001; **44**: 537–543.
55. Ratner RE, Hirsch IB, Neifing JL, Garg SK, Mecca TE and Wilson CA. Less hyperglycemia with insulin glargine in intensive insulin therapy for Type 1 diabetes. *Diabetes Care* 2000; **23**: 639–643.
56. Reaven GM and Laws A (eds). *Insulin Resistance, the Metabolic Syndrome*. 1999. Totowa, NJ: Humana.
57. Schmidt-Nielsen B. August and Marie Krogh. *Lives in Science*. 1995. New York: Oxford University Press.
58. Shah J. Erectile failure: the complication 'that dare not speak its name'. In *Diabetes Current Perspectives*, Betteridge DJ (ed.). 2000. London: Dunitz, pp. 197–208.
59. Stevens KJ, Coleman RL, Adler AI, Stratton IM, Mathews DR and Holman RR. UKPDS 66 risk factors for myocardial infarction case fatality and stroke case fatality in Type 2 diabetes. *Diabetes Care* 2004; **27**: 201–207.
60. Shaughnessy AF and Slawson DC. What happened to the valid POEMs? A survey of review articles on the treatment of Type 2 diabetes. *BMJ* 2003; **327**: 266–269.

61. Stumvoll M, Häring HU and Matthaei S. Metformin. In *Textbook of Type 2 Diabetes*, Goldstein BJ, Müller-Wieland D. 2003. London: Dunitz, pp. 87–101.
62. Vague P. Is metformin more than an oral hypoglycaemic agent? *Diabetes Metab* 2003; **29**: S5–S8.
63. Vance ML. Can growth hormone prevent aging? *N Engl J Med* 2003; **348**: 779–780.
64. Vesterdal H and Musaeus L. The nurse on the diabetes team. In *Concepts for the ideal diabetes clinic*, Mogensen CE and Standl E. 1992. Berlin: de Gruyter, pp. 65–72.
65. Wakabayashi I, Kobaba-Wakabayashi R and Masuda H. Relation of drinking alcohol to atherosclerotic risk in Type 2 diabetes. *Diabetes Care* 2002; **25**: 1223–1228.
66. Wald NJ and Law MR. A strategy to reduce cardiovascular disease by more than 80 per cent. *BMJ* 2003; **326**: 1419.
67. Wald NJ, Law MR, Morris J, Rudnicka A and Jordan R. 'Polypill' to fight cardiovascular disease: Author's reply. *BMJ* 2003; **327**: 809–810.
68. Willett WC. *The harvard medical school guide to healthy eating*. 2003. Boston, MA: Free Press.
69. Williams B. Drug treatment of hypertension. *BMJ* 2003; **326**: 61–62.
70. Witters LA. The blooming of the French lilac. *J Clin Invest* 2001; **108**: 1105–1107.
71. Wong JS and Kohner EM. Optimal methods of detecting early retinopathy and its progression. In *Concepts for the Ideal Diabetes Clinic*, Mogensen CE and Standl E (eds). 1992. Berlin: de Gruyter, pp. 269–287.
72. Wulffelé MG, Kooy A, Lehert P, Bets D, Ogterop JC, van der Burg BB, Donker AJ and Stehouwer CD. Combination of insulin and metformin in the treatment of Type 2 diabetes. *Diabetes Care* 2002; **25**: 2133–2140.

Index

Prevention of Type 2 Diabetes Edited by Manfred Ganz
 ISBN: 0-470-85733-1